W9-ADS-099

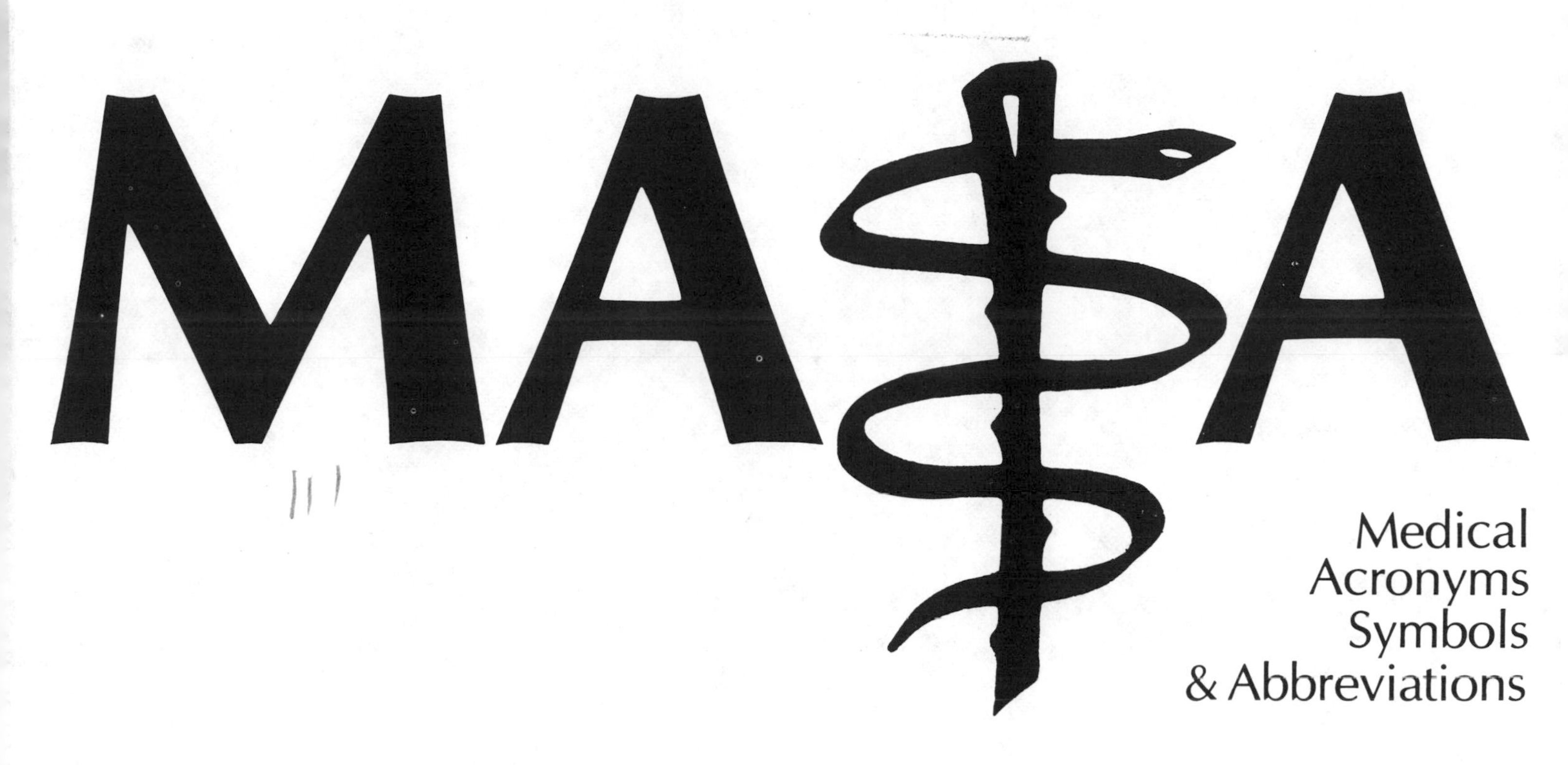

Medical Acronyms Symbols & Abbreviations

Edited by Betty Hamilton and Barbara Guidos

Neal-Schuman Publishers, Inc.

Published by Neal-Schuman Publishers, Inc.
23 Cornelia Street
New York, NY 10014

Printed and bound in the United States of America.

Library of Congress Cataloging in Publication Data

Hamilton, Betty.
MASA: medical acronyms, symbols, and abbreviations.

1. Medicine—Acronyms. 2. Medicine—Notation.
3. Medicine—Abbreviations. I. Guidos, Barbara.
II. Title. III. Title: M.A.S.A.
R123.H28 1983 610′.148 83-4191
ISBN 0-918212-72-3

Contents

Introduction

The proliferation of medical research and knowledge in recent years and the subsequent explosion of literature in the health care field have necessitated an increased use of medical shorthand in the form of acronyms, symbols, and abbreviations. Although such terminology is often used as a space-saving device, many writers do not follow the general rule of defining a term when it first appears, placing the burden of identification on the reader.

The intent of *MASA: Medical Acronyms, Symbols, and Abbreviations* is to explain abbreviations and symbols and to identify acronyms, rather than to dictate correct usage. Our listing covers all of the major specialties and subspecialties of medicine and related fields, and it includes terminology commonly used as well as that only recently introduced into the literature. Although some terms identified here are outdated, they are included because they may be found in the older literature and in medical records. Usage is often a matter of writing style, and although we have not attempted to standardize, we strongly feel that such standardization is desirable and suggest that a general committee or board be formed to meet that need.

GUIDE TO USAGE

Alphabetizing is letter-by-letter rather than word-by-word, and numerals have been ignored for the purpose of alphabetizing. Therefore, 2-D will be found under D. For the sake of consistency, the acronyms and abbreviations are presented in the singular form, unless the meaning dictates otherwise. There has been no attempt to list all of the possible forms of a word; thus, ECG may apply to either electrocardiograph, electrocardiographic, or electrocardiogram, depending on context. Acronyms for chemical compounds may represent either the salt or the acid. A stylistic variation among publishers is the use of periods and capital or lower case letters. We have followed the general trend of using primarily capital letters for the acronyms and have limited the use of periods to abbreviations of titles or ranks, such as D.R. (Diplomate of Radiology).

Like language itself, acronyms tend to undergo transition, and we have noted as many of these changes as possible. In general, when an acronym is less preferred, we have indicated that fact by referring the reader to the more commonly used acronyms with "See." For example, for Ps, which is no longer the official abbreviation, we have indicated "See P (Pseudomonas)." Since there are multiple listings under P, the specific reference is given in parentheses.

For terms that are closely related, such as HSE and HSVE, "See also" is used. If a word or phrase has more than one acronym, the alternate form is indicated by "also." When a definition is not obviously related to its acronym, as often occurs with Latin terms, the source is given in parentheses. For acronyms that have more than one possible translation (such as "computer-assisted" or "computer-aided"), the alternate form is given.

We have not included acronyms for hospitals, medical centers or medical schools, or for journals or books. Chemical symbols are included, but not those for chemical compounds, such as CO or NaCl, although chemical symbols may appear as part of an acronym, for example, FeZ.

We have endeavored to make *MASA* as comprehensive as possible so that it can be a viable research tool for all those involved in the health care field and in medical communication.

MASA: Medical Acronyms, Symbols, and Abbreviations

A

A Absidia
absolute (also abs)
absorbance
Acanthocheilonema
Acanthopis
Acarapis
Acarus
accommodation (also Acc, accom)
Acetobacter
acetum
acid
Acinetobacter
actin
Actinobacillus
Actinomyces
active (also act)
adenine
adenoma
adenosine (also Ado)
adult
Aedes
Aerobacter
age (also aet)
Alcaligenes
allergy (also Al)
alpha
alveolar gas
Amblyomma
ampere (also amp)
Ancylostoma
androsterone
angle (also ang)
Angstrom (see also nm)
annum
anode (also An)
Anopheles
antagonized
anterior (also ant)
antrectomy
area
argon (see Ar)
arterial blood
artery (also art)
Ascaris
Aspergillus
assessment (also asmt)
Asterococcus
atomic weight (also at wt)
atrium
atropine
axial
Azotobacter
before (ante)
mass number
total acidity
water (aqua) (also aq)

A I angiotensin I (also ANG I, AT I)

A II angiotensin II (also ANG II, AT II)

A_2 aortic second sound

a arteriol
asymmetry (also asym)
thermodynamic activity

AA Academy of Aphasia
acetic acid
achievement age
active alcoholic
active assistive
acupuncture analgesia
adenylic acid
adjuvant arthritis
adrenocortical autoantibody
Alcoholics Anonymous
alopecia areata
alveolar-arterial
amino acid
aminoacyl
aminoadipic acid
amyloid A
anticipatory avoidance
antigen aerosol
aortic amplitude
aortic arch
aplastic anemia
arachidonic acid
Arthrogryposis Association
ascaris antigen
ascending aorta
atomic absorption
automobile accident

A.A. Associate of Arts

A&A aid and attendance
awake and aware

aA azure A

aa of each (ana)

AAA abdominal aortic aneurysm
abdominal aortic aneurysmectomy
acquired aplastic anemia
acute anxiety attack
American Academy of Allergy (see AAAI)
American Aging Association (also AGE)
American Allergy Association
American Association of Anatomists
androgenic, anabolic agent
aromatic amino acid

aaa amalgam (amalgama)

AAAD aromatic amino acid decarboxylase

AAAHC Accreditation Association for Ambulatory Health Care

AAAI American Academy of Allergy and Immunology

AAALAC
American Association for Accreditation of Laboratory Animal Care

AAAM American Association for Automotive Medicine

AA-AMP
amino acid adenylate (adenosine monophosphate)

AAAP American Association of Avian Pathologists

AAAS American Association for the Advancement of Science

AAAT American Association of Artist-Therapist

AAATCM
American Academy of Air Traffic Control Medicine

AAB Action Against Burns
American Association of Bioanalysts
aminoazobenzene

AABB American Association of Blood Banks

AABG alpha-acetobromoglucose

AABP American Association of Bovine Practitioners

AABR Association for Advancement of the

Blind and Retarded
AABT Association for Advancement of Behavior Therapy
AAC aminoglycoside 6'-acetyltransferase
antibiotic-associated colitis
AAcadNS
American Academy of Neurological Surgeons (also AANS)
AACC American Association for Clinical Chemistry
AACCN American Association of Critical Care Nurses (also AACN)
AACDP American Association of Chairmen of Departments of Psychiatry
AACE American Association for Cancer Education
AACHP American Association for Comprehensive Health Planning
AACI Association of American Cancer Institutes
AACIA American Association for Clinical Immunology and Allergy
AACM American Academy of Compensation Medicine
AACMS American Association of Councils of Medical Staffs
AACN American Association of Colleges of Nursing
American Association of Critical Care Nurses (also AACCN)
AACO American Association of Certified Orthoptists
AACOM American Association of Colleges of Osteopathic Medicine
AACP American Academy of Cerebral Palsy
American Academy of Child Psychiatry
American Academy of Clinical Psychiatrists
American Association of Colleges of Pharmacy
AACPDM
American Academy for Cerebral Palsy and Developmental Medicine
AACPM American Association of Colleges of Podiatric Medicine
AACR American Association for Cancer Research
AACT American Academy of Clinical Toxicology
AACU American Association of Clinical Urologists
AAD alpha-1-antitrypsin deficiency
American Academy of Dermatology
aminoglycoside 6'-O-adenylyltransferase
aromatic acid decarboxylase
AADC amino acid decarboxylase
Asthma and Allergy Disease Center
AAdC anterior adductor of the coxa
AADE American Association of Dental Examiners
American Association of Diabetes Educators
$AaDO_2$ alveolar to arterial oxygen tension difference
AADP American Academy of Denture Prosthetics
amyloid A degrading protease
AADR American Academy of Dental Radiology
American Association for Dental Research
AADS American Association of Dental Schools
AAE active assistive exercise
acute allergic encephalitis
American Association of Endodontists
AAEE American Association of Electromyography and Electrodiagnosis
AAEH Association to Advance Ethical Hypnosis
AAEP American Association of Equine Practitioners
AAES Adolescent Assertion Expression Scale
AAF acetylaminofluorene (also FAA)
ascorbic acid factor
AAFA Asthma and Allergy Foundation of America
AAFC anhydro-ara-5-fluorocytidine
AAFMC American Association of Foundations for Medical Care
AAFMG American Association of Foreign Medical Graduates
AAFP American Academy of Family Physicians
American Association of Feline Practitioners
AAFPRS
American Academy of Facial Plastic and Reconstructive Surgery
AAFS Academy of Ambulatory Foot Surgery
American Association of Foot Specialists
American Association for Forensic Science
AAG alpha-1-acid glycoprotein (also AGP)
autoantigen
AAGL American Association of Gynecological Laparoscopists
AAGP American Academy of General Practice (see AAFP American Academy of Family Practitioners)
American Association for Geriatric Psychiatry
AAGS See AAGUS
AAGUS American Association of Genito-Urinary Surgeons
AAHA American Academy of Health Administration
American Animal Hospital Association
AAHC American Association of Hospital Consultants
Association of Academic Health Centers
AAHD American Association of Hospital Dentists
AAHDS American Association of Health Data Systems
AAHE Association for the Advancement of Health Education
AAHM American Association for the History of Medicine
AAHP American Association of Homeopathic Pharmacists
American Association for Hospital Planning
American Association of Hospital Podiatrists
AAHPERD
American Alliance for Health, Physical Education, Recreation, and Dance
AAI acute alveolar injury
American Association of Immunologists
AAID American Academy of Implant Dentistry
AAIH American Academy of Industrial Hygiene
AAIMS Association for the Advancement of Industrial Medicine and Surgery
AAIN acute allergic intestinal nephritis
American Association of Industrial Nurses
AAIP Association of American Indian Physicians

AAIV American Association of Industrial Veterinarians
AAIVT American Association of I.V. Therapy
AAL anterior axillary line
AALAS American Association for Laboratory Animal Science
AAM amino acid mixture
AAMA American Academy of Medical Administrators
American Association of Medical Assistants
AAMAREF
American Academy of Medical Administrators Research and Education Foundation
AAMC American Association of Marriage Counselors
American Association of Medical Clinics
Association of American Medical Colleges
AAMCH American Association for Maternal and Child Health
AAMD American Association on Mental Deficiency
AAMFC American Association of Marriage and Family Counselors
AAMFT American Association for Marriage and Family Therapy
AAMI Association for the Advancement of Medical Instrumentation
Association of Allergists for Mycological Investigations
AAMMC American Association of Medical Milk Commissions
AAMP American Academy of Maxillofacial Prosthetics
American Academy of Medical Preventics
AAMR American Academy on Mental Retardation
AAMRL American Association of Medical Record Librarians
AAMSE American Association of Medical Society Executives
AAMT American Association for Music Therapy
AAMX acetoacet-m-xylidide
AAN alpha-amino nitrogen
American Academy of Neurology (also AANeur)
American Academy of Nursing
American Association of Neuropathologists
AANA American Anorexia Nervosa Association
American Association of Nurse Anesthetists
AANeur
American Academy of Neurology (also AAN)
AANN American Association of Neurosurgical Nurses
AANNT American Association of Nephrology Nurses and Technicians
AANP American Association of Neuropathologists
AANS American Academy of Neurological Surgery
American Association of Neurological Surgeons (also AAcadNS)
AAO American Academy of Ophthalmology
American Academy of Optometry
American Academy of Osteopathy
American Academy of Otolaryngology
American Association of Ophthalmology
American Association of Orthodontists
amino acid oxidase
AAOG American Association of Obstetricians and Gynecologists
AAOGP American Academy of Orthodontics for the General Practitioner
AAOHN American Association of Occupational Health Nurses
AAO-HNS
American Academy of Otolaryngology--Head and Neck Surgery
AAOM American Academy of Occupational Medicine
American Academy of Oral Medicine
AAOMS American Association of Oral and Maxillofacial Surgeons
AAOO American Academy of Ophthalmology and Otolaryngology
AAOP American Academy of Oral Pathology
American Academy of Orthotists and Prosthetists
AAOPS American Association of Oral and Plastic Surgeons
AAOR American Academy of Oral Roentgenology
AAOS American Academy of Orthopaedic Surgeons
AAP alpha-l-antiprotease
American Academy of Pediatrics (also AAPd)
American Academy of Pedodontics
American Academy of Periodontology
American Academy of Psychoanalysis
American Academy of Psychotherapists
American Association of Pathologists
Association of Academic Physiatrists
Association for Advancement of Psychoanalysis
Association for the Advancement of Psychotherapy
Association of American Physicians
Association for Applied Psychoanalysis
AAPA American Academy of Physician Assistants
American Academy of Podiatry Administration
American Association of Pathologists' Assistants
American Association of Physical Assistants
American Association of Physician Assistants
American Association of Psychiatric Administrators
AAPB American Association of Pathologists and Bacteriologists
AAPC antibiotic-associated pseudomembranous colitis (also AAPMC)
AAPCC American Association of Poison Control Centers
AAPD American Academy of Physiologic Dentistry
AAPd American Academy of Pediatrics (also AAP)
AAPE Association of American Peroral Endoscopists
AAPH American Association of Professional Hypnologists
AAPHD American Association of Public Health Dentists
AAPHP American Association of Public Health Physicians
AAPL American Academy of Psychiatry and the Law

AAPM American Association of Physicists in Medicine
AAPMC antibiotic-associated pseudomembranous colitis (also AAPC)
AAPMR American Academy of Physical Medicine and Rehabilitation
AAPO&S American Association for Pediatric Ophthalmology and Strabismus
AAPPP American Association of Planned Parenthood Physicians
AAPRD American Academy for Plastics Research in Dentistry
AAPS American Association of Plastic Surgeons
Association of American Physicians and Surgeons
AAPSC American Association of Psychiatric Services for Children
AAPSM American Academy of Podiatric Sports Medicine
AAPSRO American Association of Professional Standards Review Organizations
AAR antigen-antiglobulin reaction
AARD American Academy of Restorative Dentistry
AAROM active assistive range of motion
AARP American Association of Retired Persons
AARS American Association of Railway Surgeons
AART American Association for Rehabilitation Therapy
American Association of Religious Therapists
American Association for Respiratory Therapy
AAS American Academy of Sanitarians
anthrax antiserum
aortic arch syndrome
Association for Academic Surgery
atomic absorption spectroscopy
AASA American Association of Surgical Assistants
AASD American Academy of Stress Disorders
Aase asparaginase
AASECT American Association of Sex Educators, Counselors and Therapists
AASGP American Association of Sheep and Goat Practitioners
AASH American Association for the Study of Headache
AASLD American Association for the Study of Liver Diseases
AASND American Association for the Study of Neoplastic Diseases
AASP American Association of Senior Physicians
American Association for Social Psychiatry
American Association of Swine Practitioners
ascending aorta synchronized pulsation
AAST American Association for the Study of Trauma
American Association for the Surgery of Trauma
AAT acute abdominal tympany
alkylating agent therapy
alpha-1-antitrypsin
American Academy of Toxicology
aminoazotoluene
AATA American Art Therapy Association
AATB American Association of Tissue Banks
AATM American Academy of Tropical Medicine
AATP American Academy of Tuberculosis Physicians
AATS American Association for Thoracic Surgery
AAU acute anterior uveitis
AAUP American Association of University Professors
AAV adeno-associated virus
AAVA American Association of Veterinary Anatomists
AAVD American Academy of Veterinary Dermatology
AAVLD American Association of Veterinary Laboratory Diagnosticians
AAVN American Academy of Veterinary Nutrition
AAVP American Association of Veterinary Parasitologists
Association of American Volunteer Physicians
AAVSB American Association of Veterinary State Boards
AAW anterior aortic wall
AAWB American Association of Workers for the Blind
AAWD American Association of Women Dentists
AAWH American Association for World Health
AAWP American Association for Women Podiatrists
AAZV American Association of Zoo Veterinarians
AB abdominal
abnormal (also abn)
abortion (also abor)
air bleed
Alcian blue
apex beat
asbestos body
asthmatic bronchitis
axiobuccal
A.B. Bachelor of Arts (also B.A.)
Ab alabamine (see At)
antibody
See abstr
A b anisotropic band
aB azure B
ab about (also abt)
ABA abscissic acid
American Board of Anesthesiology
American Burn Association
antibacterial activity
azobenzenearsonate
ABAI American Board of Allergy and Immunology
ABAN American Board of Anesthesiology
ABAS American Board of Abdominal Surgery
abbr abbreviation
ABBS American Brittle Bone Society
ABC absolute basophilic count
absolute bone conduction
acalculous biliary colic
alternative birth center
alum, blood, clay
American Blood Commission
antigen-binding capacity
artificial B cell
aspiration biopsy cytology
Association of Bendectin Children

atomic, biologic, chemical
axiobuccocervical
ABCC Atomic Bomb Casualty Commission
ABCH American Boards of Clinical Hypnosis
ABCIA American Board of Clinical Immunology and Allergy
ABCOP American Board of Certified Orthotists and Prosthetists
ABCRS American Board of Colon and Rectal Surgery
ABCS American Board of Cosmetic Surgery
ABD American Board of Dermatology
Abd abdomen
abduction
Abdom abdominal
ABDPH American Board of Dental Public Health
ABE acute bacterial endocarditis
American Board of Endodontics
ABEA American Broncho-Esophagological Association
ABEM American Board of Emergency Medicine
ABEPP American Board of Examiners in Professional Psychology
ABESPA
American Board of Examiners in Speech Pathology and Audiology
ABFP American Board of Family Practice
ABG arterial blood gas
axiobuccogingival
ABHES Accrediting Bureau of Health Education Schools
ABHP American Board of Health Physics
ABI ankle-brachial index
atherothrombotic brain infarction
ABIM American Board of Internal Medicine
ABIS American Blood Irradiation Society
ABJS Association of Bone and Joint Surgeons
ABL acid-base laboratory
African Burkitt lymphoma
alpha-beta-lipoproteinemia
angioblastic lymphadenopathy
antigen-binding lymphocyte
axiobuccolingual
ABLB alternate binaural loudness balance
ABLR American Burkitt Lymphoma Registry
ABM adjusted body mass
alveolar basement membrane
autologous bone marrow
ABMS American Board of Medical Specialties
ABMT American Board of Medical Toxicology
ABN American Board of Nutrition
abn abnormal (also AB)
ABNM American Board of Nuclear Medicine (also ABNuM)
abnor See abn
ABNS American Board of Neurological Surgery
ABNuM American Board of Nuclear Medicine (also ABNM)
ABO absent bed occupancy
American Board of Ophthalmology (also ABOP)
American Board of Opticianry
American Board of Orthodontics
American Board of Otolaryngology (also ABOT)
ABOB N^1,N^1-anhydrobis(beta-hydroxyethyl)-biguanide
ABOG American Board of Obstetrics and Gynecology
ABO-HD
ABO hemolytic disease
ABOMS American Board of Oral and Maxillofacial Surgery
ABOP American Board of Ophthalmology (also ABO)
abor abortion (also AB)
ABOS American Board of Orthopaedic Surgery
ABOT American Board of Otolaryngology (also ABO)
ABP actin-binding protein
American Board of Pathology
American Board of Pediatrics (also ABPd)
American Board of Pedodontics
American Board of Periodontology
American Board of Prosthodontics
4-aminobiphenyl
androgen-binding protein
arterial blood pressure
doxorubicin (Adriamycin), bleomycin, prednisone
ABPA allergic broncopulmonary aspergillosis
ABPD American Board of Podiatric Dermatology
ABPd American Board of Pediatrics (also ABP)
ABPH American Board of Psychological Hypnosis
ABPlS American Board of Plastic Surgery (also ABPS)
ABPM American Board of Preventive Medicine (also ABPrM)
ABPMR American Board of Physical Medicine and Rehabilitation
ABPN American Board of Psychiatry and Neurology
ABPO American Board of Podiatric Orthopedics
ABPP 2-amino-5-bromo-6-phenyl-4-pyrimidinone
ABPrM American Board of Preventive Medicine (also ABPM)
ABPS American Board of Plastic Surgery (also ABPlS)
American Board of Podiatric Surgery
ABR abortus Bang ring
absolute bed rest
American Board of Radiology
auditory brainstem response
ABRA American Blood Resources Association
abras abrasions
ABS abdominal surgery
abnormal brainstem
acrylonitrile-butadiene-styrene
acute brain syndrome
alkyl benzene sulfonate
aloin, belladonna, strychnine
American Biological Society
American Board of Surgery
anti-B serum
autoantibody
Abs absorption (also absorp)
abs absent
absolute (also A)
absc abscissa
ABSe ascending bladder septum
abs feb
absence of fever (absente febre)
absorp
absorption (also Abs)
abst See abstr
abstr abstract
ABT aminopyrine breath test
abt about (also ab)
ABTR Association for Brain Tumor Research
ABTS American Board of Thoracic Surgery
ABTX alpha-bungarotoxin
ABU American Board of Urology

aminobutyrate
asymptomatic bacteriuria

ABVD doxorubicin (Adriamycin), bleomycin, vinblastine, dacarbazine

ABW actual body weight

AC abdominal circumference
abdominal compression
absorption coefficient
absorptive cell
abuse case
accumbens
acidified complement
Acinetobacter calcoaceticus
aconitine
acromioclavicular
activated charcoal
acute
acute cholecystitis
adenocarcinoma (also ACA)
adenylate cyclase
adherent cell
adrenal cortex (also AdC)
Aesculapian Club
air changes
air conduction
alcoholic cirrhosis
allyl chloride
alternating current
ambulatory controls
anesthesia circuit
angio-cellular
anodal closure
antecubital
anterior chamber
anterior column
anterior commissure
anticoagulant
anticomplementary
anti-inflammatory (or antiphlogistic) corticoid
aortic closure
aortocoronary
arm circumference
arterial capillary
ascending colon
atriocarotid
auriculocarotid
axiocervical
doxorubicin (Adriamycin), cyclophosphamide
See ACh

A/C anterior chamber of the eye

Ac accelerator
acetate
acetyl
actinium

^{227}Ac radioactive isotope of actinium

aC arabinosylcytosine
azure C

ac before meals (ante cibum)

ACA acute cerebellar ataxia
adenine-cytosine-adenine
adenocarcinoma (also AC)
adenylate cyclase activity
American Chiropractic Association
American College of Allergists
American College of Anesthesiologists
American College of Angiology (also ACAng)
American College of Apothecaries
ammonia, copper, arsenic
anomalous coronary artery
anterior cerebral artery
anterior communicating aneurysm
anticentromere antibody
anticollagen autoantibody
automated clinical analyzer

AC/A accommodative convergence to accommodation ratio

7-ACA 7-aminocephalosporanic acid

ACACN American Council of Applied Clinical Nutrition

Acad academy

ACALD Association for Children and Adults with Learning Disabilities

ACAneS American College of Anesthetists

ACAng American College of Angiology (also ACA)

ACanS American Cancer Society (also ACS)

ACAT acyl cholesterol acyltransferase
American Center for the Alexander Technique

ACB American Council of the Blind
antibody-coated bacteria
aortocoronary bypass
arterial capillary blood

ACBFE American Council of the Blind Federal Employees

ACBG aortocoronary bypass graft

ACC adenoid cystic carcinoma
alveolar cell carcinoma
ambulatory care center
American College of Cardiology
American College of Chemosurgery
American College of Cryosurgery
anodal closure contraction
antitoxin-containing cell
articular chondrocalcinosis

Acc acceleration (also accel)
accident
accommodation (also A, accom)
accompany
according

ACCA American Clinical and Climatological Association

ACCC Association of Community Cancer Centers

accel acceleration (also Acc)

ACCH Association for the Care of Children's Health
Association of Child Care in Hospitals

AcCH See ACh

ACCl anodal closure clonus

ACCME Accreditation Council of Continuing Medical Education

AcCoA acetyl coenzyme A

accom accommodation (also A, Acc)

ACCP American College of Chest Physicians
American College of Clinical Pharmacology

accur accurately

ACD absolute cardiac dullness
acid, citrate, dextrose
actinomycin D
adult celiac disease
allergic contact dermatitis
alpha-chain disease
American College of Dentists
annihilation coincidence detection
anterior chest diameter
anticoagulant citrate dextrose
area of cardiac dullness
citric acid, trisodium citrate, dextrose

AcD alive with disease
ACE adrenocortical extract
alcohol, chloroform, ether
American Council on Education
angiotensin-converting enzyme
See AChE
ACEH acid cholesterol ester hydrolase
ACEHSA
Accrediting Commission on Education for Health Services Administration
ACEI angiotensin-converting enzyme inhibitor
ACEP American College of Emergency Physicians
ACERP American College of Emergency Room Physicians
ACF accessory clinical finding
advanced communications function
area correction factor (also CaF)
ACFn additional cost of false negatives
ACFNY Asthmatic Children's Foundation of New York
ACFO American College of Foot Orthopedists
ACFp additional cost of false positives
ACFR American College of Foot Roentgenologists
ACFS American College of Foot Specialists
American College of Foot Surgeons
ACFUCY
actinomycin D 5-fluorouracil, cyclophosphamide
ACG American College of Gastroenterology
angiocardiography
apexcardiogram
AcG accelerator globulin
ACGIH American Conference of Governmental and Industrial Hygienists
ACGME Accreditation Council for Graduate Medical Education
ACGPOMS
American College of General Practitioners in Osteopathic Medicine and Surgery
ACH achalasia
adrenocortical hormone
See ACHi
ACh acetylcholine
ACHA American College Health Association
American College of Hospital Administrators
AChE acetylcholinesterase
AChemS
American Chemical Society (also ACS)
ACHI Association for Childbirth at Home, International
ACHi arm girth, chest depth, hip width index
AChR acetylcholine receptor
AChRAb
acetylcholine receptor antibody
ACI adrenocortical insufficiency
average cost of illness
ACIF anticomplement immunofluorescence
ACIP acute canine idiopathic polyneuropathy
Advisory Committee for Immunization Practices
American College of International Physicians
ACL anterior cruciate ligament
ACLA American Clinical Laboratory Association
ACLAM American College of Laboratory Animal Medicine
ACLD Association for Children with Learning Disabilities (see ACALD)
ACLM American College of Legal Medicine
ACLS advanced cardiac life support
ACM aclacinomycin
albumin, calcium, magnesium
alveolar capillary membrane
anticardiac myosin
atom connectivity matrix
ACMC Association of Canadian Medical Colleges
ACME Automated Classification of Medical Entities
ACMF arachnoid cyst of the middle fossa
ACMP alveolar-capillary membrane permeability
ACMS Advisory Committee on Medical Science
American Chinese Medical Society
ACMV assist-controlled mechanical ventilation
ACN American College of Neuropsychiatrists
American College of Nutrition
ACNHA American College of Nursing Home Administrators
ACNM American College of Nurse-Midwives
ACNP American College of Neuropsychopharmacology
American College of Nuclear Physicians (also ACNuP)
ACNU 1-(4-amino-2-methyl-5-pyrimidinyl)-methyl-3-(2-chloroethyl)-3-nitrosourea
ACNuM American College of Nuclear Medicine
ACNuP American College of Nuclear Physicians (also ACNP)
ACO acute coronary occlusion
American College of Orgonomy
American College of Otorhinolaryngologists
American Council of Otolaryngology
anodal closing odor
ACOG American College of Obstetricians and Gynecologists
ACOHA American College of Osteopathic Hospital Administrators
ACO-HNS
American Council of Otolaryngology-Head and Neck Surgery
ACOI American College of Osteopathic Internists
ACO-M aconitase, mitochondrial
ACOMS American College of Oral and Maxillofacial Surgeons
ACOOG American College of Osteopathic Obstetricians and Gynecologists
ACOP American College of Osteopathic Pediatricians
doxorubicin (Adriamycin), cyclophosphamide, vincristine (Oncovin), prednisolone
ACopp doxorubicin (Adriamycin), cyclophosphamide, vincristine (Oncovin), predinisone, procarbazine
ACORE Advisory Council for Orthopedic Resident Education
ACOS American College of Osteopathic Surgeons
ACO-S aconitase, soluble
acous acoustics
ACP acid phosphatase (also AP)
acyl carrier protein
American College of Pathologists
American College of Physicians

American College of Podopediatrics
American College of Prosthodontists
American College of Psychiatrists
2-amino-4-chlorophenol
anodal closing picture
aspirin, caffeine, phenacetin
Association for Child Psychoanalysis
Association of Clinical Pathologists
N-amidino-3-amino-6-chloropyrazinecarboxamide

ACPA American Cleft Palate Association
ACPC 1-aminocyclopentanecarboxylic acid
ACPE American Council on Pharmaceutical Education
ACPM American College of Preventive Medicine (also ACPrM)
ACPMR American Congress of Physical Medicine and Rehabilitation (see ACRM)
ACPn American College of Psychoanalysts
ACPR American College of Podiatric Radiologists
ACPrM American College of Preventive Medicine (also ACPM)
ACPS acrocephalopolysyndactyly
ACR abnormally contracting regions
absolute catabolic rate
American College of Radiology
anticonstipation regimen
axillary count rate
Acr acriflavin
ACRM American College of Rehabilitation Medicine
American Congress of Rehabilitation Medicine
ACRMD Association for Children with Retarded Mental Development
ACS acetyl strophanthidin
acrocephalosyndactyly
acute confusional state
acute mountain sickness
ambulatory care services
American Cancer Society (also ACanS)
American Celiac Society
American Chemical Society (also AChemS)
American College of Surgeons
anodal closing sound
anticytotoxic serum
antireticular cytotoxic serum
Association of Clinical Scientists
ACSH American Council on Science and Health
ACSM American College of Sports Medicine
ACSW Academy of Certified Social Workers
ACT abdominal computerized tomogram
activated clotting time
activated coagulation time
Advanced Coronary Treatment Foundation
Alliance for Cannabis Therapeutics
antichromotrypsin
anticoagulant therapy
antrocolic transposition
Anxiety Control Training
atropine coma therapy
act active (also A)
ACTA American Cardiology Technologists Association
American Corrective Therapy Association
ACTe anodal closure tetanus
ACTH adrenocorticotropic hormone
ACTH-RF
adrenocorticotropic hormone-releasing factor
ACTN adrenocorticotrophin
ACTP adrenocorticotropic polypeptide
ACU acute care unit
agar colony-forming unit
ambulatory care unit
ACURP American College of Utilization Review Physicians
ACV acyclovir
arterial, corotid, ventricular
atherosclerotic cardiovascular
ACVD acute cardiovascular disease
ACVM American College of Veterinary Microbiologists
ACVO American College of Veterinary Ophthalmologists
ACVP American College of Veterinary Pathologists
ACVR American College of Veterinary Radiology
ACVT American College of Veterinary Toxicologists
ACWC American Council of Women Chiropractors
AD accident dispensary
active disease
acute dermatomyositis
adenoidal degeneration
admitting diagnosis
adrenal demedullated
aerosol deposition
after discharge
alcohol dehydrogenase (see ADH)
Aleutian disease
alveolar duct
Alzheimer's disease
anodal duration
antigenic determinant
appropriate disability
atopic dermatitis
autosomal dominant
average day
average deviation
axiodistal
axis deviation
diphenylchlorarsine
right ear (auris dextra) (also RE)
A.D. Associate Degree
A/D analog to digital
A&D admission and discharge
Ad adipocyte
A d anisotropic disk
ad add
let there be added (addetur)
ADA adenosine deaminase
American Dental Association
American Dermatological Association
American Diabetes Association (also ADiabA)
American Dietetic Association
ammonium dihydrogen arsenate
anterior descending artery
ADAA American Dental Assistants Association
ADAF American Dietetic Association Foundation
ADAI Alcoholism and Drug Abuse Institute
ADAMHA
Alcohol, Drug Abuse, and Mental Health Administration
ADARA American Deafness and Rehabilitation Association
ad aur
to the ear (ad aurem)
adB acceleration decibel
ADC Affective Disorders Clinic

Aid to Dependent Children
albumin, dextrose, catalase
analog to digital converter
anodal duration contraction
anterior descending coronary
antral diverticulum of the colon
average daily census
axiodistocervical

AdC adrenal cortex (also AC)

ADCC antibody-dependent cell-mediated cytotoxicity
antibody-dependent cellular cytotoxicity

ADD attention deficit disorder
average daily dose

add adduction

ad def an
to the point of fainting (ad defectionem animi)

ad deliq
to fainting (ad deliquium)

ADD-HA
attention deficit disorder with hyperactivity

ADDS American Digestive Disease Society
American Diopter and Decibel Society

ADE acute disseminated encephalitis

ADEM acute disseminated encephalomyelitis

ad feb
fever present (adstante febre)

ADFS American Dentists for Foreign Service

ADG axiodistogingival

ad grat acid
to an agreeable sourness (ad gratum aciditatem)

ad grat gust
to an agreeable taste (ad gratum gustum)

ADH Academy of Dentistry for the Handicapped
alcohol dehyrogenase
antidiuretic hormone

ADHA American Dental Hygienists' Association

adhib to be administered (adhibendus)

ADI Academy of Dentistry International
acceptable daily intake
allowable daily intake
antral diverticulum of the ileum
autosomal dominant ichthyosis

ADiabA
American Diabetes Association (also ADA)

ad int
in the meantime (ad interim)

adj adjoining
adjunct
adjutant

ADK adenosine kinase (also AK)

ADKC atopic dermatitis with keratoconjunctivitis

ADL activities of daily living

ad lib
as desired (ad libitum)

ADM Adriamycin
apparent distribution mass

AdM adrenal medulla

adm administrator
admission

admin administration

admov let there be added (admove)

ADMR average daily metabolic rate

ADMX adrenal medullectomy

ad naus
producing nausea (ad nauseum)

ADNB antideoxyribonuclease B

ad neut
neutralization (ad neutralizandum)

ADO axiodisto-occlusal

Ado adenosine (also A)

AdoMet
S-adenosylmethionine (also SAM)

ADOP doxorubicin (Adriamycin), vincristine (Oncovin), prednisone

ADP Academy of Denture Prosthetics
acute dermatomyositis and polymyositis
adenosine diphosphate
advanced pancreatitis
ammonium dihydrogen phosphate
automatic data processing
See ADM (Adriamycin)

AdP adductor pollicus

ADPA Alcohol and Drug Problems Association

ad part dolent
to the painful parts (ad partes dolentes)

ADPase
apyrase (adenosine diphosphatase)

ADPL average daily patient load

ad pond om
to the weight of the whole (ad pondus omnium)

adq adequate

ADR adverse drug reaction
airway dilation reflex

Adr See E (epinephrine)

ADRDA Alzheimer's Disease and Related Disorders Association

Adria See ADM (Adriamycin)

ADS alternate delivery system
antibody deficiency syndrome
antidiuretic substance

ADSA American Dental Society of Anesthesiology

ADSAI American Dermatologic Society of Allergy and Immunology

ad sat
to saturation (ad saturandum)

ADSE American Dental Society of Europe

adst feb
while fever is present (adstante febre)

ADT adenosine triphosphate
Alphabetischer Durchstreichtest
alternate day therapy
any desired thing

ADTA American Dance Therapy Association
American Dental Trade Association

ADTe anodal duration tetanus

ad tert vic
three times (ad tertiam vicem)

ADTN 2-amino-6,7-dihydroxy-1,2,3,4-tetrahydronapthalene

ADU acute duodenal ulcer

ad us according to custom (ad usum)

ad us ext
for external use (ad usum externum)

ADV adenovirus
adventitia

Adv advisory

adv advanced
against (adversum)

ad 2 vic
for two doses (ad duas vices)

A5D5W 5% alcohol, 5% dextrose in water

ADX adrenalectomized

AE above elbow
Accurate Empathy
acetyleugenol
activation energy
adrenal epinephrine
adult erythrocyte
alcohol embryopathy
androstanediol
antitoxin unit (antitoxineinheit)
aryepiglottic
Ae at the age of (aetatis)
AEC adenylate energy charge
at earliest convenience
Atomic Energy Commission
S-(2-aminoethyl)L-cysteine
AED antiepileptic drug
AEDiol
5-androstanediol
AEDP automated external defibrillator pacemaker
AEEGS American Electroencephalographic Society
AEF allogenic effect factor
aryepiglottic fold
AEG air encephalogram
aeg the patient (aeger)
AEI arbitrary evolution index
atrial emptying index
AEM analytic electron microscope
AEP acute edematous pancreatitis
artificial endocrine pancreas
auditory evoked potential
average evoked potential
AEpS American Epilepsy Society (also AES)
AEq age equivalent
aeq equal (aequales)
AER active E-rosette
agranular endoplasmic reticulum
aided equilization response
albumin excretion rate
aldosterone excretion rate
apical ectodermal ridge
auditory evoked response
average electroencephalic response
average evoked response
AerosMA
Aerospace Medical Association (also AMA)
AERP atrial effective refractory period
AES American Encephalographic Society
American Endodontic Society
American Endoscopic Society
American Epidemiological Society
American Epidermological Society
American Epilepsy Society (also AEpS)
American Equilibration Society
AET 2-aminoethylisothiuronium
aet age (aetas) (also A)
at the age of (aetatis)
AETT acetyl ethyl tetramethyl Tetralin
AEV avian erythroblastosis virus
AEVH Association for Education of the Visually Handicapped
AF acid fast
activity front
albumose-free
aldehyde fuchsin
alleged father
2-aminofluorene
amniotic fluid
anchoring fibril
anteflexion
antibody forming
aortic flow
Arthritis Foundation
artificially fed
ascitic fluid
atrial fibrillation
atrial fusion
attenuation factor
audiofrequency
auricular fibrillation
2AF 2-aminofluorene
AFA alcohol-formalin-acetic acid
Allergy Foundation of America
American Fracture Association
AFAHC American Foundation for Alternative Health Care
AFAR American Foundation for Aging Research
AFB acid fast bacillus
American Foundation for the Blind
AFB_1 aflatoxin B_1
AFC antibody-forming cell
AFCI acute focal cerebral ischemia
AFCR American Federation for Clinical Research
AFDC Aid to Families with Dependent Children
AFDO Association of Food and Drug Officials
aff afferent
having an infinity for (affinis)
AFG auditory figure ground
AFH American Foundation for Homeopathy
anterior facial height
AFI amaurotic familial idiocy
AFIP Armed Forces Institute of Pathology
AFL atrial flutter
AFLP acute fatty liver of pregnancy
AFN afunctional neutrophil
AFO ankle-foot orthosis
AFOS Armed Forces Optometric Society
AFP alpha-fetoprotein
anterior faucial pillar
AFPD American Federation of Physicians and Dentists
AFPE American Foundation for Pharmaceutical Education
AFPPG American Foundation for Psychoanalysis and Psychoanalysis in Groups
AFRD acute febrile respiratory disease
AFRI acute febrile respiratory illness
AFS acid-fast smear
American Fertility Society
American Fracture Society
AFT_3 absolute free triiodothyronine
AFT_4 absolute free thyroxine
AFTA American Family Therapy Association
AFTER Ask a Friend to Explain Reconstruction
AFV amniotic fluid volume
AFX atypical fibroxanthoma
AG antiglobulin
antigravity
Association for Gnotobiotics
atrial gallop
axiogingival
A/G albumin to globulin ratio
Ag antigen
silver (argentum)
^{105}Ag radioactive isotope of silver
^{110}Ag radioactive isotope of silver
^{111}Ag radioactive isotope of silver
AGA accelerated growth area
American Gastroenterological Association
appropriate for gestational age

N-acetylglutamate (also NAG)
AGAS N-acetylglutamate synthetase (also NAGS)
AGBA Alexander Graham Bell Association
AGC automatic gain control
AGCT Army General Classification Test
AGD Academy of General Dentistry
agar gel diffusion
AGE American Aging Association (also AAA)
angle of greatest extension
AGEA American Gastro-Enterological Association (see AGA--American Gastroenterological Association)
AGEPC acetyl glyceryl ether phosphorylcholine
AGerS American Geriatrics Society (also AGS)
AGF angle of greatest flexion
AGG agammaglobulinemia
aggravated
agg agglutination (also AGL)
aggregate
aggred feb
while the fever is coming on (aggrediente febre)
AGH American Guild of Hypnotherapists
agit shake (agita)
agit a sum
shake before taking (agita ante sumendum)
agit a us
shake before using (agita ante usum)
agit b
shake well (agita bene)
agit vas
the vial being shaken (agitato vase)
AGL acute granulocytic leukemia
agglutination (also agg)
aminoglutethimide
AGMK African green monkey kidney
AGMKC African green monkey kidney cell
AGML acute gastric mucosal lesion
AGN acute glomerulonephritis
AGP agar gel precipitation
alpha-l-acid glycoprotein (also AAG)
AGPA American Group Practice Association
American Group Psychotherapy Association
AGPP Association for Group Psychoanalysis and Process
AGS adrenogenital syndrome
American Geriatrics Society (also AGerS)
American Gerontology Society
American Gynecological Society
antiglucagon
AGT abnormal glucose tolerance
activity group therapy
antiglobulin test
agt agent
AGTH adrenoglomerulotropin
AGTT abnormal glucose tolerance test
AGU aspartylglycosaminuria
AGV antiline gentian violet
AH abdominal hysterectomy
accidental hypothermia
acetohexamide
acid hydrolysis
acute hepatitis
adult home
alcoholic hepatitis
amenorrhea and hirsutism
aminohippurate
anterior hypothalamus
antihyaluronidase
arterial hypertension
axillary hair
hyperopic astigmatism (also aha, ASH)
Ah ampere hour
AHA acetohydroxamic acid
acquired hemolytic anemia
American Healing Association
American Heart Association
American Hospital Association
American Hypnotists' Association
antiheart antibody
arylhydrocarbon-hydroxylase
autoimmune hemolytic anemia
aha hyperopic astigmatism (also AH, ASH)
See alt hor
AHAF American Health Assistance Foundation
AHAT arylhydroxamic acid N,O-acyltransferase
AHC acute hemorrhagic conjunctivitis
AHCA American Health Care Association
AHCC Academy of Health Care Consultants
AHCTL N-acetylhomocipteinethiolactone
AHD arteriosclerotic heart disease
atherosclerotic heart disease
autoimmune hemolytic disease
AHF American Health Foundation
American Hepatic Foundation
American Hospital Formulary
antihemophilic factor
Argentine hemorrhagic fever
AHFS American Hospital Formulary Service
AHG aggregated human globulin
antihemolytic globulin
antihemophilic globulin
antihuman globulin
AHGG aggregated human gamma globulin
antihuman gamma globulin
AHGS acute herpetic gingivostomatitis
AHH alpha-hydrazine analogue of histidine
arylhydrocarbon hydroxylase
Association for Holistic Health
AHL apparent half-life
AHLE acute hemorrhagic leukoencephalitis
AHLS antihuman lymphocyte serum
AHMA American Holistic Medical Association
antiheart muscle autoantibody
AHP acute hemorrhagic pancreatitis
after hyperpolarization
air at high pressure
Assistant House Physician
AHPA American Health Planning Association
AHPR Academy of Hospital Public Relations
AHQ Association for Healthcare Quality
AHRF American Hearing Research Foundation
AHS American Hearing Society
Assistant House Surgeon
AHSA American Human Serum Association
AHSN Assembly of Hospital Schools of Nursing
AHT antihyaluronidase titer
augmented histamine test
autogenous hamster tumor
AHTN Association of Hospital Television Networks
AHTS antihuman thymus serum
AHU arginine, hypoxanthine, uracil
AHVN American Hospital Video Network
AI accidentally incurred
aortic incompetence
aortic insufficiency
apical impulse
articular index
artificial insemination

artificial intelligence
autoimmune
axioincisal
A&I Allergy and Immunology
AIA Acupuncture International Association
allylisopropylacetamide
anti-insulin antibody
aspirin-induced asthma
automated image analysis
AIAA American Institute of Aeronautics and Astronautics
AIANNA American Indian/Alaska Native Nurses Association
AIB aminoisobutyric acid
AIBN 2,2'-azobisisobutyronitrile
AIBS American Institute of Biological Sciences
AIC aminoimidazole carboxamide
Association des Infirmières Canadiennes
AICA anterior inferior cerebellar artery
AICAR aminoiminazolecarboxyamide ribonucleotide
AICE angiotensin I converting enzyme
AID acquired immunodeficiency disease
acute infectious disease
Agency for International Development
artificial insemination, donor
autoimmune disease
average interocular difference
AIDA Association of Independent Doctors in Addiction
AIDS acquired immunodeficiency syndrome
AIE acetylisoeugenol
acute inclusion body encephalitis
AIEP amount of insulin extractable from the pancreas
AIF anti-inflammatory
A-IGP activity-interview group psychotherapy
AIH American Institute of Homeopathy
artificial insemination, homologous
artificial insemination, husband
AIHA American Industrial Hygiene Association
autoimmune hemolytic anemia
AIHC American Industrial Health Council
AIHP American Institute of the History of Pharmacy
AIL angioimmunoblastic lymphadenopathy
AILD alveolar-interstitial lung disease
angioimmunoblastic lymphadenopathy with dysproteinemia
AIM Academy of Internal Medicine
Aid for International Medicine
assessment of interactive mode
AIMC American Institute of Medical Climatology
AIMD abnormal involuntary movement disorder
AIME American Institute of Mining and Metallurgical Engineers
AIMS Abnormal Involuntary Movement Scale
Arthritis Impact Measurement Scales
Association for International Medical Study
AIN acute interstitial nephritis
American Institute of Nutrition
A Insuf See AI (aortic insufficiency)
AIOPI Association of Information Officers in the Pharmaceutical Industry
AIP acute intermittent porphyria
aldosterone-induced protein
American Institute for Psychoanalysis
annual implementation plan
average intravascular pressure
AIPCM American Institute of Primary Care Medicine
AIPS American Institute of Pathologic Science
AIR aminoimidazole ribonucleotide
Average Impairment Rating
AIREN American Institute for Research and Education in Naturopathy
AIRS Amphetamine Interview Rating Scale
AIS Abbreviated Injury Scale
anti-insulin serum
AISI American Iron and Steel Institute
AIT Academy for Implants and Transplants
AIU absolute iodine uptake
AIUM American Institute of Ultrasound in Medicine
AIVR accelerated idioventricular rhythm
AIVV anterior internal vertebral vein
AJ ankle jerk
AJC American Joint Committee for Cancer Staging and End-Results Reporting
AJCC American Joint Committee on Cancer
AK above the knee
adenosine kinase (also ADK)
adenylate kinase
AKA above knee amputation
alcoholic ketoacidosis
alpha-allokainic acid
also known as
antikeratin antibody
AKF Aga Khan Foundation
AL absolute latency
acinar lumina
acute leukemia
adaptation level
amyloid L
annoyance level
argininsuccinate lysate
axiolingual
furaltadone
lethal antigen
See ad lib
Al allergy (also A)
aluminum
^{26}Al radioactive isotope of aluminum
ALA American Laryngological Association
American Longevity Association
American Lung Association
aminolevulinic acid
anterior lip of the acetabulum
ALa axiolabial
Ala alanine
ALAD abnormal left axis deviation
aminolevulinic acid dehydrase
ALaG axiolabiogingival
ALaL axiolabiolingual
ALAS delta-aminolevulinic acid synthetase
ALAT alanine transferase
See ALT (alanine transaminase)
alb albumin
white (albus)
ALC absolute lymphocyte count
approximate lethal concentration
avian leukosis complex
axiolinguocervical
alc alcohol
ALCA anomalous left coronary artery
ALCEQ Adolescent Life Change Event Questionnaire
alcoh See alc

alc r alcohol rub
ALD adrenoleukodystrophy
alcoholic liver disease
aldosterone
anterior latissimus dorsi
Ald aldolase
ALDH aldehyde dehydrogenase
ALE allowable limits of error
ALF acute liver failure
American Liver Foundation
anterior long fiber
ALFA aluminum formaldehyde
ALG antilymphoblastic globulin
antilymphocyte globulin
axiolinguogingival
ALH anterior lobe hormone
anterior lobe of the hypophysis (also ALP--anterior lobe of the pituitary)
ALIMDA
Association of Life Insurance Medical Directors of America
Alk alkaline
Alk phos
alkaline phosphatase (also ALP, AP)
ALL acute lymphoblastic leukemia
acute lymphocytic leukemia
Airlifeline
ALLO atypical Legionella-like organism
ALM alveolar lining material
American Leprosy Missions
ALME acetyl-lysine methyl ester
ALMI anterior lateral myocardial infarct
ALMV anterior leaflet of the mitral valve
ALN anterior lymph nodes
ALO axiolinguo-occlusal
ALOS average length of stay
ALP alkaline phosphatase (also Alk phos, AP)
anterior lobe of the pituitary (also ALH--anterior lobe of the hypophysis)
antilymphocyte plasma
argon laser photocoagulation
ALPS Aphasia Language Performance Scales
ALROS American Laryngological, Rhinological, and Otological Society
ALS advanced life support
afferent loop syndrome
amyotrophic lateral sclerosis
antilymphatic serum
antilymphocytic serum
antiviral lymphocyte serum
ALSD Alzheimer-like senile dementia
ALSSOA
Amyotrophic Lateral Sclerosis Society of America
ALT alanine aminotransferase (SGPT)
alanine transaminase
alt alternate
altitude
other (alter)
alt dieb
every other day (alternis diebus)
ALTEE acetyl-L-tyrosine ethyl ester
alt hor
every other hour (alternis horis)
alt noc
every other night (alternis nocte)
ALV ascending lumbar vein
avian leukosis virus
alv alveolar
ALVAD abdominal left ventricular assist device
alv adst
when the bowels are constipated (alvo adstricta)
alv deject
alvine dejections (alvi dejectiones)
ALVT aortic and left ventricular tunnel
ALW arch, loop, whorl
AM acrylamide
actomysin
adult monocyte
aerospace medicine
alveolar macrophage
alveolar mucosa
ametropia
amperemeter
amplitude modulation
anovular menstruation
anterior mitral
arithmetic mean
aviation medicine
axiomesial
before noon (ante meridiem)
meter angle
mixed astigmatism
myopic astigmatism (also ASM)
A.M. Master of Arts
Am American
americium
^{241}Am radioactive isotope of americium
am amplitude (also amp)
AMA actual mechanical advantage
Aerospace Medical Association (also AerosMA)
against medical advice
American Medical Association
antimitochrondial antibody
Australian Medical Association
AMA-ERF
American Medical Association Education and Research Foundation
AMAL Aeromedical Acceleration Laboratory
AMAP as much as possible
AMAT amorphous material
AMB amphotericin B
Amb ambulance
ambulatory
AMBOP American Board of Oral Pathology
AMC 7-amino-4-methylcourmarin
antibody-mediated cytotoxicity
arm muscle circumference
arthrogryposis multiplex congenita
axiomesiocervical
AMCA American Mosquito Control Association
AMCHA trans-4-(aminomethyl)cyclohexanecarboxylic acid
AMCN anteromedial caudate nucleus
AMD acid maltase deficiency
actinomycin D
adrenomyelodystrophy
Aleutian mink disease
alpha-methyldopa
Association for Macular Diseases
axiomesiodistal
AMDA Airline Medical Directors Association
AMDGF alveolar macrophage-derived growth factor
AMDS Association of Military Dental Surgeons
AME amphotericin B methyl ester
AMEEGA
American Medical Electroencephalographic Association
AMEL Aeromedical Equipment Laboratory

AMESLAN American sign language
AMG antimacrophage globulin
axiomesiogingival
AMGP Association of Medical Group Psychoanalysts
AMH anti-Mullerian hormone
automated medical history
mixed astigmatism with myopia predominating
AMHA Association of Mental Health Administrators
AMHCA American Mental Health Counselors Association
AMHF American Mental Health Foundation
AMHT automated multiphasic health testing
AMHV age at minimal height velocity
AMHVR age at minimal height velocity return
AMI acute myocardial infarction
amitriptyline
anterior myocardial infarction
Association of Medical Illustrators
axiomesioincisal
AMIS Aspirin Myocardial Infarction Study
AMJA American Medical Joggers Association
AML acute monocytic leukemia
acute mucosal lesion
acute myeloblastic leukemia
acute myelocytic leukemia
acute myelogenous leukemia
anterior mitral leaflet
AMLC adherent macrophage-like cell
autologous mixed lymphocyte culture
AMLR autologous mixed lymphocytic reaction
autologous mixed lymphocyte response
AMLS antimouse lymphocyte serum
AMM agnogenic myeloid metaplasia
amm ammonia
AMML acute myelomonocytic leukemia
AMN adrenomyeloneuropathy
anterior median nucleus
AMO axiomesio-occlusal
amo See amor
AMOL See AML (acute monocytic leukemia)
amor amorphous
AMP acid mucopolysaccharide
adenosine monophosphate
ampicillin
average mean pressure
amp ampere (also A)
amplitude (also am)
ampule
amputation
AMPAC American Medical Political Action Committee
AMPD 2-amino-2-methyl-1-propandiol
AMPH amphetamine
AMPRA American Medical Peer Review Association
AMPS abnormal mucopolysacchariduria
acid mucopolysaccharide
AMPT alpha-methyl-p-tyrosine
AMR acoustic muscle reflex
AMRA American Medical Record Association
AMRDC Association of Medical Rehabilitation Directors and Coordinators
AMRI anteromedial rotatory instability
AMRL Aerospace Medical Research Laboratory
AMRSHF Adrenal Metabolic Research Society of the Hypoglycemia Foundation
AMS acute mountain sickness
aggravated in military service
American Meteorological Society
American Microbiological Society
antimacrophage serum
Army Medical Service
auditory memory span
automated multiphasic screening
ams amount of a substance
AMSA acridinylamino-methane-sulfon-m-anisidide
American Medical Society on Alcoholism
American Medical Students' Association
AmSECT American Society of Extracorporeal Technology
AMSPDC Association of Medical School Pediatric Department Chairmen
AMSUS Association of Military Surgeons of the United States
AMT alpha-methyltyrosine
American Medical Technologists
amethopterin
4'-aminomethyl-4,5',8-trimethylpsoralen (also ATMD)
aminomethyltrioxsalen
amitriptyline
Anxiety Management Training
amt amount
AMTA American Massage and Therapy Association
AMTP alpha-methyltryptophan
AMU atomic mass unit
AMV assisted mechanical ventilation
avian myeloblastosis virus
AMWA American Medical Women's Association
American Medical Writers' Association
AMX amoxicillin
Amy amylase
AN acanthosis nigricans
administratively necessary
ala nasi
aminonucleoside
amyl nitrate
anorexia nervosa
autonomic neuropathy
avascular necrosis
normal atmosphere
6-AN 6-aminonicotinamide
An actinon
anatomy response
aniridia
anisometropia
anode (also A)
ANA acetylneuraminic acid
American Naprapathic Association
American Narcolepsy Association
American Neurological Association
American Nurses' Association
antinuclear antibody
aspartyl naphthylamide
ANAD antinicotinamide adenine dinucleotidase
ANAE alpha-naphthyl acetate esterase
anal analgesic
analysis
ANAP agglutination negative, absorption positive
anat anatomy
ANC absolute neutrophil count
Army Nurse Corps
AnCC See ACC (anodal closure contraction)
AND administratively necessary days

ANDA Abbreviated New Drug Application
AnDTe anodal duration tetanus
Anes anesthesia
anesth
See Anes
an ex anode excitation
ANF alpha-naphthoflavone
American Nurses' Federation
American Nurses' Foundation
antineuritic factor
antinuclear factor
ANG I angiotensin I (also A I, AT I)
ANG II
angiotensin II (also A II, AT II)
ang angiogram
angle (also A)
ANGOS Air National Guard Optometric Society
ANHA American Nursing Home Association
ANHS American Natural Hygiene Society
ANIT alpha-naphthylisothiocyanate
ANL acute nonlymphocytic leukemia (also ANLL)
ANLL acute nonlymphoblastic leukemia
acute nonlymphocytic leukemia (also ANL)
ANM auxiliary nurse midwife
ann annual
AnOC See AOC (anodal opening contraction)
ANOVA analysis of variance
ANP acute necrotizing pancreatitis
ANRC American National Red Cross
ANS American Neurological Society
American Nuclear Society
8-anilino-1-naphthalenesulfonate
anterior nasal spine
antineutrophilic serum
arteriolonephrosclerosis
atrial depolarization not sensed
autonomic nervous system
ans answer
ANSI American National Standards Institute
ANT aminoglycoside 2'-O-nucleotidyltransferase
2-amino-5-nitrothiazol
antimycin
ANT III
See AT III
ant anterior (also A)
antag antagonistic
ant ax line
anterior axial line
anti antidote
ant jentac
before breakfast (ante jentaculum)
ant pit
See AP (anterior pituitary)
ant prand
before dinner (ante prandium)
ANTR apparent net transfer rate
ant sup sp
anterior superior spine
ANTU alpha-naphthylthiourea
ANUG acute necrotizing ulcerative gingivitis
AO abdominal aorta
acid output
acridine orange
anodal opening
aortic opening
Arbeitsgemeinschaft Osteosynthesefragen
ascending aorta
atrioventricular valve opening
auriculoventricular valve opening
average optical density
avoidance of others
axio-occlusal
A/O alert and oriented
Ao aorta
AOA American Ontoanalytic Association
American Optometric Association
American Orthopaedic Association
American Orthopsychiatric Association
American Osteopathic Association
average orifice area
AOAA aminooxoacetic acid
AOAC Association of Official Analytical Chemists
AOAO American Osteopathic Academy of Orthopedics
AOAS American Osteopathic Academy of Sclerotherapy
AOB alcohol on breath
AOC American Orthoptic council
anodal opening contraction
AOCA American Osteopathic College of Anesthesiologists
AOCD American Osteopathic College of Dermatology
AOCl anodal opening clonus
AOCP American Osteopathic College of Pathologists
American Osteopathic College of Proctology
AOCR American Osteopathic College of Radiology
AOCRM American Osteopathic College of Rehabilitation Medicine
AOD arterial occlusive disease
arterial oxygen desaturation
AODM adult-onset diabetes mellitus
AODT Animal and Opposite Drawing Technique
AOE Association of Optometric Educators
AOEHI American Organization for the Education of the Hearing Impaired
AOF American Optometric Foundation
AOFS American Orthopedic Foot Society
AOHA American Osteopathic Hospital Association
AOM acute otitis media
azoxymethane
A.O.M.
Master of Obstetric Art
AOMA American Occupational Medical Association
copolymer of maleic acid and alpha-oelfin
AoMP aortic mean pressure
AOO anodal opening odor
AOP Academy of Orthomolecular Psychiatry
acetoxypregnenolone
anodal opening picture
aortic pressure
AOPA American Orthotic and Prosthetic Association
AoPW aortic posterior wall
AOQL average outgoing quality limit
AOR auditory oculogyric reflex
AORN Association of Operating Room Nurses
AOrPA American Ortho-Psychiatric Association
AORT Association of Operating Room Technicians
aort regurg
aortic regurgitation
aort sten
aortic stenosis

AOS American Ophthalmological Society
American Orthodontic Society
American Otological Society (also AOtS)
anodal opening sound
AOSA American Optometric Student Association
AOSED Association of Osteopathic State Executive Directors
AOSSM American Orthopaedic Society for Sports Medicine
AOT accessory optic tract
Association of Occupational Therapists
AOTA American Occupational Therapy Association
AOTe anodal opening tetanus
AOtS American Otological Society (also AOS)
AOV See ANOVA
AoV aortic valve
AP abdominal-perineal
Academy of Periodontology
acid phosphatase (also ACP)
acinar parenchyma
action potential
active pepsin
acute phase
acute pneumonia
adolescent population
after parturition
alkaline phosphatase (also Alk phos, ALP)
aminopeptidase
aminopyrine
angina pectoris
animal passaged
antepartum
anterior pituitary
anteroposterior
antiparkinsonian
antipyrine
antral peristalsis
aortic pressure
aortic pulmonary
apical pulse
appendix
area postrema
arterial pressure
artificial pneumothorax
aspiration pneumonitis
Association for Psychotheatrics
association period
atherosclerotic plaque
axiopulpal
A-P analytic-psychologic
A&P anterior and posterior
assessment and plans
auscultation and percussion
4-AP 4-aminopyridine
ap apothecary
before meals (ante prandium)
prior to (a priori)
APA aldosterone-producing adenoma
Ambulatory Pediatric Association
American Pancreatic Association
American Paralysis Association
American Podiatry Association
American Psychiatric Association
American Psychoanalytic Association (also APsychoA)
American Psychological Association (also APsychA)
American Psychopathological Association (also APsychpthA)
American Psychotherapy Association
aminopenicillanic acid
antiparietal antibody
antipernicious anemia factor
See APhA
See APTA
6-APA 6-aminopenicillanic acid
APAA American Physician Art Association
APAP Association of Physician Assistant Programs
N-acetyl-p-aminophenol
APArc arcuate nucleus
APB abductor pollicis brevis
atrial premature beat
auricular premature beat
APC acetylsalicylic acid, phenacetin, caffeine
adenoidal, pharyngeal, conjunctival
alternative patterns of complement
antigen-presenting cell
Association of Pathology Chairmen
atrial premature contraction
APCC activated prothrombin complex concentrate
acetylsalicylic acid, phenacetin, caffeine, codeine
APCD adult polycystic kidney disease (also APKD)
APCF aquapentacyanoferrate
APD action potential duration
acute polycystic disease
adult polycystic disease
atrial premature depolarization
APDA American Parkinson Disease Association
APdS American Pediatric Society (also APS)
APE airway pressure excursion
aminophylline, phenobarbital, ephedrine
anterior pituitary extract
APF acidulated phosphate fluoride
anabolism-promoting factor
animal protein factor
antiperinuclear factor
APFRI American Physical Fitness Research Institute
APFS Association of Podiatrists in Federal Service
APGL alkaline phosphatase in granular leukocytes
APGO Association of Professors of Gynecology and Obstetrics
APH alcohol-positive history
American Printing House for the Blind
amikacin phosphotransferase
aminoglycoside 3'-O-phosphotransferase
antepartum hemorrhage
anterior pituitary hormone
aph aphasia
APHA American Protestant Hospital Association
American Public Health Association
APhA American Pharmaceutical Association
APHI Animal and Plant Health Inspection Service
APHP antipseudomonas human plasma
APhysthA
American Physiotherapy Association
API atmospheric pressure instrument
APIC Association for Practitioners in Infection Control
APIM Association Professionnelle Internationale des Medecins
APKD adult polycystic kidney disease (also APCD)

APL abductor pollicis longus
accelerated painless labor
acute promyelocytic leukemia
anterior pituitary-like
APM Academy of Physical Medicine
Academy of Psychosomatic Medicine
alternating pressure mattress
anterior papillary muscle
anteroposterior movement
aspartame
Association of Professors of Medicine
Association for Psychoanalytic Medicine
APMR Association for Physical and Mental Retardation
APN average peak noise
APNPS N^4-acetyl-N'-(p-nitrophenyl)sulfanilamide
APO adductor pollicis obliquus
aphoxide (also TEPA)
apomorphine
Apo apolipoprotein
APOCA Association of Psychiatric Outpatients Centers of America
APON Association of Pediatric Oncology Nurses
APORF acute postoperative renal failure
APP Academy of Pharmacy Practice
acute phase protein
alum precipitated pyridine
aqueous procaine penicillin
automated physiologic profile
avian pancreatic polypeptide
app appendix
APPA American Professional Practice Association
American Psychopathological Association
appar apparatus
apparent
APPG aqueous procaine penicillin G
appl appliance
applied
applan
flattened (applanatus)
APPPA Association of Philippine Practicing Physicians in America
appr approximate (also approx)
approx
approximate (also appr)
appt appointment
APPY appendectomy
APR abdominal-perineal resection
acute phase reactant
amebic prevalence rate
anterior pituitary reaction
auropalpapebral reflex
APrS American Proctologic Society (also APS)
APRT adenine phosphoribosyltransferase
APS Academy of Pharmaceutical Sciences
acute physiology score
adenosine phosphosulfate
American Pain Society
American Paraplegia Society
American Pediatric Society (also APdS)
American Physiological Society
American Proctologic Society (see ASCRS) (also APrS)
American Prosthodontic Society
American Psychiatric Society
American Psychological Scoiety
American Psychosomatic Society (also APsychosomS)
antiprostaglandin serum
Association of Pediatric Surgeons
APSA American Pediatric Surgical Association
APsaA American Psychoanalytic Association
APSS Association for the Psychophysiological Study of Sleep
APsychA
American Psychological Association (also APA)
APsychoA
American Psychoanalytic Association (also APA)
APsychosomS
American Psychosomatic Society (also APS)
APsychpthA
American Psychopathological Association (also APA)
APT alum-precipitated toxoid
Association for Poetry Therapy
APTA American Physical Therapy Association
aneurysm of persistent trigeminal artery
APTC Ambulatory Psoriasis Treatment Center
APTO Association for Psychiatric Treatment of Offenders
APTT activated partial thromboplastin time
APTX acute parathyroidectomy
APUD amine precursor uptake and decarboxylation
APV abnormally posterior vector
APW artificial pond water
AQ accomplishment quotient
achievement quotient
aphasia quotient
aq water (aqua) (also A)
aq ad water to (aquam ad)
aq astr
frozen water (aqua astricta)
aq bull
boiling water (aqua bulliens)
aq cal
warm water (aqua calida)
aq comm
common water (aqua communis)
aq dest
distilled water (aqua destillata)
aq ferv
hot water (aqua fervens)
aq fluv
river water (aqua fluvialis)
aq frig
cold water (aqua frigida)
aq mar
sea water (aqua marina)
aq niv
snow water (aqua nivalis)
aq pluv
rain water (aqua pluvialis)
aq pur
pure water (aqua pura)
aq tep
lukewarm water (aqua tepida)
AQVN average quasivalence number
AR achievement ratio
actinic reticuloid
active resistive
acute rejection
airway reactivity
airway resistance
alarm reaction
alcohol related
allergic rhinitis

amplitude ratio
analytic reagent
androgen receptor
aortic regurgitation
apical-radial
Argyll Robertson
artificial respiration
assisted respiration
atrial regurgitation
at risk
atrophic rhinitis
attack rate
autosomal recessive
See ars

Ar argon (also A)
^{37}Ar radioactive isotope of argon
ARA Academy of Rehabilitative Audiology
American Rheumatism Association
Ara arabinose
Ara-A adenine arabinoside
Ara-C cytosine arabinoside
Ara-C-HU cytosine arabinoside and hydroxyurea
ARAMIS American Rheumatism Association Medical Information System
ARAPP$_3$ arylazido aminoproprionyl adenosine triphosphate
ARAS ascending reticular activating system
ARC Addiction Research Center
American Red Cross
anomalous retinal correspondence
antigen reactive cell
Association for Retarded Citizens
ARCI Addiction Research Center Inventory
ARCO antigen reactive cell opsonization
ARCOS Automated Reports and Consolidated Orders System
ARCRT American Registry of Clinical Radiography Technologists
ARD acute respiratory disease
adult respiratory distress
allergic respiratory disease
anorectal dressing
ARDMS American Registry of Diagnostic Medical Sonographers
ARDS acute respiratory distress syndrome
adult respiratory distress syndrome
ARE active resistive exercise
ARF acute renal failure
acute respiratory failure
acute rheumatic fever
Adjective Rating Form
American Rehabilitation Foundation
Arthritis and Rheumatism Foundation (see AF--Arthritis Foundation)
ARFC active rosette-forming cells
Arg arginine
See Ag (silver)
ARHA American Rural Health Association
ARI Acne Research Institute
acute respiratory infection
ARIMA autoregressive integrated moving average
ARIS Anturane Reinfarction Italian Study
ARL average remaining lifetime
ARM aerosol rebreathing method
anorectal manometry
arteria radicularis magna
artificial rupture of the membranes
ARMA American Registry of Medical Assistants
ARMH Academy of Religion and Mental Health
Association for Rural Mental Health
ARN Association of Rehabilitation Nurses
ARNMD Association for Research in Nervous and Mental Disease
ARNP Advanced Registered Nurse Practitioner
ARO Association for Research in Ophthalmology
AROM active range of motion
ARP Alcohol Recovery Program
assay reference plasma
at risk period
ARPT American Registry of Physical Therapists
ARRS American Roentgen Ray Society
ARRT American Registry of Radiologic Technologists
ARS acquiescent response scale
American Radium Society
American Rhinologic Society
antirabies serum
ars arsphenamine
ARS-A arylsulfatase A (also ASA)
ARS-B arylsulfatase B (also ASB)
ARS-C arylsulfatase C (also ASC)
ART Accredited Record Technician
Anturane Reinfarction Trial
autologous reactive T-cell
automated reagin test
art artery (also A)
ARTI acute respiratory tract illness
artic articulation
artif artificial
ARVD arrhythmogenic right ventricular dysplasia
ARVO Association for Research in Vision and Ophthalmology
AS Academy of Science
acetylstrophanthidin
acidified serum
active sarcoidosis
active sleep
Adams-Stokes
adolescent suicide
aerosol steroid
affective style
alveolar sac
alveolar space
amyloid substance
andosterone sulfate
ankylosing spondylitis
annulospiral
antisocial
antistreptolysin
antral spasm
aortic stenosis
aqueous solution
aqueous suspension
arteriosclerosis
asthma astrocyte
atherosclerosis
atrial sense
atrial septum
left ear (auris sinistra) (also LE)
A.S. Associate of Science
12(9)AS 12(9)-anthroyl stearate
As arsenic
^{72}As radioactive isotope of arsenic
^{74}As radioactive isotope of arsenic
^{76}As radioactive isotope of arsenic
^{77}As radioactive isotope of arsenic

A_s atmosphere, standard
as See ast
ASA acetylsalicylic acid
Acoustical Society of America
active systemic anaphylaxis
Adams-Stokes attack
American Schizophrenia Association
American Society of Anesthesiologists
American Standards Association
American Stomatological Association
American Surgical Association
argininosuccinic acid
arylsulfatase A (also ARS-A)
5-ASA 5-amino salicylic acid
Asa arsenate
ASAAD American Society for Advancement of Anesthesia in Dentistry
ASAC acidified serum, acidified complement
ASA-G guaiacolic acid ester of acetylsalicylic acid
ASAHP American Society of Allied Health Professions
ASAIO American Society for Artificial Internal Organs
ASAL argininosuccinic acid lyase
ASAnes American Society of Anesthetists
ASAP American Society for Adolescent Psychiatry
asap as soon as possible
ASAPlS American Society of Aesthetic Plastic Surgery (also ASAPS)
ASAPS American Society for Aesthetic Plastic Surgery (also ASAPlS)
ASAS American Society of Abdominal Surgery
argininosuccinic acid synthetase
ASAT See AST (aspartate aminotransferase)
ASB American Society of Bacteriologists
arylsulfatase B (also ARS-B)
asymptomatic bacteriuria
ASBC American Society of Biologic Chemists
ASBMR American Society for Bone and Mineral Research
ASBP American Society of Bariatic Physicians
ASC acetylsulfanilyl chloride
adenosine-coupled spleen cell
altered state of consciousness
American Society of Cytology
antigen-sensitive cell
arylsulfatase C (also ARS-C)
ASCAD arteriosclerotic coronary artery disease
ASCB American Society for Cell Biology
ASCC American Society of Colposcopy and Colpomicroscopy
American Society for the Control of Cancer
ASCCP American Society for Colposcopy and Cervical Pathology
ASCE American Society of Childbirth Educators
ASCH American Society of Clinical Hypnosis
ASCH-ERF American Society of Clinical Hypnosis--Education and Research Foundation
ASCI American Society for Clinical Investigation
ASCLT American Society of Clinical Laboratory Technicians
ASCMS American Society of Contemporary Medicine and Surgery
ASCN American Society for Clinical Nutrition
ASCO American Society of Clinical Oncology
American Society of Contemporary Ophthalmology
Association of Schools and Colleges of Optometry
ASCP American Society of Clinical Pathologists
American Society of Consultant Pharmacists
ASCPT American Society for Clinical Pharmacology and Therapeutics
ASCRS American Society of Colon and Rectal Surgeons
ASCT autologous stem cell transplantation
ASCVD arteriosclerotic cardiovascular disease
atherosclerotic cardiovascular disease
ASD aldosterone secretion defect
Alzheimer's senile dementia
American Society of Dermatopathology
atrial septal defect
ASDA American Student Dental Association
ASDC American Society of Dentistry for Children
Association of Sleep Disorders Center
ASDR American Society of Dental Radiographers
American Society of Diagnostic Radiology
ASDS American Society for Dermatologic Surgery
ASE American Society of Echocardiography
American Society for Electrotherapy
ASEP American Society for Experimental Pathology (See AAP--American Association of Pathologists)
ASES Adult Self-Expression Scale
ASET American Society of Electroencephalographic Technologists
asex asexual
ASF aniline, sulfur, formaldehyde
asialofetium
ASFO American Society of Forensic Odontology
ASG advanced stage group
American Society of Genetics
Army Surgeon General
ASGBI Association of Surgeons of Great Britain and Ireland
ASGD American Society for Geriatric Dentistry
ASGE American Society for Gastrointestinal Endoscopy
ASGP&P American Society of Group Psychotherapy and Psychodrama
ASGTP American Society for Group Therapy and Psychodrama
ASH Academy of Scientific Hypnotherapy
Action on Smoking and Health
aldosterone stiumlating hormone
American Society of Hematology
ankylosing spinal hyperostosis
asymmetric septal hypertrophy
hyperopic astigmatism (also AH, aha)
hypertropic astigmatism
ASHA American School Health Association
American Social Health Association
American Speech-Language-Hearing Association
ASHCSP American Society for Hospital Central Service Personnel

ASHD arteriosclerotic heart disease
atrial septal heart disease
ASHE American Society for Hospital Engineering
ASHFSA American Society for Hospital Food Service Administrators
ASHG American Society of Human Genetics
ASHI Association for the Study of Human Infertility
ASHMET American Society for Health Manpower Education and Training
ASHN acute sclerosing hyaline necrosis
ASHNS American Society for Head and Neck Surgery
ASHP American Society of Hospital Pharmacists
ASHPA American Society for Hospital Personnel Administration
ASHPMM American Society for Hospital Purchasing and Materials Management
ASHPR American Society for Hospital Public Relations
ASHPREF American Society of Hospital Pharmacists Research and Education Foundation
ASHRM American Society for Hospital Risk Management
ASHT American Society of Hand Therapists
ASI Addiction Severity Index
ASIA American Spinal Injury Association
ASIF Association for the Study of Internal Fixation
ASII American Science Information Institute
ASIM American Society of Internal Medicine
ASIS anterior superior iliac spine
ASK antistreptokinase
ASL ankylosing spondylitis lung
antistreptolysin
average speech level
ASLAP American Society of Laboratory Animal Practitioners
ASLC acute self-limited colitis
ASLM American Society of Law and Medicine
ASLO antistreptolysin-O (also ASO)
ASLT antistreptolysin-O test (also ASOT)
ASM airway smooth muscle
American Society for Microbiology
myopic astimatism (also AM)
ASMA antismooth muscle antibody
ASMC arterial smooth muscle cell
ASMCHCCD Association of State Maternal and Child Health and Crippled Children's Directors
ASMDT American Society of Master Dental Technologists
ASME Association for the Study of Medical Education
ASMI anteroseptal myocardial infarct
ASMS American Society of Maxillofacial Surgeons
ASMT American Society for Medical Technology
asmt assessment (also A)
ASN alkali soluable nitrogen
American Society of Nephrology
Asn asparagine
ASNR American Society of Neuroradiology
ASNSA American Society for Nursing Service Administrators
ASNuM American Society of Nuclear Medicine
ASO American Society of Orthodontists
antistreptolysin-O (also ASLO)
arteriosclerosis obliterans
ASOOA American Society of Ophthalmologic and Otolaryngologic Allergy
ASOPRS American Society of Ophthalmological Plastic and Reconstructive Surgery
ASOR asialo-orosomucoid
ASOS American Society of Oral Surgeons
ASOT antistreptolysin-O test (also ASLT)
ASP American Society of Parasitologists
American Society of Pharmacognosy
antisocial personality
area systolic pressure
Asp aspartic acid
asp asparaginase
aspirate
ASPA American Society of Physician Analysts
American Society of Podiatric Assistants
ASPAT antistreptococcal polysaccharide A test
ASPD American Society of Podiatric Dermatology
ASPDM American Society of Psychosomatic Dentistry and Medicine
ASPE American Society of Psychopathology of Expression
ASPEN American Society for Parenteral and Enteral Nutrition
ASPET American Society for Pharmacology and Experimental Therapeutics
ASPH Association of Schools of Public Health
ASpHearA American Speech and Hearing Association (see also ASHA)
ASPL American Society for Pharmacy Law
ASPM American Society of Paramedics
American Society of Podiatric Medicine
ASPN American Society for Pediatric Neurosurgery
ASPO American Society for Psychoprophylaxis in Obstetrics
ASPR American Society for Psychical Research
ASPRS American Society of Plastic and Reconstructive Surgeons
ASPS American Society of Pre-Dental Students
ASQ Anxiety Scale Questionnaire
ASR aldosterone secretion rate
atrial septal resection
ASRA American Society of Regional Anesthesia
ASRT American Society of Radiologic Technologists
ASS anterior superior spine
argininosuccinate synthetase
ASSAl American Society for the Study of Allergy
ASSArthr American Society for the Study of Arthritis
ASSFN American Society for Stereotactic and Functional Neurosurgery
ASSH American Society for Surgery of the Hand
ASSLD American Association for the Study of Liver Diseases
assn association
ASSO American Society for the Study of Orthodontics
assoc associate

Asst assistant
AST angiotensin sensitivity test
aspartate aminotransferase (SGOT)
aspartate transaminase
Association of Surgical Technologists
audiometry sweep test
ast astigmatism
ASTA American Surgical Trade Association (see HIDA--Health Industry Distributors Association)
ASTDD Association of State and Territorial Dental Directors
ASTDN Association of State and Territorial Directors of Nursing
asth asthenopia
ASTHO Association of State and Territorial Health Officials
ASTM American Society for Testing Materials
American Society of Tropical Medicine
ASTMH American Society of Tropical Medicine and Hygiene
ASTO See ASLO
as tol
as tolerated
ASTPHND
Association of State and Territorial Public Health Nutrition Directors
ASTR American Society of Therapeutic Radiologists
ASTZ antistreptozyme
ASV anodic stripping voltammetry
antisnake venom
avian sarcoma virus
ASVIP atrial-synchronous ventricular-inhibited pacemaker
ASVO American Society of Veterinary Ophthalmology
ASVPP American Society of Veterinary Physiologists and Pharmacologists
ASW artificial seawater
asw artificially sweetened
Asx See Asn
See Asp
ASXRT American Society of X-Ray Technicians
asym asymmetry (also a)
AT achievement test
adaptive thermogenesis
air temperature
air trapping
anaerobic threshold
anionic trypsinogen
antitrypsin
antral transplantation
applanation tension
ataxia telangiectasia
atraumatic
atropine
autoimmune thrombocytopenia
axonal terminal
old tuberculin (Alt Tuberculin)
AT I angiotensin I (also A I, ANG I)
AT II angiotensin II (also A II, ANG II)
AT III
antithrombin III
AT_{10} dihydrotachysterol
At astatine
at airtight
ampere turn
atomic
ATA alimentary toxic aleukia
American Thyroid Association
American Tinnitus Association
aminotriazole
antithyroid antibody
anti-Toxoplasma antibody
Association for Transpersonal Anthropology
atmosphere, absolute (also ata)
aurintricarboxylic acid
ata atmosphere, absolute (also ATA)
ATB atypical tuberculosis
ATBAC 3,4,5-trimethoxybenzoyl-epsilon-aminocaproic acid (also TBACA)
ATCC American Type Culture Collection
ATCS active trabecular calcification surface
anterior tibial compartment syndrome
ATD Alzheimer-type dementia
antithyroid drug
asphyxiating thoracic dystrophy
ATE acute toxic encephalopathy
adipose tissue extract
autologous tumor extract
ATEE acetyltyrosine ethyl ester
ATEM analytic transmission electron microscope
ATEN atenolol
A tetra P
adenosine tetraphosphate
ATFC alternative temporal forced choice
at fib
See atr fib
ATG antithymocyte globulin
antithyroglobulin
ATHF allo-tetrahydrocortisol
AThorS
American Thoracic Society (also ATS)
AThS American Therapeutic Society
ATL Achilles tendon lengthening
adult T cell leukemia
anterior tricuspid leaflet
ATLA adult T cell leukemia antigen
ATLS advanced trauma life support
ATLV adult T cell leukemia virus
ATM abnormal tubular myelin
acute transverse myelitis
atm atmosphere
ATMCH Association of Teachers of Maternal and Child Health
ATMD 4'-aminomethyl-4,5',8-trimethylpsoralen (also AMT)
atmos See atm
ATN acute tubular necrosis
ATNC atraumatic normocephalic
at no atomic number (also Z)
ATNR asymmetric tonic neck reflex
ATP adenosine triphosphate
autoimmune thrombocytopenic purpura
ATPase
adenosine triphosphatase
ATPD ambient temperature and pressure, dry
ATPM Association of Teachers of Preventive Medicine (also ATPrM)
ATPrM Association of Teachers of Preventive Medicine (also ATPM)
ATPS ambient temperature and pressure, saturated
ATPTX acute thyroparathyroidectomy
ATR Achilles tendon reflex
attenuated total reflection
atr fib
atrial fibrillation
ATrS American Trauma Society (also ATS)
ATS American Thermographic Society
American Thoracic Society (also AThorS)

American Trauma Society (also ATrS)
antitetanic serum
antithymocyte serum
anti-T serum
anxiety tension state
arteriosclerosis
atherosclerosis

ATT arginine tolerance time
aspirin tolerance time

att attending

ATU allylthiourea

AtV arteriovenous
assisted ventilation
atrioventricular

at vol
atomic volume

at wt atomic weight (also A)

ATX Anemonia sulcata toxin

ATx adult thymectomy

AU Angstrom unit
antitoxic unit
arbitrary unit
atomic unit
azauridine (also AZU)
both ears (aures unitas)
each ear (auris uterque)

Au Australian
gold (aurum)

^{195}Au radioactive isotope of gold

^{198}Au radioactive isotope of gold

^{199}Au radioactive isotope of gold

AUA American Urological Association
Association of University Anesthetists

AuAg Australian antigen

AUC area under the curve

AUD arthritis of unknown diagnosis

aud auditory

AUFS absorbance units full scale

AUG acute ulcerative gingivitis
adenine, uracil, guanine
adenine, uridine, guanosine

AUI Alcohol Use Inventory

AUL acute undifferentiated leukemia

AUM asymmetric unit membrane

AUO amyloid of unknown origin

AuP Australian antigen protein

AUPHA Association of University Programs in Health Administration

AUPO Association of University Professors of Ophthalmology

AUR Association of University Radiologists

aur auricle

aur fib
auricular fibrillation

AuSH Australian serum hepatitis

aux auxiliary

AV antevert
antivirion
aortic valve
arteriovenous
assisted ventilation
atrioventricular
audiovisual
augmented vector
auriculoventricular
doxorubicin (Adriamycin), vincristine

A/V artery to vein ratio

av average (also avg)
avoirdupois (also avdp)

AVA antiviral antibody
aortic valve area
aortic valve atresia
arteriovenous anastomosis

AVB atrioventricular block

AVBR automated ventricular brain ratio

AVC aberrant ventricular conduction
Academy of Veterinary Cardiology
automatic volume control

AVCS atrioventricular conduction system

AVD aortic valve disease
apparent volume of distribution
arteriovenous difference
atrioventricular dissociation

AVDA American Venereal Disease Association

$AVDO_2$ arteriovenous oxygen content difference

AvDP average diastolic pressure

avdp avoirdupois (also av)

AVF antiviral factor
arteriovenous fistula

avg average (also av)

AVH acute viral hepatitis

AVHD acquired valvular heart disease

AVI air velocity index

AVJ atrioventricular junction

AVJR atrioventricular junctional rhythm

AVJT atrioventricular junctional tachycardia

AVL anterior vein of the leg

AVM arteriovenous malformation
atrioventricular malformation

AVMA American Veterinary Medical Association

AVN arbitrary value unit
atrioventricular node

AVO atrioventricular opening

AVP antiviral protein
arginine vasopressin

AVR anomalous venous return
aortic valve replacement

AVr antiviral regulator

AVRB added viscous resistance to breathing

AVRP atrioventricular refractory period

AVS American Vacuum Society
aneurysm of membranous ventricular septum
aortic valve stenosis
Association for Voluntary Sterilization

AVSD atrioventricular septal defect

AVSV aortic valve stroke volume

AVT arginine-vasotocin

AVTB absolute volume of trabecular bone

AV3V anteroventral third ventricle

AVZ avascular zone

AW alcohol withdrawal
aluminum wafer
alveolar wall
alveolar wash
anterior wall
atomic warfare

A&W alive and well

A3W crystalline amino acid solution

awa as well as

AWBM alveolar wall basement membrane

AWF adrenal weight factor

AWHS American Women's Hospitals Service

AWI anterior wall infarction

AWMA American Women's Medical Association

AWMI anterior wall myocardial infarction

AWOL absent without leave

AWRU active wrist rotation unit

AWU atomic weight unit

AWV Association for Women Veterinarians

AX alloxan

ax axillary
axis
axon

AXL axillary lymphoscintigraphy
AZ acetazolamide
azathioprine
A-Z Aschheim-Zondek
az nitrogen (azote)
AZA 5-azacytidine
AZG azaguanine
AZR alizarin red
AZT Aschheim-Zondek test
AZU azauridine (also AU)

B

B Bacillus
bacitracin
bacterium (also bact)
Bacteroides
Balantidium
balneum (also BAL)
barometric (also bar)
Bartonella
base
baseline
Basidiobolus
bath
Baume (also Be)
behavior (also beh)
Benoist
Bertiella
bicuspid
black
Blastomyces
blood (also bl)
body
boils at
bone
Bordetella
born
boron
Borrelia
brother (also br, bro)
Brucella
Brugia
buccal
corticosterone (compound B)
gauss
b barn
BA background activity
bacterial agglutination
basilar artery
basket axon
benzanthracene
benzyl alcohol
benzylamine
betamethasone acetate
bile acid
biologic activity
blocking antibody
blood agar
bone age
boric acid
bovine albumin
brachial artery
bronchial asthma
bronchoalveolar
buccoaxial
buffered acetone
butyric acid
sand bath (balneum arenae) (also bal are)
B.A. Bachelor of Arts (also A.B.)
B/A backache
Ba barium
^{131}Ba radioactive isotope of barium
^{133}Ba radioactive isotope of barium
^{140}Ba radioactive isotope of barium
ba basophil (also baso)
BAA benzoyl arginine amide
BAAR British Acupuncture Association and Research
BAC bacterial antigen complex
blood alcohol concentration
blood alcohol content
buccoaxiocervical
BACON bleomycin, doxorubicin (Adriamycin), lomustine (CCNU), vincristine (Oncovin), nitrogenmustard
BACOP bleomycin, doxorubicin (Adriamycin), cyclophosphamide, vincristine (Oncovin), prednisone
BACT carmustine (BCNU), Ara-C, cyclophosphamide, 6-thioguanine
bact bacteriologist
bacteriology
bacterium (also B)
BADS British Association of Dermatology and Syphilology
BAE bovine aortic endothelium
BaE barium enema
BAEE benzoyl arginine ethyl ester
BAEP brainstem auditory evoked potential
BAER brainstem auditory evoked response
BAG buccoaxiogingival
BAI basilar artery insufficiency
BAIB beta-aminoisobutyric acid
BAIF bile acid independent fraction
BAL bath (balneum) (also B)
blood alcohol level
British anti-Lewisite
bronchoalveolar lavage
bal balance
bal are
sand bath (balneum arenae) (also BA)
BALB binaural alternate loudness balance
bal cal
hot bath (balneum calidum)
bal coen
mud bath (balneum coenosum)
BALF bronchoalveolar lavage fluid
bal frig
cold bath (balneum frigidum)
bal lact
milk bath (balneum lacteum)
bal mar
seawater bath (balneum maris) (also bm)
bal pneu
air bath (balneum pneumaticum)
bals balsam
BALT bronchus-associated lymphoid tissue
bal tep
warm bath (balneum tepidum)
bal vap
steam bath (balneum vaporis) (also BV)
BAM bronchoalveolar macrophage
BAME benzoyl arginine methyl ester
BAN British approved name
BANA benzoyl-L-arginyl-2-naphthylamine
BANS back, arm, neck, and scalp
BAO basal acid output

BAP basic adaptive process
Behavior Activity Profile
blood agar plate
brachial artery pressure
4-BAP 4-benzamidopiperidine
BaP benzo a pyrene
BAPN beta-aminoproprionitrile
BAPNA N-alpha-benzoyl-dl-arginine-p-nitroanilide
BAPS bovine albumin phosphate saline
BAQ Brain-Age Quotient
bar barometric (also B)
BARN bilateral acute retinal necrosis
BARP British Association of Radiology and Physiotherapy
BAS British Anatomical Society
bas basilar
BASH body acceleration synchronous with the heartbeat
baso basophil (also ba)
BAT Basic Aid Training
benzilic acid 3-alpha-tropanyl ester (also BETE, BTE)
best available technology
brown adipose tissue
BAU British Association Unit
BAVIP bleomycin, doxorubicin (Adriamycin), vinblastine, dacarbazine, prednisone
BAW bronchoalveolar washing
BAWP butan-1-ol-acetic acid, water, pyridine
BB blood bank
blue bloater
both bones
breakthrough bleeding
breast biopsy
brush border
buffer base
bundle branch
Bureau of Biologics
BBA born before arrival
BBB blood-brain barrier
blood buffer base
bundle branch block
BBC bromobenzylcyanide
BBF bronchial blood flow
BBG big big gastrin
BBM brush border membrane
BBN broad band noise
n-butyl-n-butanol nitrosamine
BBP butyl benzyl phthalate
BBS bashful bladder syndrome
bombesin (also BN)
BBT basal body temperature
BB/W BioBreeding/Worcester
BC backcross
background counts
bactericidal concentration
basal cell
basket cell
battle casuality
bicarbonate
biotin carboxylase
birth control
blood cardioplegia
blood center
blood culture
bone conduction
Bowman's capsule
brachiocephalic
buccocervical
buffy coat
B.C. Bachelor of Chemistry
Bachelor of Surgery (Chirurgiae Baccalaureus) (also B.CH.)
bc back care
BCA Blue Cross Association
breast cancer antigen
BCAA branched chain amino acid
BCAC Breast Cancer Advisory Center
BCAT brachiocephalic arterial trunk
BCB brilliant cresyl blue
BCBR bilateral carotid body resection
BCC basal cell carcinoma
biliary cholesterol concentration
birth control clinic
BCCE 3-carbomethoxy-beta-carboline
BCCP biotin carboxyl-carrier protein
BCD bleomycin, cyclophosphamide, dactinomycin
BCDDP Breast Cancer Detection Demonstration Project
BCDSP Boston Collaborative Drug Surveillance Program
BCE basal cell epithelioma
B cell enriched
BCF basophil chemotactic factor
bioconcentration factor
breast cyst fluid
BCG bacille Calmette-Guerin
ballistocardiogram
bicolor guaiac
bromcresol green
BCH basal cell hyperplasia
basal cell hypoplasia
B.Ch. Bachelor of Surgery (Chirurgiae Baccalaureus) (also B.C.)
Bchl bacteriochlorophyll
BCIA Biofeedback Certification Institute of America
BCKA branched chain keto acids
BCL basic cycle length
BCLS basic cardiac life support
BCM body cell mass
BCME bis (chloromethyl) ether
BCMF bleomycin, cyclophosphamide, methotrexate, 5-fluorouracil
BCNS basal cell nevus syndrome
BCNU carmustine (1,3-bis-(2-chloroethyl)-1-nitrosourea)
BCO biliary cholesterol output
BCOP carmustine (BCNU) cyclophosphamide, vincristine (Oncovin), prednisone (also BCVP)
BCOPP carmustine (BCNU), cyclophosphamide, vincristine (Oncovin), procarbazine, prednisone
BCP birth control pill
bromcresol purple
butylcyclohexyl trioxoperhydropyrimidine
BCP-D bromcresol purple desoxycholate
BCPS battery-charging power supply
BCR B cell reactivity
bulbocavernosus response
BCS battered child syndrome
Budd-Chiari syndrome
BCT brachiocephalic trunk
BCVP carmustine (BCNU), cyclophosphamide, vincristine, prednisone (also BCOP)
BCVPP carmustine (BCNU), cyclophosphamide, vinblastine, procarbazine, prednisone
BCYE buffered charcoal yeast extract
BD base deficit
base of prism down

beclomethasone dipropionate
behavior disorder
Behcet's disease
benzidine (also Bzd)
bile duct
birth date
block design
brain damage
brain death
bronchodilator
buccodistal

B_1D N-benzyldaunorubicin
B_2D N,N-dibenzyldaunorubicin
bd band
board
See bid
BDA British Dental Association
British Dermatological Association
BDAE Boston Diagnostic Aphasia Examination
BDB bis-diazotized benzidine
BDE bile duct examination
bile duct exploration
BDG bilirubin diglucuronide
buffered desoxycholate glucose
BDI Beck Depression Inventory
BDID bystander dominates initial dominant
BDL bile duct ligation
BDM benzphetamine demethylase
BDMP Birth Defects Monitoring Program
BDP beclomethasone dipropionate
bilateral diaphragm paralysis
BDR background diabetic retinopathy
B.D.S.
Bachelor of Dental Surgery
bds to be taken twice a day (bis die sumendum)
B.D.Sc.
Bachelor of Dental Science
BE Bacillen emulsion
bacterial endocarditis
barium enema
Barrett's esophagus
base excess
below elbow
bovine enteritis
bronchoesophagology
Be Baume (also B)
beryllium
^{7}Be radioactive isotope of beryllium
^{10}Be radioactive isotope of beryllium
BEA below elbow amputation
BEAM brain electric activity mapping
BEE basal energy expenditure
BEEP both end-expiratory pressure
bef before
beg begin
beh behavior (also B)
BEHA bis(2-ethylhexyl) adipate
BEHP bis(2-ethylhexyl) phthalate
BEI backscatter electron imaging
butanol extractable iodine
BEIR biologic effects of ionizing radiation
BEL bovine embryonic lung
BELIR beta-endorphin-like immunoreactivity
benz benzidine
BEPI beta-endorphin immunoreactivity
BER basic electric rhythm
See BSER
BERA brainstem electric response audiometry
brainstem evoked response audiometry
BESM bovine embryo skeletal muscle
BET benign epithelial tumor
bet between (also bi)
BETA 2-benzoxyethyltrimethyl ammonium
BETE benzilic acid 3-alpha-tropanyl ester (also BAT, BTE)
BEV baboon endogenous virus
bleeding esophageal varices
BeV billion electron volts
BF Barren Foundation
bentonite flocculation
bile flow
blastogenic factor
blister fluid
blocking factor
blood flow
Bolivian hemorrhagic fever
bouillon filtrate
breast feed
buccofacial
buffered
B/F black female
bound to free ratio
BFD bias flow down
BFDI bronchodilation following deep inspiration
BFDT Bekesy Functionality Detection Test
BFE blood flow energy
BFO balanced forearm orthesis
ball-bearing forearm orthesis
buccofacial obturator
BFP biologic false positive
BFPR biologic false positive reaction
biologic false positive reactor
BFR blood flow rate
bone formation rate
buffered Ringer's
BFS blood fasting sugar
BFT bentonite flocculation test
biofeedback training
bladder flap tube
BFU burst-forming unit
BFU-E burst-forming unit, erythroid
BFU-M/E
burst-forming unit, myeloid/erythroid
BG Basenji-Greyhound
big gastrin
blood glucose
bone graft
buccogingival
B-G Bordet-Gengou
BGA Behavior Genetics Association
BGAg blood group antigen
BGCA bronchogenic carcinoma
BGG bovine gamma globulin
BGH bovine growth hormone
BGLB brilliant green lactose broth
BGP beta-glycerophosphatase
BGS British Geriatrics Society
BGSA blood granulocyte-specific activity
BGT basophil granulation test
Bender Gestalt Test
bungarotoxin (also BuTx)
BGTT boarderline glucose tolerance test
BH benzalkonium and heparin
borderline hypertensive
brain hormone
breath holding
bronchial hyperactivity
bronchial hyperreactivity
bundle of His
BH2 dihydrobiopterin
BH4 tetrahydrobiopterin

BHA benign hilar adenopathy
bilateral hilar adenopathy
bound hepatitis antibody
butylated hydroxyanisole
BHAT Beta-Blocker Heart Attack Trial
BHB beta-hydroxybutyrate
butoxybenzyl hyoscyaminium bromide
BHC benzene hexachloride
BHCDA Bureau of Health Care Delivery and Assistance
BHD BCNU, hydroxyurea, dacarbazine
BHDV BCNU, hydroxyurea, dacarbazine, vincristine
BHF British Heart Foundation
BHI Better Hearing Institute
biosynthetic human insulin
brain-heart infusion
BHIB beef-heart infusion broth
BHIRS brain-heart infusion and rabbit serum
BHK baby hamster kidney
BHL bilateral hilar lymphadenopathy
biologic half-life
BHM Bureau of Health Manpower
BHN Brinell hardness number
BHP Bureau of Health Professions
BHS beta-hemolytic Streptococcus
breath-holding spell
BHT breath hydrogen test
butylated hydroxytoluene (also DBPC)
BHU basic health unit
B.Hyg.
Bachelor of Hygiene
BI background interval
bactericidal index
bacteriologic index
base of prism in
Braille Institute
brain injured
burn index
Bi bismuth
^{206}Bi radioactive isotope of bismuth
^{207}Bi radioactive isotope of bismuth
^{210}Bi radioactive isotope of bismuth
bi between (also bet)
bilateral (also bil, bilat)
BIA Biogenic Institutes of America
bib drink (bibe)
bic biceps
bicarb
bicarbonate
BICROS
bilateral contralateral routing of signals
BID brought in dead
bid twice a day (bis in die)
BIDLB block in the posteroinferior division of the left branch
BIH benign intracranial hypertension
bihor during two hours (bihorium)
bi isch
between ischial
BIL basal insulin level
bil bilateral (also bi, bilat)
bilirubin
BIL/ALB
bilirubin to albumin ratio
bilat bilateral (also bi, bil)
bilat SLC
bilateral short leg case
bilat S&O
bilateral salpingo-oophorectomy
bin twice a night (bis in nocte)
biol biology
BIP Background Interference Procedure
bacterial intravenous protein
bismuth iodoform paraffin
bismuth iodoform petrolatum
brief infertile period
BIPM Bureau International des Poides et Mesures
BIPP bismuth iodoform paraffin paste
bismuth iodoform petrolatum paste
BIR British Institute of Radiology
BIS Brain Information Service
bis twice
BISG Bockus International Society of Gastroenterology
BISP between ischial spines
BIT between trochanters
BIU barrier isolation unit
biw biweekly
BJ Bence-Jones
biceps jerk
BJM bones, joints, muscles
BJP Bence-Jones protein
BK bekanamycin
below knee
bradykinin
Bk berkelium
bk back
BKA below-knee amputation
BK-A basophil kinin of anaphylaxis
bkfst breakfast
bkly back lying
BKS beekeeper serum
BL bacterial levan
baralyme
baseline
Bessey-Lowry
blind loop
blood loss
boarderline lepromatous
bronchial lavage
buccolingual
Burkitt's lymphoma
butyrolactone
bl bland
bleeding
blood (also B)
blue
BLa buccolabial
BLAVA British Laboratory Animals Veterinary Association
BLB black light blue
black light bulb
Boothby, Lovelace, Bulbulian
BLC beef liver catalase
bl cult
blood culture
BLD basal cell liquefactive degeneration
beryllium lung disease
BLE both lower extremities
BLEP Breast Lesion Evaluation Project
BLFD buccolinguofacial dyskinesia
BLG beta-lactoglobulin
BLM basolateral membrane
black lipid membrane
bleomycin
buccolinguomasticatory
BLN bronchial lymph nodes
bl pr blood pressure (also BP)
BLRA beta-lactamase resistant antimicrobial
BLROA British Laryngological, Rhinological, and Otological Association

BLS basic life support
BLST Bankson Language Screening Test
BLT blood clot lysis time
blood test
blood type
BLU Beesey-Lowry unit
BLV blood volume
bovine leukemia virus
BM basal metabolism
basement membrane
Bergersen medium
betamethasone
biomedical
Bird Mark
blood monocyte
body mass
bone marrow
bowel movement
breast milk
buccomesial
B.M. Bachelor of Medicine
B/M black male
bm seawater bath (balneum maris) (also bal mar)
BMA British Medical Association
BMAP bone marrow acid phosphatase
BMC blood mononuclear cell
bone marrow cell
bone mineral content
BMCS Bureau of Motor Carrier Safety
BMD bone marrow depression
BME basal minimal Eagle's
beta-mercaptoethanol
BMET biomedical equipment technician
BMG benign monoclonal gammopathy
BMI bicuculline methiodide
body mass index
bmk birthmark
BML bone marrow lymphocytosis
BMLM basement membranelike material
BMMP benign mucous membrane pemphigoid
BMN bone marrow necrosis
BMNR bone marrow neutrophil reserve
BMP bone morphogenetic protein
BMPI bronchial mucous proteinase inhibitor
BMQA Board of Medical Quality Assurance
BMR basal metabolic rate
BMRC British Medical Research Council
BMS betamethasone
B.M.S.
Bachelor of Medical Science (also B.M.Sc.)
B.M.Sc.
Bachelor of Medical Science (also B.M.S.)
BMT basement membrane thickness
benign mesenchymal tumor
bone marrow transplant
BMZ basement membrane zone
BN bombesin (also BBS)
brachial neuritis
bronchial nodes
Brown-Norway
bucconasal
BNA Basle Nomina Anatomica
BNB blood-nerve barrier
BNDD Bureau of Narcotics and Dangerous Drugs
BNF British National Formulary
BNGF beta-nerve growth factor
BNLI British National Lymphoma Investigation
BNO bladder neck obstruction
BNPA binasal pharyngeal airway
BNU N-butyl-N-nitrosourea
BO base of prism out
body odor
bowel obstruction
bowels open
bucco-occlusal
B&O belladonna and opium
bo bowel
BOA born on arrival
British Orthopaedic Association
BOD biochemical oxygen demand
biologic oxygen demand
Bureau of Drugs
Bod Bodansky
BOEA ethyl biscoumacetate
BOFA beta-oncofecal antigen
BOHB beta-hydroxybutyrate
bol pill (bolus)
BOM bilateral otitis media
Bureau of Medicine
BOMA bilateral otitis media, acute
BONP bleomycin, vincristine (Oncovin), procarbazine (Natulan), prednisolone
BOP bromo-oxy-progesterone
N-nitrosobis (2-oxopropyl) amine
bot botany
BOW bag of waters
BP back pressure
basic protein
bathroom privileges (also BRP)
bed pan
behavior pattern
benzpyrene
bioequivalence problem
biparietal
birth place
blood pressure (also bl pr)
body plethysmography
British Pharmacopoeia (also BPh)
bronchopleural
buccopulpal
bullous pemphigoid
bypass
bp boiling point
BPA Bauhinia purpura agglutinin
Black Psychiatrists of America
British Paediatric Association
burst-promoting activity
BPAP benzoyl-phenylalanyl-alanyl-proline
BPAS benzoyl-p-aminosalicylic acid
British Pregnancy Advisory Service
BPB bromphenol blue
BPC Behavior Problem Checklist
bile phospholipid concentration
British Pharmaceutical Codex
bronchial provocation challenge
BPD biparietal diameter
blood pressure decrease
broncopulmonary dysplasia
BPEC bipolar electrocoagulation
BPF bronchopleural fistula
BPG bypass graft
BPH benign prostatic hyperplasia
benign prostatic hypertrophy
BPH_4 tetrahydrobiopterin
BPh British Pharmacopoeia (also BP)
buccopharyngeal
Bph bacteriopheophytin
BPI Basic Personality Inventory
beef-pork insulin
blood pressure increase
BPL benzylpenicilloyl-polylysine

beta-propiolactone
bone phosphate of lime

BPM beats per minute
bipiperidyl mustard
births per minute
breaths per minute

BPO basal pepsin output
benzylpenicilloyl
bile phospholipid output

BPO-HSA
benzylpenicilloyl human serum albumin

BPP bovine pancreatic polypeptide
breast parenchymal pattern

BPR blood production rate

BPRS Brief Psychiatric Rating Scale
Brief Psychiatric Reacting Scale

BPS Behavioral Pharmacology Society
Board of Pharmaceutical Specialties
bovine papular stomatitis

BPV benign paroxysmal vertigo
benign positional vertigo
bioprosthetic valve
bovine papilloma virus

Bq becquerel

BR baseline recovery
bathroom
bed rest
bedside rounds
benzodiazepine receptor
bilirubin
bowel rest
brachialis
breathing rate
British (or Birmingham) Revision
bronchitis
bronchus

Br bromine
See B (Brucella)

^{77}Br radioactive isotope of bromine

^{82}Br radioactive isotope of bromine

br boiling range
brachial (also brach)
branch
breath
broiled
brother (also B, bro)

BRA beta-resorcylic acid
brain

BRAC basic rest-activity cycle

brach brachial (also br)

BRAO branch retinal artery occlusion

BrAP brachial artery pressure

BRAT bananas, rice, apples, toast
bananas, rice cereal, applesauce, tea

BRBC bovine red blood cell
burro red blood cell

BRBPR bright red blood per rectum

BRD bladder retraining drills

BRDU bromodeoxyuridine

Brd Ur
See BRDU

BRET bretylium tosylate

BRF Brain Research Foundation

BRH benign recurrent hematuria
Bureau of Radiological Health

BRIC benign recurrent intrahepatic cholestasis

Brit British

BRM biologic response modifier
biuret reactive material

BRMP Biological Response Modification Program

BRO bromocriptine
bronchoscopy

bro brother (also B, br)

bronch
bronchoscope

BRP bathroom privileges (also BP)
bilirubin production

BRR baroreceptor reflex response

BRS British Roentgen Society

BrU bromouracil

BRVO branch retinal vein occlusion

BS bedside
Behcet's syndrome
bile salt
blood sugar
Bloom's syndrome
borderline schizophrenia
bowel sounds
breaking strength
breath sounds

B.S. Bachelor of Science (also B.Sc.)
Bachelor of Surgery

B-S Bjork-Shiley

BSA benzene sulfonic acid
Biofeedback Society of America
Blind Service Association
Blue Shield Association
body surface area
bovine serum albumin
bowel sounds active

BSB body surface burned

BSBC buffer-soluble binding component

BSC bedside care
bedside commode
bile salt concentration
Biological Stain Commission

B.Sc. Bachelor of Science (also B.S.)

BSD baby soft diet

BSDLB block in the anterosuperior division of the left branch

BSE Bacillus species enzyme
breast self-examination (also SBE)

BSER brainstem electric response
brainstem evoked response

BSF back scatter factor

BSI bound serum iron
British Standards Institution

BSICF bile salt independent canalicular fraction

BSID Bayley Scales of Infant Development

BSN barium sodium niobate
bowel sounds normal

B.S.N.
Bachelor of Science in Nursing

BSO bilateral salpingo-oophorectomy
bile salt output

BSP body segment parameter
sulfobromophthalein (also SBP)

BSPM body surface potential map

BSQ Behavior Style Questionnaire

BSR blood sedimentation rate
bowel sounds regular

BSRI Bem Sex Role Inventory

BSS balanced salt (or saline) solution
black silk suture

BSSE bile salt stimulated esterase

BSSI Basic School Skills Inventory

BSSL bile salt stimulated lipase

BST Bacteriuria Screening Test
biceps semitendinosus
blood serologic test
brief stimulus therapy

BT	base of tongue
	bedtime
	bitemporal
	bladder tumor
	bleeding time
	blood transfusion
	blue tetrazolium
	body temperature
	borderline tuberculoid
	brain tumor
	breast tumor
BTB	breakthrough bleeding
	bromothymol blue
BTBL	bromothymol blue lactose
BTC	basal temperature chart
BTE	benzilic acid 3-alpha-tropanyl ester (also BAT,BETE)
BTEE	benzoyl-L-tyrosine ethyl ester
BTFS	breast tumor frozen section
BTG	beta-thromboglobulin
BThU	See BTU
BTL	bilateral tubing ligation
BTP	biliary tract pain
BT-PABA	N-benzoyl-L-tyrosine-p-aminobenzoic acid
BTPD	body temperature, pressure, dry
BTPS	body temperature, pressure, saturation
BTR	Bezold-type reflex
BTRS	Behavior Therapy and Research Society
BTS	bithional sulfoxide
BTSG	Brain Tumor Study Group
BTTP	British Testicular Tumour Panel
BTU	British thermal unit
BTX	bactrachotoxin
	benzene, toluene, xylene
BU	base of prism up
	Bodansky unit
	5-bromouracil
	burn unit
bu	butyl
BUA	blood uric acid
BUD	budesonide
BUE	both upper extremities
	built-up edge
bull	let it boil (bulliat)
BuM	butyl-2-acetoxyethyl-2'-chloroethyl-amine
BUN	blood urea nitrogen
BUO	bilateral ureteral occlusion
Bur	bureau
BURD	See BRDU
BUS	Bartholin, urethral, Skene
BUT	breakup time
but	butter
BuTx	bungarotoxin (also BGT)
BV	billion volts
	biologic value
	blood vessel
	blood volume
	bronchovesicular
	buccoversion
	steam bath (balneum vaporis) (also bal vap)
BVD	biventricular hypertrophy
	bovine viral diarrhea
BVDU	E-5-(2-bromovinyl)-2'-deoxyuridine
BVE	blood vessel endothelium
	blood volume expansion
BVH	biventricular hypertrophy
BVI	Better Vision Institute
	blood vessel invasion
BVO	branch vein occlusion
	brominated vegetable oil
BVP	Bonhoeffer van der Pol
	blood volume pulse
BVR	baboon virus replication
BVRT	Benton Visual Retention Test
BVS	blanked ventricular sense
BVU	bromisovalum
BW	below waist
	biologic warfare
	birth weight
	body water
	body weight
BWS	battered woman syndrome
Bx	biopsy
BYE	Barile-Yaguchi-Eveland
BZ	benzodiazepine
	benzoyl
BZA	benzylamine
Bzd	benzidine (also BD)
BZQ	benzquinamide

C

C	Calymmatobacterium
	Campylobacter
	Candida
	candle
	canine (secondary dentition)
	capacitance
	carbohydrate (also carbo)
	carbon
	cathode
	Catholic
	Caucasian
	Caulobacter
	Celsius
	centigrade
	certified (also cert)
	cervical
	chest (also ch)
	Chilomastix
	Chlamydia
	chloramphenicol
	cholesterol (also CHO, chol)
	Chromobacterium
	Cimex
	Citrobacter
	Cladosporium
	clear
	clearance
	Clonorchis
	clonus (also Cl)
	Clostridium
	closure (also cl)
	clubbing
	Coccidioides
	coefficient (also coeff)
	color sense
	complement
	compliance
	compound (also comp, cpd)
	concentration (also conc)
	condyle
	constant
	contact
	contraction

control
cortex
Corynebacterium
coulomb
Coxiella
creatine
Cryptococcus
cubic (also cu)
Culex
curie (also Ci)
cuspid (secondary dentition)
cuticular
cylinder
cytidine (also Cyd)
cytosine (also Cyt)
gallon (congius) (also cong, gal)
hundred (centum)
large calorie (also Cal)
rib (costa)

C1...C7
cervical nerve 1 through 7
cervical vertebra 1 through 7

C1...C9
first through ninth component of complement

^{14}C radioactive isotope of carbon

c about (circa) (also ca)
canine (primary dentition)
capillary blood
cuspid (primary dentition)
small calorie (also cal)

$\bar{c}$ with (cum)

c' coefficient of portage

CA cancer
Candida albicans
caproic acid
carbonic anhydrase
carcinoma
cardiac arrest
cardiac arrhythmia
carotid artery
cathecholamine
cathode (also K, KA, Ka)
cellulose acetate
cervicoaxillary
chemotactic activity
cholic acid
chronologic age
citric acid
coefficient of absorption
cold agglutinin
collagenolytic activity
commissural associated
common antigen
community acquired
conceptual age
conditioned abstinence
conditioned air
coronary artery
corpora allata
corpus amylacea
cortisone acetate
Cranial Academy
cricoid arch
croup associated
cytosine arabinoside (also Ara-C)
cytotoxic antibody

C&A Clinitest and Acetest

Ca calcium
carmustine

^{45}Ca radioactive isotope of calcium

^{47}Ca radioactive isotope of calcium

ca about (circa) (also c)

CAA chloroacetaldehyde
computer-assisted (or aided) assessment

CAAHA Council on Arteriosclerosis of the American Heart Association

CAB cellulose acetate butyrate
coronary artery bypass

CABB cord artery buffer base

CABG coronary artery bypass graft

CABOP cyclophosphamide, doxorubicin (Adriamycin), bleomycin, vincristine (Oncovin), prednisone

CaBP calcium-binding protein

CAC cardiac accelerator center
carotid artery canal
cefacetrile
circulating anticoagulant

CACX cancer of the cervix

CAD cadaver
computer-assisted (or aided) diagnosis
coronary artery disease
cyclophosphamide, doxorubicin (Adriamycin), dacarbazine
cytosine arabinoside, daunorubicin

CADL Communicative Abilities in Daily Living

CaDTe See CDTe

CAE coronary artery embolization

CaEDTA
calcium disodium edetate

CAER caerulein

CAF Cooley's Anemia Foundation
cyclophosphamide, doxorubicin (Adriamycin), 5-fluorouracil

CaF correction of area factor (also ACF)

CAG cholangiogram
chronic atrophic gastritis
coronary angiogram

CAGE Cut, Annoyed, Guilty, Eye-opener

CAH central alveolar hypoventilation
chronic active hepatitis
chronic agressive hepatitis
combined atrial hypertrophy
congenital adrenal hyperplasia
congenital adrenogenital hyperplasia

CaHA calcium hydroxylapatite

CAHC chronic active hepatitis with cirrhosis

CAHCT Center for Assessment Health Care Technology

CAHD coronary atherosclerotic heart disease

CAI computer-assisted (or aided) instruction

CAL chronic airflow limitation
computer-assisted (or aided) learning

Cal large calorie (also C)

cal small calorie (also c)

C_{alb} albumin clearance

calc calculate

cal ct
calorie count

CALD chronic active liver disease

calef warm (calefactus)

CALGB Cancer and Leukemia Group B

CALLA common acute lymphocytic leukemia antigen

CAM calf aortic microsome
carminomycin
cell adhesion molecule
chorioallantoic membrane
computer-assisted (or aided) myelography
contralateral axillary metastasis

CAMA Civil Aviation Medical Association

CAMEO cyclophosphamide, doxorubicin (Adriamycin), methotrexate, etoposide, vincristine (Oncovin)
CAmg cortical amygdaloid nucleus
CAMP computer-assisted (or aided) menu planning
cyclophosphamide, doxorubicin (Adriamycin), methotrexate, procarbazine
cAMP cyclic adenosine monophosphate
CaM-RITC
calmidulin and tetramethylrhodamine isothiocyanate
CAMS computer-assisted (or aided) monitoring system
can cannabis
canc cancel
CANS central auditory nervous system
CAO chronic airway (or airflow) obstruction
cyclophosphamide, doxorubicin (Adriamycin), vincristine (Oncovin) (also CAV)
CaO_2 arterial oxygen content
CaOC See COC (cathode opening contraction)
CAOD coronary artery occlusive disease
CAOM chronic adhesive otitis media
CAP captopril
catabolite activator protein
cellulose acetate phthalate
central apical portion
chloroacetophenone
chronic alcoholic pancreatitis
College of American Pathologists
compound action potential
cyclic AMP-binding protein
cyclophosphamide, doxorubicin (Adriamycin), cisplatin
cyclophosphamide, doxorubicin (Adriamycin), prednisolone
cap capacity
capsule (also capsul)
let him take (capiat)
CAPD Citizens Alliance to Prevent Drug Abuse
continuous ambulatory peritoneal dialysis
CAPIS Canadian Association of Plastic Surgery
cap moll
soft capsule (capsula mollis)
CAPP Child Amputee Prosthetic Program
Clinical Appraisal of Psychosocial Problems
CaPPD See CPPD (calcium pyrophosphate dihydrate)
CAPPS Current and Past Psychopathology Scales
capsul
capsule (also cap)
CAR Canadian Association of Radiologists
conditioned avoidance response
carbo carbohydrate (also C)
card cardiology
CARE Clinical Assessment Research and Education
CARF Commission on Accreditation of Rehabilitation Facilities
CARS childhood autism rating scale
Children's Affective Rating Scale
CARTOS
computer-assisted (or aided) reconstruction by tracing of serial sections
CAS carbohydrate-active steroid
casein
cerebral arteriosclerosis
Chemical Abstracts Service
Children's Aid Society
CASA computer-assisted (or aided) self-assessment
CASH corticoadrenal-stimulating hormone
CASHD coronary atherosclerosis heart disease
CASS Collaborative Study of Coronary Artery Surgery
CAST Children of Alcoholism Screening Test
C-AST cytoplasmic aspartate aminotransferase
CAT catalase
catecholamine
cellular atypia
Children's Apperception Test
chloramphenicol-3-O-acetyltransferase
choline acetyltransferase
computed abdominal tomography
computer-assisted (or aided) tomography
computerized axial tomography (see also CT)
cytosine arabinoside, doxorubicin (Adriamycin), 6-thioguanine
cat catalyst
cataract
cath cathartic
catheter
CAUSN Canadian Association of University Schools of Nursing
CAV lomustine (CCNU), doxorubicin (Adriamycin), vinblastine
congenital absence of the vagina
congenital adrenal virilism
cyclophosphamide, cytosine arabinoside, vincristine
cyclophosphamide, doxorubicin (Adriamycin), vincristine (also CAO)
cav cavity
CAVC complete atrioventricular canal
CAVD completion, arithmetic, vocabulary, directions
$C(a\text{-}VDO_2)$
arteriovenous oxygen difference
CAW central airways
CAZ ceftazidime
CB carbenicillin
carbonated beverage
catheterized bladder
chronic bronchitis
circumflex branch
coccobacillus
color blind
conjugated bilirubin
contrast bath
coroco-brachialis
cytochalasin B
C.B. See B.Ch.
C/B chest-back
Cb columbium
CBA chronic bronchitis with asthma
competitive-binding assay
cost benefit analysis
CBB Coomassi brilliant blue
CBC cannabichromene
cerebrobuccal connective
child behavior characteristics
complete blood count
CBCN carbenicillin
CBD cannabidiol
carotid body denervation
closed bladder drainage
common bile duct
community-based distribution

CBDC chronic bullous disease of childhood
CBDE common bile duct exploration (see also CDE)
CBDL chronic bile duct ligation
CBDS Carcinogenesis Bioassay Data System
CBF cerebral blood flow
Children'a Blood Foundation
ciliary beat frequency
coronary blood flow
CBG cannabigeral
corticosteroid-binding globulin
cortisol-binding globulin
CBH chronic benign hepatitis
cutaneous basophil hypersensitivity
CBL circulating blood lymphocyte
cord blood leukocyte
Cbl cobalamin
CBM capillary basement membrane
CBMT capillary basement membrane thickness
CRMW capillary basement membrane width
CBN cannabinol
central benign neoplasm
CBOC completion of bed occupancy care
CBR chemical, bacteriologic, radiologic
chronic bed rest
complete bed rest
CBS chronic brain syndrome
conjugated bile salts
CBSA chlorobenzenesulfonamide
CBSU chlorobenzenesulfonyluria
CBT cognitive behavior therapy
computed body tomography
CBV capillary blood flow velocity
central blood volume
cerebral blood volume
Coxsackie B virus
CBW chemical, biologic warfare
CBX computer-based examination
CBZ carbamazepine
Cbz carbobenzoxy (benzyloxycarbonyl) (also Z)
CBZO carbamazepine-exoxide
CC Cajal Club
calcaneo-cuboid
cardiac catheterization
cardiac cycle
carotid-cavernous
case coordinator
caval catheterization
chest circumference
chief complaint
cholecalciferol
chondrocalcinosis
ciliated cell
clinical course
closing capacity
closing volume
coefficient of correlation
colorectal cancer
commission certified
contractile component
cord compression
coronary collaterals
corpus callosum
costochondral
creatine clearance (also CrCl)
critical condition
crus communis
cup cell
current complaint
cytochrome C
Cc concave
cc cubic centimeter (also ccm, cm^3, cu cm)
CCA chick cell agglutination
chimpanzee coryza agent
choriocarcinoma
chromated copper arsenate
circumflex coronary artery
colitis colon antigen
common carotid artery
CCAT conglutinating complement absorption test
CCB Carroll Center for the Blind
CCBC Council of Community Blood Centers
CCBV central circulating blood volume
CCC cathodal closure contraction
Certificate of Clinical Competence
chronic calculary cholecystitis
citrated calcium carbimide
comprehensive care clinic
consecutive case conference
critical care complex
CCCCP Comprehensive Community Cardiovascular Control Program
CCCl cathodal closure clonus
CCCP carbonylcyanide-m-chlorophenylhydrazone
CCCS condom catheter collecting system
CCCU comprehensive cardiovascular care unit
CCD charge coupled device
childhood celiac disease
cortical collecting duct
cumulative cardiotoxic dose
CCE clubbing, cyanosis, and edema
countercurrent electrophoresis
CCF carotid cavernous fistula
cephalin cholesterol flocculation
compound comminuted fracture
congestive cardiac failure
CCFA Children's Cancer Fund of America
cycloserine-cefoxitin-fructose agar
CCG cholecystogram
CCGC capillary column gas chromatography
CCGG cytosine-cytosine-guanine-guanine
CCH chronic cholestatic hepatitis
Consumer Coalition for Health
CCh carbamylcholine
CCHD Committee to Combat Huntington's Disease
cyanotic congenital heart disease
CCHS congenital central hypoventilation syndrome
CCI chronic coronary insufficiency
corrected count increment
CCK cholecystokinin
CCKLI cholecystokinin-like immunoreactivity
CCK-PZ
cholecystokinin-pancreozymin (also PZ-CCK)
CCLI composite clinical and laboratory index
CCM congestive cardiomyopathy
contralateral competing message
critical care medicine
cyclophosphamide, lomustine (CCNU), methotrexate
ccm cubic centimeter (also cc, cm^3, cu cm)
CCMSU clean catch midstream urine
CCMU critical care medicine unit
CCN caudal central nucleus
coronary care nursing
critical care nursing
CCNU lomustine (1-(2-chloroethyl)-3-cyclohexyl-1-nitrosourea)
CCOC Council on Clinical Optometric Care
CCOF chromosomally competent ovarian failure

CCOP Community Clinical Oncology Program
CCP chronic calcifying pancreatitis
ciliocytophthoria
Crippled Children's Programs
CCPD continuous cyclic peritoneal dialysis
crystalline calcium pyrophosphate dihydrate
CCPDS centralized cancer patient data system
CCPR crypt cell production rate
C_{cr} creatinine clearance
CCRS carotid chemoreceptor stimulation
CCS casualty clearing station
cholecystosonography
Crippled Children Services
CCSA central chemosensitive area
CCSG Children's Cancer Study Group
CCT carotid compression tomography
central conduction time
chocolate-coated (covered) tablet
composite cycle therapy
cranial computed tomography
crude coal tar
cyclocarbothiamine
CCTe cathodal closure tetanus
CCTG Coccidioidomycosis Cooperative Treatment Group
CCU cardiac care unit
cardiovascular care unit
coronary care unit
critical care unit
CCVD chronic cerebrovascular disease
Ccw chest wall compliance
ccw counterclockwise
CD cadaver donor
Caesarian delivered
carbon dioxide
cardiac disease
cardiac dullness
cardiac dysrhythmia
cardiovascular disease
caudal (also cd)
cefaloridine
celiac disease
central deposition
character disorder
chemotactic difference
circular dichroism
colloid droplet
common duct
communicable disease
communication deviance
complete diagnosis
conduct disorder
conjugata diagonalis
consanguineous donor
constant drainage
contagious disease
control diet
convulsive disorder
convulsive dose
copying drawings
covert dyskinesia
Crohn's disease
curative dose
cutdown
cystic duct
Czapek-Dox
C/D cigarettes per day
cup to disk ratio
CD_{50} median curative dose
Cd cadmium
color denial
^{109}Cd radioactive isotope of cadmium
^{115}Cd radioactive isotope of cadmium
cd candela
caudal (also CD)
coccygeal (also coc)
cord
CDA cesium dihydrogen arsenate
chenodeoxycholic acid
complement-dependent antibody
congenital dyserythropoietic anemia
CDAA chlorodiallylacetamide
CDAI Crohn's disease activity index
CDC calculated date of confinement
cancer detection center
capillary diffusion capacity
cardiac diagnostic center
Centers for Disease Control
chenodeoxycholate
child development clinic
complement-dependent cytotoxicity
Crohn's disease of the colon
CDCA chenodeoxycholic acid
CDCF Clostridium difficile culture filtrate
CDCI Civilian Doctors Careers Index
CDD certificate of disability for discharge
critical degree of deformation
CDDO Coalition of Digestive Disease Organizations
CDDP cis-diamminedichloroplatinum
CDE canine distemper encephalitis
common duct exploration (see also CBDE)
CDEC 2-chlorallyl diethyldithiocarbamate
CDFR cumulative duration of the first remission
CDH chronic disease hospital
congenital diaphragmatic hernia
congenital dislocated hip
congenital dysplasia of the hip
CDI cell directed inhibitor
Children's Diagnostic Inventory
CDILD chronic diffuse interstitial lung disease
CDL Copying Drawings with Landmarks
CDLE chronic discoid lupus erythematosus
cDNA complementary deoxyribonucleic acid
CDNB 1-chloro-2,4-dinitrobenzene
CDP chlordiazepoxide
chronic destructive periodontitis
Coronary Drug Project
cytidine diphosphate
CDPA Coronary Drug Project Aspirin Study
CDPC cytidine diphosphocholine
CDPS common duct pigment stones
CDR Chronological Drinking Record
computed digital radiography
CDRS-R Children's Depression Rating Scale--Revised
CDS Christian Dental Society
Communication Disorders Specialist
cumulative duration of survival
CDSC Communicable Diseases Surveillance Center
CDSS Clinical Decision Support System
CDT carbon dioxide therapy
Certified Dental Technician
Clostridium difficile toxin
combined diphtheria tetanus
CDTe cathode duration tetanus
CDTF Clinical Dialysis and Transplant Forum
CDV canine distemper virus
CDZ chlordiazepoxide

CE California encephalitis
cardiac enlargement
Carpentier-Edwards (also C-E)
cell extract
chick embryo
chloroform and ether
cholesterol ester
cholinesterase
chromatoelectrophoresis
ciliated epithelial
columnar epithelium
constant error
constant estrus
contractile element
converting enzyme
crude extract
C-E Carpentier-Edwards (also CE)
C&E consultation and examination
Ce cerium
^{139}**Ce** radioactive isotope of cerium
^{141}**Ce** radioactive isotope of cerium
^{143}**Ce** radioactive isotope of cerium
^{144}**Ce** radioactive isotope of cerium
CEA carcinoembryonic antigen
cholinesterase
cost effectiveness analysis
crystalline egg albumin
CEAP Clinical Efficacy Assessment Project
CEBD controlled extrahepatic biliary drainage
CEC cefacolor
contractile electrical complex
Council for Exceptional Children
CECF Children's Eye Care Foundation
CECT contrast-enhanced computed tomography
CED cefradine
Council on Education of the Deaf
CEE chick embryo extract
CEEC calf esophagus epithelial cell
CEEV Central European encephalitis virus
CEF chick embryo fibroblast
CEG chronic erosive gastritis
CEH cholesterol ester hydrolase
CEI convertive enzyme inhibitor
corneal epithelial involvment
CEL Committee for an Extended Lifespan
Cel See C (Celsius)
CELOV chicken embryo lethal orphan virus
cent See C (centigrade)
See cm (centimeter)
CEO chloroethylene oxide
CEP congenital erythropoietic porphyria
cortical evoked potential
counterelectrophoresis
CEPB Carpentier-Edwards porcine bioprosthesis
CEPH Council on Education for Public Health
ceph floc
cephalin flocculation
CER conditioned emotional response
conditioned escape response
control electrical rhythm
cortical evoked response
Cer ceramide
CERA continuous electrical response activity
cert certified (also C)
CES Center for Epidemiologic Studies
central excitatory state
CES-D Center for Epidemiologic Studies--Depression Scale
CET cephalothin (also CF--cefalotin)
controlled environment treatment
CETA Comprehensive Employment Training Act
CEU continuing education unit
CEX cephalexin
CEZ cefazolin
CF carbolfuchsin
cardiac failure
carotid foramen
carrier free
case file
cationized ferritin
cefalotin (also CET--cephalothin)
characteristic frequency
chemotactic factor
chest and left leg
Chiari-Frommel syndrome
choroid fissure
Christmas factor
citrovorum factor
climbing fiber
clotting factor
colicinogenic factor
collected fluid
colonization factor
color and form
complement fixation
completely follicular
contractile force
cough frequency
coupling factor
count fingers
cystic fibrosis
C/F colored female
CFII Cohn fraction II
Cf californium
cf bring together (confero)
centrifugal force
compare (confer)
CFA clofibric acid
colonization factor antigen
colony-forming assay
complement-fixing antibody
complete Freund adjuvant
cryptogenic fibrosing alveolitis
CFA/I colonization factor antigen I
CFC capillary filtration coefficient
chlorofluorocarbon
colony-forming cells
continuous flow centrifugation
CFCCT Committee for Freedom of Choice in Cancer Therapy
CFCL continuous flow centrifugation leukapheresis
CFC-S colony-forming cells-spleen
CFD craniofacial dysostosis
CFDA carboxy-fluorescein-diacetate
CFF critical flicker frequency
critical fusion frequency
Cystic Fibrosis Foundation
CFI Cancer Federation, Inc.
cardiac function index
chemotactic factor inactivator
CFM chlorofluoromethane
CFMA Council for Medical Affairs
CFN cefonicid
CFP cefoperazone
chronic false positive
cyclophosphamide, fluorouracil, prednisone
cystic fibrosis of the pancreas
cystic fibrosis patients
cystic fibrosis protein
CFPD critical frequency of photic driving

CFR case fatality rate
cefadroxil
Code of Federal Regulations
CFRS Clinical Frequencies Recording System
CFS call for service
Canada Fitness Survey
cancer family syndrome
cefsulodin
Code of Federal Regulations
craniofaciostenosis
CFT clinical full time
complement fixation test
complement fixing titer
CFU colony-forming unit
CFU-C colony-forming unit-culture
CFU-E colony-forming unit-erythroid
CFU-F colony-forming unit-fibroblast
CFU-GM
colony-forming unit-granulocyte macrophage
CFU-M colony-forming unit-megakaryocyte
CFU-S colony-forming unit-spleen
colony-forming unit-stem
CFWM cancer-free white mouse
CFY Clinical Fellowship Year
CFZ capillary-free zone
CG calcium gluconate
central gray
cholylglycine
chorionic gonadotropin (also CGT)
chronic glomerulonephritis (also CGN)
cingulate gyrus
colloidal gold
control group
cryoglobulinemia
phosgene (choking gas)
cg center of gravity
centigram
CGA catabolite gene activator
CGD chronic granulomatous disease
CGFH congenital fibrous histiocytoma
CGH chorionic gonadotrophic hormone
CGI Clinical Global Impressions
clinical global inventory
CGL chronic granulocytic leukemia
clorgyline
CGM central gray matter
cgm See cg (centigram)
cCMP cyclic guanosine monophosphate
CGN chronic glomerulonephritis (also CG)
CGP chorionic growth hormone prolactin
circulating granulocyte pool
CGRS Clinician's Global Rating Scale
CGS catgut suture
centimeter-gram-second
Community Guidance Service
CGT chorionic gonadotropin (also CG)
CGTT cortisone glucose tolerance test
CH case history
casein hydrolysate
Chinese hamster
chloral hydrate
chlorpheniramine
cholesterol
chronic hepatitis
chronic hypertension
common hepatic
complete healing
congenital hypothyroidism
continuous heparization
crown-heel
CH_{50} total hemolytic complement
Ch^1 Christchurch chromosome
cH hydrogen ion concentration
ch chest (also C)
child
chronic
CHA Catholic Hospital Association
common hepatic artery
congenital hypoplastic anemia
continuous heated aerosols
cyclohexylamine
N^6-cyclohexyladenosine
ChAcT choline acetyltransferase
CHAD cyclophosphamide, hexamethylmelamine, doxorubicin (Adriamycin), cisplatin (DDP)
CHAID chi-square automatic interaction detection
CHAL chronic haloperidol
CHAMPUS
Civilian Health and Medical Programs of the Uniformed Services
CHAP Child Health Assessment Program
Chart paper (charta)
CHAT choline acetyltransferase
CHB complete heart block
Ch.B. Bachelor of Surgery (Chirurgiae Baccalaureus)
CHC community health center
CHCC Commonwealth Health Care Corporation
CHD childhood disease
congenital heart disease
congenital hip disease
constitutional hepatic dysfunction
coronary heart disease
Ch.D. Doctor of Surgery (Chirurgiae Doctor)
CHE cholesterol ester
ChE cholinesterase
CHEAR National Foundation for Children's Hearing Education and Research
chem chemical
CHESS Cornell High Energy Synchrotron Source
CHEST Chick Embryotoxicity Screening Test
Chex-Up
cyclophosphamide, hexamethylmelamine, 5-fluorouracil, cisplatin
CHF congenital hepatic fibrosis
congestive heart failure
cyclophosphamide, hexamethylmelamine, 5-fluorouracil
chg change
CHH cartilage hair hypoplasia
CHI closed head injury
creatinine-height index
CHINA chronic infectious neuropathic agent
chronic infectious neurotropic agent
CHIP cis-dichloro-transdihydroxy-bis (isopropylamine) platinum
Comprehensive Hospital Infections Project
Chl chlorophyll
chl chloroform
Ch.M. Master of Surgery (Chirurgiae Magister)
CHO Chinese hamster ovary
cholesterol (also C, chol)
chorea
cyclophosphamide, hydroxydaunorubicin, vincristine (Oncovin)
CHOI considered characteristic of osteogenesis imperfecta
CHOICE
Center for Humane Options in Childbirth Experiences

chol cholesterol (also C, CHO)
CHOP cyclophosphamide, hydroxydaunorubicin, vincristine (Oncovin), prednisone
CHOP-BLEO
cyclophosphamide, hydroxydaunorubicin, vincristine (Oncovin), prednisone, bleomycin
CHOR cyclophosphamide, hydroxydaunorubicin, vincristine (Oncovin), radiation
CHP capillary hydrostatic pressure
child psychiatry
comprehensive health planning
coordinating hospital physician
Chp clinohypersthene
chpx chickenpox
CHQ chlorquinol
CHR Crick-Harper-Raper
Chr See C (Chromobacterium)
chr chronic
c hr candle hour
curie hour
CHRIS Cancer Hazards Ranking and Information System
CHRS cerebro-hepato-renal syndrome
CHS Chediak-Higashi syndrome
chondroitin sulfate
contact hypersensitivity
CHT contralateral head turning
CHVP cyclophosphamide, hydroxydaunorubicin, VM-26, prednisone
CI cardiac index
cardiac insufficinecy
cellular immunity
cerebral infarction
chemical ionization
chemotactic index
chemotherapeutic index
chronically infected
ciclacillin
clinical impression
clinical investigator
clonus index
closure index
coefficient of intelligence
colloidal iron
colony inhibition
Color Index
confidence interval
contamination index
continuous infusion
coronary insufficiency
crystalline insulin
cytotoxic index
Ci curie (also C)
CIA canine inherited ataxia
Collegium Internationale Allergologicum
cib food (cibus)
CIBD chronic inflammatory bowel disease
CIBHA congenital inclusion body hemolytic anemia
CIC cardiac inhibitor center
circulating immune complex
CICA cervical internal carotid artery
Committee on International Collaborative Activities
CICU cardiac intensive care unit
coronary intensive care unit
CID Center for Infectious Diseases
central integrative deficit
chick infective dose
combined immunodeficiency disease
cytomegalic inclusion disease
CIDAC Cancer Information Dissemination Analysis Center
CIDS cellular immunodeficiency syndrome
CIE countercurrentimmunoelectrophoresis
counterimmunoelectrophoresis
crossed immunoelectrophoresis (also CIEP)
CIE-C counterimmunoelectrophoresis-colorimetric
CIE-D counterimmunoelectrophoresis-densitometric
CIEP crossed immunoelectrophoresis (also CIE)
CIF clone-inhibiting factor
CIg cytoplasmic immunoglobulin
CIH Certificate in Industrial Health
CIIA common internal iliac artery
CIIP chronic idiopathic intestinal pseudo-obstruction
CIIT Chemical Industry Institute of Toxicology
CIL Cancer Information Line
CIM cimetidine
cortically inducted movement
CIMS chemical ionization mass spectrometry
clinical information scale
Conflict in Marriage Scale
CIN cervical intraepithelial neoplasm
cinoxacin
cinromide
C_{in} inulin clearance
CINE chemotherapy-induced nausea and vomiting
CINP Collegium Internationale Neuropsychopharmacologicum
CIOF chromosomally incompetent ovarian failure
CIOMS Council for International Organizations on Medical Sciences
CIP Carcinogen Information Program
chronic inflammatory polyneuropathy
CIPC chloroisopropyl carbanilate
CIPD chronic inflammatory demylinating polyradiculoneuropathy
chronic intermittent peritoneal dialysis
CIPF clinical illness promotion factor
CIR Committee of Interns and Residents
cir circuit
circumference
Circ circumcision
circ circulation
CIRID Center for Interdisciplinary Research on Immunologic Diseases
CIRM Centro Internazionale Radio-Medico
CIS Cancer Information Service
carcinoma in situ
central inhibitory state
cit citrate
cito disp
dispense quickly (cito dispensetur)
CIV Chilo iridescent virus
common iliac vein
CJD Creutzfeldt-Jakob disease
CK chicken kidney
contralateral knee
creatine kinase
ck check
CKC cold knife conization
CKG cardiokymograph
CKMB creatine kinase MB
ckw clockwise

CL capillary lumen
cardinal ligament
center line
centralis lateralis
chemiluminescence
chest and left arm
cholelithiasis
clamp lamp
clear liquid
cleft lip
complex loading
composite lymphoma
confidence level
contact lens
continence line
corpus luteum
cricoid lamina
criterion level
Crithidia luciliae
critical list
cutis laxa
cycle length
C_L lung compliance
Cl chlorine
clonus (also C)
See C (Clostridium)
^{36}Cl radioactive isotope of chlorine
^{38}Cl radioactive isotope of chlorine
cl centiliter
clavicle
clinic
closure (also C)
CLAH congenital lipoid adrenal hyperplasia
CLAO Contact Lens Association of Ophthalmologists
CLAS congenital localized absence of skin
Congress of Lung Association Staff
classif
classification
CLB chlorambucil
CLBBB complete left bundle branch block
CLC Charcot-Leyden crystal
CLD chronic liver disease
chronic lung disease
congenital limb deficiency
cld cleared
colored
CLDM clindamycin (also CM)
cldy cloudy
CLE centrilobular emphysema
CLED cystine-lactose-electrolyte deficient
CLEHA Conference of Local Environmental Health Administrators
CLEP College Level Examination Program
CLF cardiolipin fluorescence antibody
Children's Liver Foundation
clin clinical
CLIP corticotrophin-like intermediate lobe peptide
CLL cholesterol lowering level
cholesterol lowering lipid
chronic lymphatic leukemia
chronic lymphocytic leukemia
chronic lymphoproliferative disease
CLMA Clinical Laboratory Management Association
Cl_2MDP
dichloromethylene diphosphate
CLO cod liver oil
CLOF clofibrate
CLON clonazepam
CLP chymotrypsin-like protein
CLSH corpus luteum-stimulating hormone
CLSL chronic lymphosarcomatous leukemia
CLT clot-lysis time
clotting time
ClVPP chlorambucil, vinblastine, procarbazine, prednisone
CLX cloxacillin
CM capreomycin
carboxymethyl
cardiac muscle
cardiomyopathy
cell membrane
centrum medianum
cerebral mantle
cervical mucus
chemotactic migration
chylomicron
circular muscle
clindamycin (also CLDM)
clinical medicine
coccidioidal meningitis
cochlear microphonic
community meeting
conditioned medium
continuous murmur
contrast media
costal margin
cow's milk
cytoplasmic membrane
C.M. Master in Surgery (Chirurgiae Magister)
C/M counts per minute
See B/M
Cm curium
maximum clearance
^{242}Cm radioactive isotope of curium
^{244}Cm radioactive isotope of curium
cM centimorgan
cm centimeter
tomorrow morning (cras mane)
cm^2 square centimeter
cm^3 cubic centimeter (also cc, ccm, cu cm)
CMA Canadian Medical Association
Candida metabolic antigen
Certified Medical Assistant
chronic metabolic acidosis
CMA-A Certified Medical Assistant--Administrative
CMA-A/C
Certified Medical Assistant--Administrative/Clinical
CMA-C Certified Medical Assistant--Clinical
CMAmg corticomedial amygdaloid nucleus
CMAP compound muscle action potential
CMB carbolic methylene blue
CMC carboxymethyl cellulose
carpometacarpal
cell-mediated cytotoxicity
chronic mucocutaneous candidiasis (also CMCC)
critical micelle concentration
CMCC chronic mucocutaneous candidiasis (also CMC)
CMCHCI
Center for Medical Consumers and Health Care Information
CMCHS Civilian-Military Contingency Hospital System
CMD count median diameter
CME cervical mucous extract
continuing medical education
crude marijuana extract
cystoid macular edema

CME-AMA
Council on Medical Education of the American Medical Association
CMF calcium and magnesium free
chondromyxoid fibroma
cortical magnification factor
cyclophosphamide, methotrexate, 5-fluorouracil
CMFAVP
cyclophosphamide, methotrexate, 5-fluorouracil, doxorubicin (Adriamycin), vincristine, prednisone
CMFE calcium and magnesium free plus EDTA
CMFP cyclophosphamide, methotrexate, 5-fluorouracil, prednisone
CMFT cyclophosphamide, methotrexate, 5-fluorouracil, tamoxifen
CMFVAT
cyclophosphamide, methotrexate, 5-fluorouracil, vincristine, doxorubicin (Adriamycin), testosterone
CMFVP cyclophosphamide, methotrexate, 5-fluorouracil, vincristine, prednisone
CMG canine myasthenia gravis
congenital myasthenia gravis
cooked meat glucose
cyanmethemoglobin
cystometrogram
CMGN chronic membranous glomerulonephritis
CMHC community mental health center
CMHI Community Mental Health Ideology
CMI carbohydrate metabolism index
cell-mediated immunity
circulating microemboli index
computer-managed instruction
Cornell Medical Index
CMID cytomegalic inclusion disease
c/min cycles per minute
CMIR cell-mediated immune response
CMJ carpometacarpal joint
CML cell-mediated lymphocytotoxicity
cell-mediated lympholysis
chronic myelocytic leukemia
chronic myelogenous leukemia
chronic myeloid leukemia
chronic myeloproliferative disease
count median length
cross midline
CMM cutaneous malignant melanoma
cmm cubic millimeter (also cu mm, mm^3)
CMME chloromethyl-methylether
CMMS Columbia Mental Maturity Scale
CMN caudal mediastinal node
cystic medial necrosis
CMNAA cystic medial necrosis of the ascending aorta
CMO calculated mean organism
cardiac minute output
card made out
CMOMC cell meeting our morphologic criteria
C-MOPP
cyclophosphamide, mechlorethamine, vincristine (Oncovin), procarbazine, prednisone
CMP chondromalacia patellae
cytidine monophosphate
CMR cerebral metabolic rate
common mode rejection
crude mortality rate
CMRG cerebral metabolic rate of glucose
CMRL cerebral metabolic rate of lactate
$CMRO_2$ cerebral metabolic rate of oxygen
CMRR common mode rejection ratio
CMRW Coalition for the Medical Rights of Women
CMS Center for Management Systems
cervical mucous solution
chromosome modification site
click murmur syndrome
cms to be taken tomorrow morning (cras mane sumendus)
CMSS Council of Medical Specialty Societies
CMT California mastitis
chronic motor tic
CMTD Charcot-Marie-Tooth disease
CMU chlorophenyldimethylurea
complex motor unit
CMV controlled mechanical ventilation
cytomegalovirus
CN caudate nucleus
charge nurse
clinical nursing
cochlear nucleus
congenital nephrosis
congenital nystagmus
cranial nerve
cyanogen
Cn color naming
cn tomorrow night (cras nocte)
CNA Canadian Nurses' Association
chlornaltrexamine
CNAP cochlear nucleus action potential
CNATS Canadian Nurses' Association Testing Service
CNBr cyanogen bromide
CNC clinical nursing conference
CND cannot determine
CNDC chronic nonspecific diarrhea of childhood
CNE chronic nervous exhaustion
concentric needle electrode
could not establish
CNEMG concentric needle electromyography
CNF Canadian Nurses' Foundation
congenital nephrotic syndrome
CNH central neurogenic hyperapnea
community nursing home
CNHD congenital nonspherocytic hemolytic disease
CNHI Committee for National Health Insurance
CNHS Coalition for a National Health Service
CNI Community Nutrition Institute
CNM Certified Nurse-Midwife (also CNW)
CNP Child Neurology Program
community nurse practitioner
continuous negative pressure
cranial nerve palsy
CNPV continuous negative pressure ventilation
CNRS Canadian Nurses' Respiratory Society
Centre National de la Recherche Scientifique
citrated normal rabbit serum
CNRU Clinical Nutrition Research Unit
CNS central nervous system
clinical nurse specialist
computerized notation system
Congress of Neurological Surgeons
cns to be taken tomorrow night (cras nocte sumendus)
CNT could not test
current night terrors
CNV contingent negative variation
CNW Certified Nurse-Midwife (also CNM)

CO candidal onychomycosis
cardiac output
castor oil
community organization
corneal opacity
crossover
C/O check out
complained of
Co cobalt
coenzyme
^{56}Co radioactive isotope of cobalt
^{57}Co radioactive isotope of cobalt
^{58}Co radioactive isotope of cobalt
^{60}Co radioactive isotope of cobalt
COA calculated opening area
Canadian Orthopaedic Association
CoA coenzyme A
COAD chronic obstructive airway disease
coag coagulation
COAP cyclophosphamide, vincristine (Oncovin), cytosine arabinoside, prednisone
COATS Comprehensive Occupational Assessment and Training System
COC cathodal opening contraction
combination oral contraceptive
coc coccygeal (also cd)
cochl spoonful (cochleare)
cochl amp
heaping spoonful (cochleare amplum)
cochl mag
tablespoonful (cochleare magnum)
cochl med
dessert spoonful (cochleare medium)
cochl parv
teaspoonful (cochleare parvum)
COCl cathodal opening clonus
coct boiling (coctio)
COD cause of death
chemical oxygen demand
CODAP Client Oriented Data Acquisition Process
COE Council on Optometric Education
coeff coefficient (also C)
COEPS cortically originating extrapyramidal system
COF cut-off frequency
COG clinical obstetrics and gynecology
cognitive
COHb carboxyhemoglobin
COL CircOlectric
Col collagen
col colony
color
column
strain (cola)
colat strained (colatus)
COLD chronic obstructive lung disease
colet let it be strained (coletur)
coll collective
colloidal
collat
collateral
collun
nose wash (collunarium)
collut
mouth wash (collutorium)
collyr
eye wash (collyrium)
COM chronic otitis media
cyclophosphamide, vincristine (Oncovin), methotrexate
cyclophosphamide, vincristine (Oncovin), semustine (methyl-CCNU)
COMB cyclophosphamide, vincristine (Oncovin), semustine (methyl-CCNU), bleomycin
comb combine
COMF cyclophosphamide, vincristine (Oncovin), methotrexate, 5-fluorouracil
comf comfortable
COMLA cyclophosphamide, vincristine (Oncovin), methotrexate, leucovorin, cytosine arabinoside
comm communication
COMP cyclophosphamide, vincristine (Ovcovin), methotrexate, prednisolone
comp compare
compound (also C, cpd)
compress
COMS chronic organic mental syndrome
COMT catechol-O-methyltransferase
CON certificate of need
CONA Canadian Orthopaedic Nurses' Association
Con A concanavalin A
conc concentration (also C)
concis
cut (concisus)
cond condensed
conductivity
conf conference
cong congenital
gallon (congius) (also C, gal)
cons conserve
consultant
consperg
sprinkle (conspergere)
cont bruised (contusus)
contain
continue
contag
contagious
conter
rub together (contere)
cont rem
let the medicine be continued (continuentur remedium)
conv convalescent
conventional
COP capillary osmotic pressure
circumoval precipitin
colloid osmotic pressure
cyclophosphamide, vincristine (Oncovin), prednisone (also CVP)
COP-BLAB
cyclosphamide, vincristine (Oncovin), prednisone, bleomycin, doxorubicin (Adriamycin), procarbazine
COPC Community-Oriented Primary Care
COPD chronic obstructive pulmonary disease
COPE Committee on Patient Education
COphS Canadian Ophthamological Society
COPP cyclophosphamide, vincristine (Oncovin), procarbazine, prednisone
COPRO coproporphyria (also CP)
coq boil (coque)
coq in s a
boil in sufficient water (coque in sufficiente aqua)
coq s a
boil properly (coque secundum artem)
COR conditioned orientation reflex
CoR Congo red (also CR)
cor correct

CORA conditioned orientation reflex audiometry
CORE Coordinated Operating and Reporting Entities
corr correspondence
COrS Clinical Orthopaedic Society
cort bark (cortex)
cortical
COS Canadian Ophthalmological Society
clinically observed seizure
Clinical Orthopaedic Society
cos cosine
COT content of thought
continuous oxygen therapy
critical off-time
cot cotangent
COTe cathodal opening tetanus
COTH Council of Teaching Hospitals
COtS Canadian Otolaryngological Society
COVD College of Optometrists in Vision Development
CP candle power
capillary pressure
carbamoylphosphate
cardiac pool
cardiopulmonary
cardiopulmonary performance
cefapirin
cell passaged
cerebellopontine
cerebral palsy
ceruloplasmin
cervical probe
chemically pure
chest pain
child psychiatry
child psychology
chloramphenicol
chloroquine and primaquine
chronic pancreatitis
chronic pyelonephritis
cicatricial pemphoid
circular polarization
cleft palate
closing pressure
combining power
constant pressure
coproporphyria (also COPRO)
cor pulmonale
cortical plate
Corynebacterium parvum
costal plaque
C peptide
creatine phosphate
cuprophane
cyclophosphamide, prednisone
cystosarcoma phyllodes
C&P cystoscopy and pyelogram
Cp peak concentration
phosphate clearance
cp centipoise
CPA carboxypeptidase A
cardiopulmonary arrest
carotid phonoangiography
cerebellopontine angle
chlorophenylalaline
chronic pyrophosphate arthropathy
circulating platelet aggregates
cyproterone acetate
CPAF chlorpropamide-alcohol flush
Cpah clearance, para-aminohippuric acid
CPAI central principal axis of inertia
CPAP continuous (or constant) positive airway pressure
CPB cardiopulmonary bypass
competitive protein binding
CPBA competitive protein binding assay
CPBV cardiopulmonary blood volume
CPC cerebral palsy clinic
cetylpyridinium chloride
Child Protection Center
chronic passive congestion
clinicopathologic conference
committed progenitor cell
CPCN capitated primary care network
CPCR cardiopulmonary cerebral resuscitation
CPCS clinical pharmacokinetics consulting service
CPD calcium pyrophosphate deposition (also CPPD)
calcium pyrophosphate dihydrate (also CPPD)
cephalopelvic disproportion
childhood polycystic disease
chronic peritoneal dialysis
citrate, phosphate, dextrose
contagious pustular dermatitis
critical point drying
cpd compound (also C, comp)
CPDD Committee on Problems of Drug Dependence
CPE cardiogenic pulmonary edema
chronic pulmonary emphysema
complex partial epilepsy
corona penetrating enzyme
Council on Podiatry Education
cytopathic effect
cytopathogenic effect
C Ped Certified Pedorthist
CPF clot-promoting factor
CPH Certificate in Public Health
chronic persistent hepatitis
CPHA Canadian Public Health Association
Commission on Professional and Hospital Activities
CPHLD Conference of Public Health Lab Directors
CPHSRR
Committee for the Protection of Human Subjects from Research Risk
CPHV Conference of Public Health Veterinarians
CPI California Psychological Inventory
constitutional psychopathia inferior
coronary prognostic index
CPIB chlorophenoxyisobutrate
CPIP chronic pulmonary insufficiency of prematurity
CPK creatine phosphokinase
CPL conditioned pitch level
C/PL cholesterol to phospholipid ratio
CPM central pontine myelinolysis
cognitive-perceptual-motor
Coloured Progressive Matrices
continuous passive motion
lomustine (CCNU), procarbazine, methotrexate
cpm counts per minute
CPMAS cross polarization and magic angle spinning
CPMI central principal moments of inertia
CPMP computer-patient management problems
CPMS chronic progressive multiple sclerosis
CPN carboxypeptidase N

chronic polyneuropathy
chronic pyelonephritis
CPNM corrected perinatal mortality
CPQ Children's Personality Questionnaire
CPP canine pancreatic polypeptide
carboxy terminus of propressophysin
cerebral perfusion pressure
Collaborative Perinatal Project
Conditioned Place Preference
cyclopentenophenanthrene
CPPB continuous (or constant) positive pressure breathing
CPPD calcium pyrophosphate deposition (also CPD)
calcium pyrophosphate dihydrate (also CPD)
CPPT Coronary Primary Prevention Trial
CPPV continuous (or constant) positive pressure ventilation
CPR cardiopulmonary reserve
cardiopulmonary resuscitation
centripetal rub
cerebral-cortex perfusion rate
chlorophenol red
cortisol production rate
cumulative patency rate
customary, prevailing, and reasonable
CPRAM controlled partial rebreathing anesthesia method
CPRS Children's Psychiatric Rating Scale
Comprehensive Psychiatric Rating Scale
CPS Canadian Psychoanalytic Society
carbamoylphosphate synthetase
cardioplegic perfusion solution
Child Personality Scale
clinical performance score
clinical pharmacokinetic service
coagulase-positive staphylococci
cumulative probability of success
3-CPS 3-carbethoxypsoralen
cps counts per second
cycles per second
CPSC Consumer Product Safety Commission
CPSI Children's Perception of Support Inventory
CPT carnitine palmitoyltransferase
carotid pulse tracing
chest physiotherapy
choline phosphotransferase
clinical pharmacokinetics team
cold pressor test
continuous performance task
continuous performance test
current procedural terminology
cytidine diphosphate choline-1-2-diacylglycerol
CPTX chronic parathyroidectomy
CPU caudate putamen
central processing unit
CPV canine parvovirus
CPZ chlorpromazine
CQ chloroquine
chloroquine-quinine
circadian quotient
conceptual quotient
CQA Concurrent Quality Assurance
CQE Comprehensive Qualifying Examination
CR calcification rate
calculus removed
calorie restricted
cardiorespiratory
cathode ray
chest and right arm
chief resident
chronic rejection
clinical research
clot retraction
colon resection
colorectal
complete remission
complete responders
conditioned reflex
conditioned response
Congo red (also CoR)
continuous reinforcement
controlled respiration
conversion rate
cooling rate
correct response
critical ratio
crown-rump
Cr chromium
creatinine (also creat)
^{51}Cr radioactive isotope of chromium
cr tomorrow (cras)
CRA central retinal artery
CRABP cellular retinoic acid-binding protein
CRACA Council on Roentgenology of the American Chiropractic Association
cran cranial
CRAO central retinal artery occlusion
CRASH Center for Reproductive and Sexual Health
crast for tomorrow (crastinus)
CRBBB complete right bundle branch block
CRBC chicken red blood cell
CRBP cellular retinol-binding protein
CRC clinical research center
concentrated red blood cell
cross-reacting cannabinoids
CrCl creatinine clearance (also CC)
CRD childhood rheumatic disease
child restraint device
chorioretinal degeneration
chronic renal disease
chronic respiratory disease
complete reaction of degeneration
creat creatinine (also Cr)
CREOG Council on Resident Education in Obstetrics and Gynecology
crep crepitation
CREST calcinosis, Raynaud's phenomenon, esophhageal dysfunction, sclerodactyly, telangiectasis in scleroderma
CRF case report form
chronic renal failure
continuous reinforcement
corticotropin-releasing factor
CRH corticotropic-releasing hormone
CRI Cardiac Risk Index
chronic renal insufficiency
Composite Risk Index
cross-reactive idiotype
crit critical
CRL crown-rump length
CRM contralateral remote masking
cross-reacting material
crown-rump measurement
CRMC Center for Research for Mothers and Children
CRNA Certified Registered Nurse Anesthesist
CRNHP Concerned Relatives of Nursing Home Patients
CRO cathode ray oscilloscope

CROS contralateral routing of signal
CRP chronic relapsing pancreatitis
confluent, reticulate papillamatosis
corneoretinal potential
coronary rehabilitation program
C-reactive protein
CRPA C-reactive protein antiserum
CRPF chloroquine-resistant Plasmodium falciparum
contralateral renal plasma flow
CRPR Child Rearing Practices Report
CRS Chinese restaurant syndrome
colon-rectal surgery
compliance of the respiratory system
congenital rubella syndrome
CRSP comprehensive renal scintillation procedure
CRST calcinosis, Raynaud's phenomenon, sclerodactylia, telangiectasis
CRT cardiac resuscitation team
cathode ray tube
chromium release test
CRU cardiac rehabilitation unit
clinical research unit
CRV central retinal vein
cr vesp
tomorrow evening (cras vespere)
CRVF congestive right ventricular failure
CRVO central retinal vein occlusion
CRVS California Relative Value Scale
CRWAD Conference of Research Workers in Animal Diseases
cryo cryoprecipitate
crys crystal
CS calf serum
carcinoid syndrome
cardiogenic shock
carotid sheath
carotid sinus
celiac sprue
central service
central supply
cerebrospinal
cesarean section
chemical sympathectomy
chest strap
chondroitin sulfate
chorionic somatomammotropin
cigarette smoker
cigarette smoke solution
citrate synthase
clinical stage
Cockayne's syndrome
colistin
completed suicide
concentrated strength
conditioned stimulus
contact sensitivity
continuing smoker
continuous stripping
control serum
convalescent status
coronary sinus
corpus striatum
Corson and Stoughton
corticosteroid
current smoker
current strength
Cushing's syndrome
cycloserine
C&S culture and sensitivity
C_S static compliance
Cs case
cell surface antigen
cesium
consciousness
standard clearance
^{131}Cs radioactive isotope of cesium
^{132}Cs radioactive isotope of cesium
^{134}Cs radioactive isotope of cesium
^{137}Cs radioactive isotope of cesium
c/s cycles per second
CSA canavaninosuccinic acid
chondroitin sulfate A
colony-stimulating activity
cross-sectional area
CsA cyclosporin A (also CyA)
CSAA Child Study Association of America
CSAD cystein sulfinic acid decarboxylase
CSATP Child Sexual Abuse Treatment Program
CSAVP cerebral subarachnoid venous pressure
CSAVR Council of State Administrators of Vocational Rehabilitation
CSB Cheyne-Stokes breathing
Controlled Substance Board
CSBF coronary sinus blood flow
CSC cigarette smoke condensate
Continued Stay Certification
coup sur coup
CSCD Center for Sickle Cell Disease
CSCR Central Society for Clinical Research
CSD cat scratch disease
combined system disease
craniospinal defect
critical stimulus duration
CSDH Council of Societies in Dental Hypnosis
CSE ceramide phosphinicoethanolamine
cholestyramine
C/SEC Cesareans/Support, Education, and Concern
CSER cortical somatosensory evoked response
CSF Canadian Schizophrenia Foundation
cerebrospinal fluid
circumferential shortening fraction
colony-stimulation factor
coronary sinus flow
CSFP cerebrospinal fluid pressure
CSF-WR
cerebrospinal fluid-Wassermann reaction
CSGBI Cardiac Society of Great Britain and Ireland
CSGBM collagenase solubilized glomerular basement membrane
CSGUS Clinical Society of Genito-Urinary Surgeons
CSH chronic subdural hematoma
Cold Spring Harbor
cortical stromal hyperplasia
CSI Calculus Surface Index
cavernous sinus infiltration
CSICU cardiac surgical intensive care unit
CSII continuous subcutaneous insulin infusion
CSIIP continuous subcutaneous insulin infusion pump
CSIS clinical supplies and inventory system
CSL cardiolipon synthetic lecithin
CSM carotid sinus massage
cerebrospinal meningitis
cornmeal, soybean, milk
CSMA Chemical Specialties Manufacturers Association
CSMG Center for Study of Multiple Gestation
CSMP Continuous System Modelling Program

CSN carotid sinus nerve
CSNRT corrected sinus node recovery time
CSNS carotid sinus nerve stimulation
CSO common source outbreak
CSOM chronic serous otitis media
chronic suppurative otitis media
CSP carotid sinus pressure
Cooperative Statistical Program
Crawford Small Parts
CSPH Canadian Society of Hospital Pharmacists
CSR central supply room
Cheyne-Stokes respiration
continued stay review
corrected sedimentation rate
corrected survival rate
cortisol secretion rate
cumulative survival rate
CSRT corrected sinus node recovery time
CSS Cancer Surveillance System
carotid sinus stimulation
cranial sector scan
cysteine-S-sulfate
CST Compton scatter tomography
contraction stress test
convulsive shock therapy
CSTDPHE
Conference of State and Territorial Directors of Public Health Education
CSU casualty staging unit
catheter specimen of urine
central statistical unit
CSW current sleepwalker
CT calcitonin
cardiothoracic
carotid tracing
carpal tunnel
cationic trysinogen
cellular therapy
center thickness
cerebral thrombosis
cerebral tumor
chemotaxis
chemotherapy
chloramine T
chlorothiazide
cholera enterotoxin
cholera toxin
chordae tendineae
chronic thyroiditis
chymotrypsin
circulation time
classic technique
clotiamine
coated tablet
cognitive therapy
collecting tubule
combined tumor
compressed tablet
computed tomography
connective tissue
continued treatment
continuous flow tub
contraction time
Coombs' test
corneal transplant
coronary thrombosis
corrected transposition
corrective therapy
cortical thickness
co-trimoxazole
cough threshold
crest time
crutch training
cytotechnologist
cytotoxic therapy
C/T compression to traction ratio
crossmatch to transfusion ratio
C_{T-1824}
clearance of Evans blue
CTA Canadian Tuberculosis Association
chemotactic activity
cystine trypticase agar
Cta catamenia
CTAB cetyltrimethylammonium bromide (also CTBA)
CTAC cetyltrimethylammonium chloride
CTAL cortical thick ascending limb
CTAP connective tissue activating peptide
CTBA cetrimonium bromide (also CTAB)
CTC chlortetracycline
cultured T cell
CTCL cutaneous T cell leukemia
cutaneous T cell lymphoma
CTD carpal tunnel decompression
congenital thymic dysplasia
connective tissue disease
CTE calf thymus extract
CTEM conventional transmission electron microscope
CTF cefotiam
Colorado tick fever
CTG cardiotocography
C/TG cholesterol to triglyceride ratio
CTGA complete transposition of the great arteries
CTH ceramide trihexoside
CTHBP Citizens for the Treatment of High Blood Pressure
CTL cytotoxic T lymphocyte
CTLD chlorthalidone
CTLL cytotoxic T lymphocyte line
CTLSO cervicothoracolumbosacral orthosis
CTM continuous tone masking
CTMM computed tomographic metrizamide myelography
CTN computed tomography number
ctn cotangent
CTP California Test of Personality
cytidine triphosphate
C-TPN cyclic total parenteral nutrition
CTPP cerebral tissue perfusion pressure
CTPV coal tar pitch volatiles
CTPVO chronic thrombotic pulmonary vascular obstruction
CTR cardiothoracic ratio
clotrimazole
ctr center
CTS carpal tunnel syndrome
composite treatment score
Computerized Tomography Society
contralateral threshold shift
corticosteroid
CTT central tegmental tract
computerized transaxial tomography
CTU centigrade thermal unit
CTV cervical and thoracic vertebrae
CTW central terminal of Wilson
cotton textile worker
CTX cefotaxime
cerebrotendinous xanthomatosis
chemotoxins
cyclophosphamide (Cytoxan)
CTZ chemoreceptor trigger zone

chlorothiazide
CU cardiac unit
clinical unit
contact urticaria
convalescent unit
Cu copper
^{61}Cu radioactive isotope of copper
^{64}Cu radioactive isotope of copper
^{67}Cu radioactive isotope of copper
cu cubic (also C)
CUA Canadian Urological Association
CuB copper band
CUC chronic ulcerative colitis
cu cm cubic centimeter (also cc, ccm, cm^3)
CUE cumulative urinary excretion
cu ft cubic foot
CUG cystourethrogram
CUHP Council of Urban Health Providers
CuHVL copper half value layer
cu in cubic inch
cuj of which (cujus)
cuj lib
of any you desire (cujus libet)
cult culture
cu mm cubic millimeter (also cmm, mm^3)
CUPS carcinoma of unknown primary site
cur curative
current
curat dressing (curatio)
CURE Center for Ulcer Research and Education
CUS contact urticaria syndrome
CUSPF China-United States Peoples Friendship
cu yd cubic yard
CV cardiovascular
cell volume
central venous
cerebrovascular
cervical vertebrae
Chikungunya virus
closing volume
coefficient of variation
color vision
concentrated volume
conducting vein
conduction velocity
conjugata vera
consonant vowel
contrast ventriculography
conventional ventilation
conversational voice
corpuscular volume
Coxsackie virus
crystal violet
curriculum vitae
cutaneous vasculitis
cv tomorrow evening (cras vespere)
CVA cardiovascular accident
cerebrovascular accident
cervicovaginal antibody
costovertebral angle
cresyl violet acetate
cyclophospamide, vincristine, cytarabine
CVA-BMP
cyclophosphamide, vincristine, doxorubicin (Adriamycin), carmustine (BCNU), methotrexate, procarbazine
CVAH congenital virilizing adrenal hyperplasia
CVAT costovertebral angle tenderness
CVC central venous catheter
CVCT cardiovascular computed tomography
CVD cardiovascular disease
cerebrovascular disease
cerebrovascular disorder
collagen vascular disease
color vision deviant
cvd curved
CVF cardiovascular failure
cardiovascular Fick
cervicovaginal fluid
cobra venom factor
CVG contrast ventriculography
CVH cervicovaginal hood
combined ventricular hypertrophy
CVHD chronic valvular heart disease
CVI cardiovascular incident
cerebrovascular insufficiency
CVID common variable immunodeficiency
CVL clinical vascular laboratory
CVO central vein occlusion
central venous oxygen
circumventricular organs
obstetric conjugate diameter (conjugata vera obstetrica)
CvO_2 mixed venous oxygen content
CVP cardioventricular pacing
cell volume profile
central venous pressure
cyclophosphamide, vincristine, prednisone (also COP)
CVR cardiovascular renal
cardiovascular resistance
cardiovascular respiratory
cardiovascular review
cerebrovascular resistance
CVRD cardiovascular renal disease
CVRR cardiovascular recovery room
CVS CAM Vision Stimulator
cardiovascular surgery
cardiovascular system
clean-voided specimen
CVSF conduction velocity of slower fibers
CW cardiac work
case work
cell wall
chemical warfare
chemical weapon
chest wall
children's ward
continuous wave
cotton wool
crutch walking
C/W consistent with
cw clockwise
CWD cell wall deficient
CWDF cell wall deficient form
CWF Cornell Word Form
CWI cardiac work index
CWP childbirth without pain
coal workers' pneumoconiosis
CWPEA Childbirth Without Pain Education Association
CWS cell wall skeleton
cold water soluable
comfortable walking speed
cwt hundredweight
CX cefalexin
cerebral cortex
cloxacillin
critical experiment
Cx cervix
circumflex
complex

convex
CXM cefuroxime
cyclohexamide
CXR chest x-ray
CY See CTX (cyclophosphamide)
Cy cyanogen
cyst
cytarabine
CyA cyclosporin A (also CsA)
cyath glassful (cyathus)
cyath vin
wine glassful (cyathus vinarius)
CYC See CTX (cyclophosphamide)
Cyclo See CTX (cyclophosphamide)
Cyd cytidine (also C)
CYE charcoal yeast extract
cyl cylinder
cylindrical lens
CYNAP cytotoxicity negative, absorption positive
Cys cysteine
cystine
Cyt cytosine (also C)
Cyt Ox
cytochrome oxidase
CYVADIC
cyclophosphamide, vincristine, doxorubicin (Adriamycin), dacarbazine (DTIC)
CZ cefazolin
CZD cefazedone
CZI crystalline zinc insulin
CZP clonazepam

D

D date
daughter
day
dead space gas
death
Debye
deciduous (also dec)
density
dermatology (also Derm, DM)
Dermatophagoides
detail response
deuterium
dextrorotatory
diagnosis (also DG, diag, DX)
diastole
didymium
died
Dientamoeba
diffusing capacity
dihydrouridine
diopter
Diphyllobothrium
Diplococcus
distal (also dist)
dominant
dorsal
down
Dracunculus
Drosophila
dual
duration
dwarf
sulfisomidine
unit of vitamin D potency
1-D one-dimensional
2-D two-dimensional
3-D three-dimensional
2,4-D 2,4-dichlorophenoxyacetic acid
D1...D12
dorsal vertebrae 1 through 12 (see T1...T12)
d deuteron
diarrhea
divorced
doctor (also Dr)
dose
give (da)
let it be given (detur) (also det)
rare-detail response
right (dexter) (also dex)
DA Dark Agouti
degenerative arthritis
delayed action
dental assistant
developmental age
diabetic acidosis
diphenylchlorarsine
direct agglutination
disability assistance
dopamine (also DM)
drug addict
ductus arteriosus
D.A. Diplomate in Anesthetics
D/A digital to analog ratio
discharge and advise
DAA dehydroacetic acid
desalanine-desasparagine
DAAB 1,2-diacetamidobenzene
DAAO D-amino acid oxidase
DAB days after birth
diaminobenzidine
dimethylaminoazobenzene
3,2'-dimethyl-4-aminobiphenyl
DABA diaminobenzanilide
DAC diazacholesterol
Division of Ambulatory Care
DACA dissecting aneurysm of the coronary artery
DACL Depression Adjective Check Lists
DACM N-(7-dimethylamino-4-methylcoumarinyl)-malemide
DAD diffuse alveolar damage
dispense as directed
DADA diisopropylamine dichloroacetate (also DIEDI, DIPA)
DADDS diacetyldiaminodiphenylsulfone
DADPS dapsone (4,4'-diaminodiphenyl sulfone) (also DDS)
DAE diving air embolism
DAF delayed auditory feedback
DAG diacylglycerol
DAH disorderd action of the heart
D.A.I.
Diplomate in Allergy and Immunology
DALA delta-aminolevulinic acid
DAM degraded amyloid
diacetlymonoxime
discriminant analytic model
DAMA discharge against medical advice
DAMP 2-(4,4'diacetoxydiphenylmethyl)pyridine
dAMP deoxyadenylic acid
DANB Dental Assisting National Board
DANS 1-dimethylaminophthalene-5-sulphonyl acid

DAO diamine oxidase
DAP data acquisition processor
delayed after polarization
depolarizing afterpotential
diaminopimelic acid
dihydroxyacetone phosphate
direct agglutination pregnancy
Draw-a-Person
dynamic aortic patch
DAPI 4'6-diamidino-2-phenylindole
DAPT amiphenazole (2,4-diamino-5-phenyl-thiazole)
direct agglutination pregnancy test
DAR dual asthmatic reaction
DARF direct antiglobulin rosette-forming
DARP drug abuse rehabilitation program
DAS Death Anxiety Scale
dextroamphetamine sulfate
DASE Denver Articulation Screening Examination
DAT daunomycin, Ara-C, 6-thioguanine
delayed-action tablet
dementia of the Alzheimer type
Dental Aptitude Test
diet as tolerated
differential agglutination test
differential agglutination titer
Differential Aptitude Test
dipeptidyl aminopeptidase
diphtheria antitoxin
direct antiglobulin test
DATC S-2,3-dichloroallyl diisopropylthio-carbamate
DATD diallyl tartardiamide
DATTA Diagnostic and Therapeutic Technology Assessment
DAVA delta-aminovaleric acid
DAW dispense as written
DAWN Drug Abuse Warning Network
DB Baudelocque's diameter
date of birth
dextran blue
diabetic
diagonal band
direct bilirubin
disability
distobuccal
Dolichos biflorus
double blind
dry bulb
duodenal bulb
Db dubhium
dB decibel
DBA dibenzanthracene
dBA decibel A
DBBS Division of Biomedical and Behavioral Sciences
DBC dibenzcozamide
dye-binding capacity
DBCL dilute blood clot lysis
DBCP dibromochloropropane
DBD definite brain damage
DBE 1,2-dibromoethane
DBED N,N'-dibenzylethylenediamine
DBH dopamine beta-hydroxylase
DBI development-at-birth index
DBM decarboxylase base Moeller
diabetic management
diazobenzyloxymethyl
dibromomannitol
DBMC 4,6-di-tert-butyl-m-cresol
dystrophica bullosa Mendes da Costa
DBMG beta-mandelo-nitrile glucuronide
DBMS data base management system
DBO distobucco-occlusal
DBP demineralized bone powder
diastolic blood pressure
dibutylphthalate
distobuccopulpal
di-t-butyl peroxide
PBPC butylated hydroxytoluene (2,6-di-t-butyl-p-cresol) (also BHT)
DBPCl dibenzyl chlorophosphonate
DBR disordered breathing rate
DBS deep brain stimulation
despeciated bovine serum
4',5-dibromosalicylanilide
dibromsalicil
direct bonding system
Division of Biologic Standards
DBT disordered breathing time
dry bulb temperature
DC daily census
dansylcadaverine
decarboxylase
degenerating cell
Dental Corps
deoxycholate
descending colon
dextran charcoal
diagnostic center
diagnostic code
diffuse cortical
dilation catheter
diphenylcyanarsine
direct coupled
direct current
discontinue (also D/C)
distal colon
distocervical
donor's cell
dorsal column
duodenal cap
dyskeratosis congenita
D.C. Doctor of Chiropractic
D/C decrease (also dec, decr)
discharge
discontinue (also DC)
D&C dilation and curettage
DCA deoxycholate citrate agar
deoxycholic acid
deoxycorticosterone acetate (also DOCA)
dicarboxylic acid
dichloroacetate
DCAG double coronary artery graft
DCAVP desamino-6-carba-arginine-vasopressin
DCB 3,3'-dichlorobenzidine (also DCBD)
DCBD 3,3'-dichlorobenzidine (also DCB)
DCBE double contrast barium enema
DCBF dynamic cardiac blood flow
DCC dextran-coated charcoal
dicyclohexylcarbodiimide (also DCCD, DCCI)
dorsal cell column
DCc double concave
DCCD dicyclohexylcarbodiimide (also Dcc, DCCI)
DCCI dicyclohexylcarbodiimide (also Dcc, DCCD)
DCCMP daunorubicin, cyclocytidine, 6-mercaptopurine, prednisone
DCCT Diabetes Control and Complications Trial
DCD Distortion of Circle-Diamond

DCDA deuterium with cesium dihydrogen arsenate
DCDSB Division of Criteria Documentation and Standards Development
DCE desmosterol to cholesterol enzyme
DCET O,S-dicarbethoxythiamine
DCF direct centrifugal flotation
DCG desoxycorticosterone glucoside
DCH delayed cutaneous hypersensitivity
D.C.H. Diploma in Child Health
D.Ch. Doctor of Chirurgiae (Surgery)
DCHA dicyclohexylamine
DCHN dicyclohexylamine nitrite
DCI dichloroisoprenaline
dichloroisoproterenol
DCL dicloxacillin (also DX)
diffuse cutaneous leishmaniasis
DCLS deoxycholate citrate lactose saccharose
DCLSG Dutch Childhood Leukaemia Study Group
DCM decarbamoyl mitomycin
dichloromethane
dyssynergia cerebellaris myoclonica
DCMO carboxin(2,3-dihydro-5-carboxanilido-6-methyl-1,4-oxathiin
DCMP daunorubicin, cytosine arabinoside, 6-mercaptopurine, prednisone
dCMP deoxycytidylic acid
DCMX dichloro-m-xylenol
DCN delayed conditioned necrosis
4,4'dinitrocarbanilide
dorsal column nucleus
DCNA dichloronitroaniline
D.C.O.G. Diploma of the College of Obstetricians and Gynecologists
DCOVP desamino-6-carba-ornithine-vasopressin
DCP dichlorophene
Diplomate in Clinical Pathology
dynamic compression plate
DCPA dimethyl 2,3,5,6-tetrachloroterephthalate
DCPC dichlorodiphenyl methyl carbinol (also DMC)
DCPD dicalcium phosphate dihydrate
DCPM di-(p-chlorophenoxy)methane
DCPU dorsal caudate putamen
DCR dacryocystorhinostomy
direct cortical response
Division of Clinical Research
DCS decompression sickness
disease control serum
DCT direct Coombs' test
distal convoluted tubule
diurnal cortisol test
dynamic computed tomography
DCTMA desoxycorticosterone trimethylacetate
DCTPA desoxycorticosterone triphenylacetate
DCU Dental Care Unit
Diabetes Center Unit
dichloral urea
DCx double convex
DD day of delivery
delusional disorder
dependent drainage
detrusor dyssynergia
developmental disability
developmentally disabled
died of the disease
differential diagnosis
digestive disease
Di Guglielmo's disease
disk diameter
Distortion of Dots
double diffusion
dry dressing
Duchenne dystrophy
Dupuytren's disease
DD I detrusor dyssynergia, type I
DD II detrusor dyssynergia, type II
Dd unusual detail response
dD confabulated detail response
dd daily (de die)
let it be given to (detur ad)
very small detail response
DDA 2',5'-dideoxyadenosine
DDAVP desmopressin (desamino-8-D-arginine vasopressin)
DDC 3,5-diethoxycarbonyl-1,4-dihydrocollidine
diethyldithiocarbamate
dihydroxyphenylalanine decarboxylase
NN'-didansylcystine
DDD defined daily dose
degenerative disk disease
dehydroxydinaphthyl disulfide
dense deposit disease
dichlorodiphenyldichloroethane (also TDE)
DDE 2,2'-bis-(p-chlorophenyl)-1,1-dichloroethylene (dichlorodiphenyldichloroethylene)
DDIC Digestive Diseases Information Center
DDMP 2,4-diamino-5-(3',4-dichlorophenyl)-6-methylpyrimidine
DDMS degenerative dense microsphere
dDNA denatured DNA
D.D.O. Diploma in Dental Orthopedics
DDP diamminedichloroplatinum
DDPH 1,1-diphenyl-2-picrylhydrazyl
DDQ 2,3-dichloro-5,6-dicyanobenzoquinone
DDR diastolic descent rate
DDS dapsone (diaminodiphenylsulfone) (also DADPS)
disease disability scale
dystrophy-dystocia syndrome
D.D.S. Doctor of Dental Surgery
Dds detail response to small white space
D.D.Sc. Doctor of Dental Science
DDSLA Damien Dutton Society for Leprosy Aid
DDST Denver Developmental Screening Test
DDT chlorophenothane (dichlorodiphenyltrichloroethane)
DDVP dimethyldichlorovinyl phosphate
DDW double distilled water
DdW detail response elaborating the whole
DE dendritic expansion
diagnostic error
digestive energy
dihydroeugenol
dose equivalent
dream element
duodenal exclusion
duration of ejection
2-DE two-dimensional echocardiography
D&E dilation and evacuation
de edge detail
DEA dehydroepiandrosterone (also DHA, DHEA)
diethylamine
Drug Enforcement Agency
DEA-D diethylaminoethyl dextran

DEAE diethylaminoethanol
diethylaminoethyl
DEB diepoxybutane
diethylbutanediol
DEBA diethylbarbituric acid
DEBRA Dystrophic Epidermolysis Bullosa Research Association of America
DEBS dominant epidermolysis bullosa simplex
deb spis
of the proper consistency (debita spissitudo)
DEC developmental evaluation center
diethylcarbamazine
dec deciduous (also D)
decimal
decimeter
decompose
decrease (also D/C, decr)
pour off (decanta)
DECO decreasing consumption of oxygen
decoct
decoction
decr decrease (also D/C, dec)
decub decubitus
DED defined exposure dose
delayed erythema dose
de d in d
from day to day (de die in diem)
DEDIP Department of Environmental and Drug-Induced Pathology
DEDTC diethyldithiocarbamate (also DETC)
DEET diethyltoluamide
DEF decayed, extraction, filled
duck embryo fibroblast
def defecation
deficiency
deg degeneration
degree
DEGA diethylene glycol adipate
deglut
let it be swallowed (deglutiatur)
DEHA di(2-ethylhexyl) adipate
DEHFT developmental hand function test
DEHP di(2-ethylhexyl) phthalate (also DOP)
del delivery
delusion
Dem Demerol
DEN diethylnitrosamine
DEP diethylpropanediol
diethyl pyrocarbonate (also DEPA)
dep dependents
deposit
purified (depuratus)
DEPA diethylene phosphoramide
DEPC pyrocarbonic acid diethyl ester (also DEP)
DEPS distal effective potassium secretion
Dept department
DEQ Depressive Experiences Questionnaire
DER reaction of degeneration
der derive
Derm dermatology (also D, DM)
DES dermal-epidermal separation
desmosine
diethylstilbestrol
diffuse esophageal spasm
disequilibrium syndrome
DESI Drug Efficacy Study Implementation
DEST Denver Eye Screening Test
dest distilled (destillatus)
destil
distil (destilla)
DET diethyltryptamine
det let it be given (detur) (also d)
DETC diethyldithiocarbamate (also DEDTC)
det in dup
let twice as much be given (detur in duplo)
d et s
let it be given and labeled (detur et signetur)
DEUC direct electronic urethrocystometry
DEV duck embryo vaccine
duck embryo virus
dev development
deviation
DEX dexamethasone
dex right (dexter) (also d)
DF decapacitation factor
decayed and filled, permanent
degree of freedom
Dermatology Foundation
desferrioxamine (also DFX)
diabetic father
diaphragmatic function
digital fluoroscopy
discriminant function
disseminated foci
distribution factor
dome fragment
dorsiflexion
Dysautonomia Foundation
df decayed and filled, deciduous
degree of freedom
DFA direct fluorescent antibody
dorsiflexion assist
DFC deletion of final consonants
dry-filled capsule
DFD defined formula diet
DFDD difluorodiphenyldichloroethane
DFDT difluorodiphenyltrichloroethane
DFE diffuse fasciitis with eosinophilia
DFECT dense fibroelastic connective tissue
DFG direct forward gaze
DFI disease-free interval
DFM decreased fetal movement
DFMC daily fetal movement count
DFMO 2-difluoromethylornithine
DFMR daily fetal movement recording
DFO deferoxamine (also DFOM)
DFOM deferoxamine (also DFO)
DFP diastolic filling period
diisopropylfluorophosphate (also DIFP)
DFS disease-free survival
DFSP dermatofibrosarcoma protuberans
DFT discrete Fourier transforms
DFU dead fetus in utero
dideoxyfluorouridine
DFX desferrioxamine (also DF)
DG dark-ground
deoxyglucose
desglycinamide
diagnosis (also D, Diag, DX)
diastolic gallop
diglyceride
distogingival
dg decigram
DGAVP desglycinamide-arginine-vasopressin
DGCCP Dental Guidance Council for Cerebral Palsy
DGCI delayed gamma camera image
DGI disseminated gonococcal infection
DGL deglycyrrhizined liquorice
dGMP deoxyguanylic acid

DGN diffuse glomerulonephritis
D.G.O. Diplomate in Gynecology and Obstetrics
DGP deoxyglucose phosphate
DGR degranol
DGS diabetic glomerulosclerosis
DH daily habits
dehydrochloric acid
dehydrogenase
delayed hypersensitivity
dental habits
dental hygienist
Department of Health
dermatitis herpetiformis
developmental history
diffuse histiocytic
disseminated histoplasmosis
Dix-Hallpike
dorsal horn
DHA decosahexaenoic acid
dehydroacetic acid
dehydroascorbic acid
dehydroepiandrosterone (also DEA, DHEA)
dihydroalprenolol
dihydroxyacetone
docosahexaenoic acid
DHAP dihydroxyacetone phosphate
DHAS dehydroepiandrosterone sulfate
DHB dihydroxybenzoic acid
duck hepatitis B virus
7-DHC 7-dehydrocholesterol
DHCA dihydroxycoprostanoic acid
1,25 DHCC 1,25-dihydroxycholecalciferol
DHE dihydroergokryptine
dihydroergotamine
DHE-45 dihydroergotamine mesylate
DHEA dehydroepiandrosterone (also DEA, DHA)
DHEAS dehydroepiandrosterone sulfate
DHEW Department of Health, Education and Welfare (see also DHHS)
DHF dengue hemorrhagic fever
dihydrocortisol
DHFR dihydrofolate reductase
DHFS dengue hemorrhagic fever shock syndrome
D.Hg. Doctor of Hygiene (also D.Hy.)
DHGG deaggregated human gamma globulin
DHHS Department of Health and Human Services
DHI 5,6-dihydroxyindole
DHIA dehydroisoandrosterone
DHIC dihydroisocodeine
DHK dihydroergocryptine
DHL diffuse histiocytic lymphoma
DHMA dehyroxymandelic acid
DHNA 1,4-dihydroxy-2-naphthoic acid
DHO deuterium hydrogen oxide
DHODH dihydroorotate dehydrogenase
DHP dihydroxyacetone phosphate
5 DHP 5-alpha-dihydroprogesterone
5-beta-dihydroprogesterone
DHPc dorsal hippocampus
DHPG 3,4-dihydroxyphenylethylene glycol
dihydroxyphenylglycol
DHPR dihydropteridine reductase
DHR delayed hypersensitivity reaction
DHS delayed hypersensitivity
dihydrostreptomycin (also DHSM, DS, DST)
duration of hospital stay
D-5-HS 5% dextrose in Hartman's solution
DHSM dihydrostreptomycin (also DHS, DS, DST)
DHSS Department of Health and Social Security
DHT dihydrotachysterol
dihydrotestosterone
dihydrothymine
5,7-DHT 5,7-dihydroxytryptamine
DHTC dihydroteleocidin
DHTP dihydrotestosterone propionate
D.Hy. Doctor of Hygiene (also D.Hg.)
DI defective interfering
degradation index
desorption ionization
deterioration index
detrusor instability
diabetes insipidus
diaphragmatic
disability insurance
dispensing information
distal intestine
distoincisal
dorsal interosseous
Di didymium
di inside detail
DIA depolarization-induced automaticity
Drug Information Association
Di A Diego antigen
Dia diabetes
diameter
diathermy
diab diabetic
DIAC diiodothyroacetic acid
Diag diagnosis (also D, DG, Dx)
DIAGNO differential diagnosis
DIAL Developmental Indicator for the Assessment of Learning
DIAR dextran-induced anaphylactoid reaction
DIAZ diazepam
DIB butyl-3:5-diiodo-4-hydroxybenzoate
Diagnostic Interview for Borderlines
disability insurance benefit
DIC dacarbazine (5-(dimethyltrazeno)imidazole-4-carboxamide) (also DTIC)
diffuse intravascular clotting
diffuse intravascular coagulation
disseminated intravascular coagulation
disseminated intravascular coagulopathy
drug information center
DID dead of intercurrent disease
dystonia-improvement-dystonia
DIE died in Emergency Room
dieb alt on alternate days (diebus alternis)
dieb secund every second day (diebus secundis)
dieb tert every third day (diebus tertiis)
DIEDI diisopropylamine dichloroacetate (also DADA, DIPA)
DIF difkunisal
direct immunofluorescence
diff differential blood count
DIFP diffuse interstitial fibrosing pneumonitis
diisopropylfluorophosphate (also DFP)
dig let it be digested (digeratur)
D.I.H. Diploma in Industrial Health
DIHE drug-induced hepatic encephalopathy
DIL drug information log

dil dilute
DILD diffuse infiltrative lung disease
diffuse interstitial lung disease
DILE drug-induced lupus erythematosus
diluc at daybreak (diluculo)
DIM divalent iron metabolism
D.I.M.
Diplomate in Internal Medicine
dim one-half (dimidius)
DIMS disorder of initiating and maintaining sleep
DIMSA disseminated intravascular multiple systems activation
d in dup
give twice as much (detur in duplo)
d in p aeq
divided into equal parts (divide in partes aequales)
DiNPZ N,N'-dinitrosopiperazine
DIP desquamative interstitial pneumonia (or pneumonitis)
distal interphalangeal
DIPA diisopropylamine dichloroacetate (also DADA, DIEDI)
DIPJ distal interphalangeal joint
DIRD drug-induced renal disease
dir prop
proper direction (directione propria)
dis disabled
disease (also Dz)
dislocation
distance (also dist)
distribution
disc discontinue
disch discharge
DISH diffuse idiopathic skeletal hyperostosis
DISIDA
diisopropyl iminodiacetic acid
disp dispensatory
dispense
dist distal (also D)
distance (also dis)
distill
district
DIT diet-induced thermogenesis
diiodotyrosine
drug-induced thrombocytopenia
div divide
division
divorced
DJD degenerative joint disease
DJS Dubin-Johnson syndrome
DK decay
degeneration of keratinocytes
diet kitchen
diseased kidney
dog kidney
DKA diabetic ketoacidosis
DKB dibekacin
DKDP deuterium with potassium dihydrogen phosphate
DKP dibasic potassium phosphate
diketopiperazine
DL danger list
dansyl lysine
deep lobe
difference limen
diffusion lung capacity
directed listening
distolingual
Donath-Landsteiner
dl deciliter
DLA distolabial
DLAI distolabioincisal
DLB diffuse lymphoblastic lymphoma
DLC dual lumen catheter
DL_{CO} diffusing lung capacity for carbon monoxide
DL_{CO2}
diffusing lung capacity for carbon dioxide
DLE delayed light emission
dialyzable leukocyte extract
discoid lupus erythematosus
disseminated lupus erythematosus
DLF dorsolateral funiculus
DLI distolinguoincisal
DLO distolinguo-occlusal
D.L.O.
Diplomate in Laryngology and Otolaryngology
DLP delipidized serum protein
developmental learning problems
direct linear plotting
dislocation of the patella
distolinguopulpal
DLT dental laboratory technician
DLWD diffuse lymphocytic, well differentiated
DM demeclocycline
dermatology (also D, Derm)
dermatomyositis
dextromethorphan
diabetes mellitus
diabetic mother
diastolic murmur
diffuse mixed
diphenylamine arsine chloride
dopamine (also DA)
dorsamedial
dose modification
double membrane
dry matter
duodenal mucosa
dM decimorgan
dm decimeter
DMA dimethyladenosine
dimethylamine
N,N-dimethylacetamide
N,N-dimethylaniline
DMAB dimethylaminoazobenzene
dimethylaminobenzaldehyde
DMAC dimethylacetamide
DMAG Data Management Advisory Group
DMARD disease modifying antirheumatic drug
DMAS dimethylamine sulfate
DMBA dimethylbenzanthracene
DMC Data Management Center
dichlorodiphenyl methyl carbinol (also DCPC)
DMCT demethylchlortetracycline
DMD desmethyldiazepam (also DMDZ)
disease-modifying drug
Duchenne's muscular dystrophy
D.M.D.
Doctor of Dental Medicine
DMDS dimethyl disulfide
DMDT dimethoxydiphenyltrichloroethane
DMDTP dimethyldithiophosphate
DMDZ desmethyldiazepam (also DMD)
DME dimethyl ether
Director of Medical Education
drug metabolizing enzyme

Dulbecco's modified Eagle's
D.M.E.
Doctor of Medical Education
DMEM Dulbecco's minimum essential medium
Dulbecco's modified Eagle's medium
DMF decayed, missing, or filled
dimethylformamide (also DMFA)
dmf decayed, missing, or filled, deciduous
DMFA dimethylformamide (also DMF)
DMFS decayed, missing, or filled tooth surface
dmfs decayed, missing, or filled tooth surface, deciduous
DMG dimethylglycine
DMGG N'-dimethylguanylguanidine
DMH dimethylhydrazine
DMI Defense Mechanisms Inventory
desipramine
desmethylimipramine
diaphragmatic myocardial infarct
DMJ See JDM
DMKA diabetes mellitus ketoacidosis
DML distal motor latency
N-dimethyl-4-lysine
DMM disproportionate micromelia
DMN dimethylnitrosamine (also DMNA)
dorsomedial nucleus
DMNA dimethylnitrosamine (also DMN)
DMO dimethadione (5,5-dimethyloxazolidine-2,4-dione)
DMOOC diabetes mellitus out of control
DMP diffuse mesangial proliferation
dimethyl phthalate
dura mater prosthesis
DMPA depomedroxyprogesterone acetate
DMPC dimyristoyl phosphatidylcholine
DMPE dimethyoxyphenylthylamine
DMPEA See DMPE
DMPH$_4$ 6,7-dimethyl-5,6,7,8-tetrahydropterin
DMPP 1,1-dimethyl-4-phenylpiperazinium
DMPT dimethylphenyltriazene
dimethylsuberimidate
DMRD Diploma in Medical Radio-Diagnosis
DMRF dorsal medullary reticular formation
DMRT Diploma in Medical Radio-Therapy
DMS dense microsphere
dermatomyositis
dimethyl sulfoxide (also DMSO)
D.M.S.
Doctor of Medical Science (also D.M.Sc.)
dms double minute sphere
DMSA dimercaptosuccinic acid
D.M.Sc.
Doctor of Medical Science (also D.M.S.)
DMSO dimethyl sulfoxide (also DMS)
DMT Defense Mechanism Test
dermatophytosis
dimethyltryptamine
DMTT 3,5-dimethyl-2-thionotetrahydro-1,3,5-thiodiazine
DMTU dimethylthiourea
DN Deiters nucleus
dextrose/nitrogen (also D/N)
diabetic neuropathy
dibucaine number
dicrotic notch
4,6-dinitro-o-cresol (also DNOC)
Diploma in Nursing
D/N dextrose/nitrogen (also DN)
Dn dekanem
dn decinem
DNA deoxyribonucleic acid
did not answer
did not attend
DNAP deoxyribonucleic acid polymerase
DNase deoxyribonuclease
DNB dinitrobenzene
Diplomate of the National Board of Medical Examiners
dorsal noradrenergic bundle
DNBP dinitrobutylphenol
DNC did not come
dinitrocarbanilide
DNCB dinitrochlorobenzene
DND died a natural death
DNE Director of Nursing Education
DNFB dinitrofluorobenzene (also FDNB)
DNLL dorsal nucleus of lateral lemniscus
DNOC 4,6-dinitro-o-cresol (also DN)
DNOCHP
dinitro-o-cyclohexyphenol
DNP deoxyribonucleoprotein
2,6-diiodo-4-nitrophenol
dinitrophenyl
do not publish
DNPH dinitrophenylhydrazine
DNPM dinitrophenylmorphine
DNPT dinitrosopentamethylenetetramine
DNR daunorubicin (also DRB)
did not respond
do not resuscitate
dorsal nerve root
DNS dansyl (5-dimethylaminonaphthalene-1-sulfonyl)
did not show
dinoyl sebacate
Director of Nursing Services
de novo synthesis
D.N.S.
Diplomate in Neurosurgery
D5NSS 5% dextrose in normal saline solution
DNT did not test
DNTP parathion (diethyl-p-nitrophenyl monothiophosphate)
DNUA distillable nonurea adductable
DNV dorsal nucleus of the vagus
DO diamine oxidase
dissolved oxygen
disto-occlusal
doctor's orders
doxycycline
D.O. Diploma in Ophthalmology
Diplomate in Ophthalmology
Doctor of Optometry
Doctor of Osteopathy
D-O directive-organic
Do oligophrenic response
do ditto
the same as before (dictum)
DOA date of admission
date of arrival
dead on arrival
differential optical absorption
dioctyl adipate
DOAC Dubois oleic albumin complex
DOAP daunorubicin, vincristine (Oncovin), cytosine arabinoside, prednisone
DOB dangle out of bed
date of birth
doctor's order book
DOC date of conception
dead of other causes
deoxycholate

deoxycorticosterone
DOCA deoxycorticosterone acetate (also DCA)
DOCG deoxycorticosterone glucoside
DOD date of death
dead of disease
DOE date of examination
Department of Energy
deoxyephedrine hydrochloride
dyspnea on exertion (also ED)
DOES disorders of excessive sleepiness (or somnolence)
DOET dimethoxyethyl amphetamine
DOG deoxy-D-glucose
DOH Department of Health
dol dolorimetric unit of pain intensity
DOM dimethoxymethyl amphetamine (also STP)
Dom domoic acid
DOMA dihydroxymandelic acid
DON diazo-oxonorleucine
don alv sol fuerit
until the bowels are open (donec alvus soluta fuerit)
DOP di(2-ethylhexyl) phthalate (dioctyl phthalate) (also DEHP)
DOPA dihydroxyphenylalanine
DOPAC 3,4-dihydroxyphenylacetic acid
DOPC determined osteogenic precursor cell
DOPE disease-oriented physician education
DOPEG 3,4-dihydroxyphenylglycol
DOPS diffuse obstructive pulmonary syndrome
dihydroxyphenylserine
DORV double outlet right ventricle
DOS day of surgery
D.O.S.
Diplomate in Orthopedic Surgery
DOSS dioctyl sodium sulfosuccinate (also DSS)
DOT Diploma of Occupational Therapy
DOTES Dosage Record and Treatment Emergent Symptom Scale
DOX doxorubicin (also ADM--Adriamycin; DXR)
DP deep pulse
definitive procedure
degree of polymerization
dementia praecox
dense plate
developed pressure
diaphragmatic plaque
diastolic pressure
dichloromethylene diphosphonate
diffuse precipitation
diffusion pressure
digestible protein
directional preponderance
disability pension
discriminating power
displaced person
distopulpal
donor's plasma
dorsalis pedis
D-penicillamine (also DPA)
driving pressure
D.P. Doctor of Pharmacy
Doctor of Podiatry
2,4-DP
2,4-dichlorophenoxypropionic acid
dp with proper direction (directione propria)
DPA diphenolic acid
diphenylamine
dipropylacetate
D-penicillamine (also DP)
D-phenylalanine
dynamic physical activity
propanil (N-(3,4-dichlorophenyl) propanamide)
D.P.A.
Diplomate in Pathology
DPB days postburn
DPC delayed primary closure
DPD diffuse pulmonary disease
DPDA phosphorodiamidic anhydride
DPDL diffuse, poorly differentiated lymphocytic lymphoma
DPE Death Personification Exercise
DPF days postfarrowing
DPFR diastolic pressure-flow relationship
DPG diphosphoglycerate
DPGN diffuse proliferative glomerulonephritis
DPH Department of Public Health
diaphragm
diphenylhydantoin
Diploma in Public Health
D.P.H.
Doctor of Public Health (also Dr.P.H.)
DPI daily permissible intake
dietary protein intake
(3,4-dihyroxy-phenylamino)-2-imidazoline
drug prescribing index
DPL dipalmitoyl lecithin
distopulpolingual
DPM Diploma in Psychological Medicine
dipyridamole
D.P.M.
Diplomate in Physical Medicine
Doctor of Podiatric Medicine
dpm disintegrations per minute
DPMC Directive to Provide Maximum Care
D.P.M.R.
Diplomate in Physical Medicine and Rehabilitation
DPN dermatosis papalosa nigra
diphosphopyridine nucleotide
DPN+ oxidized diphosphopyridine nucleotide
DPNH reduced diphosphopyridine nucleotide
DPNT N,N'-dinitrosopentamethylene tetramine
DPPC dipalmitoyl phosphatidylcholine
DPPD diphenyl-para-phenylenediamine
DPPR Drug Product Problem Reporting
DPR doctor population ratio
D.PR. Diplomate in Proctology
DPS dermatan polysulfate
dimethylpolysiloxane
Director of Professional Services
D.P.S.
Diplomate in Plastic Surgery
dps disintegration per second
DPSE Division of Physical Science and Engineering
DPT diphosphothiamine
diphtheria, pertussis, tetanus
dipropyltryptamine
DPTA diethylenetriamine pentaacetic acid (also DTPA)
DPTI diastolic pressure time index
DPTP diphtheria, pertussis, tetanus, poliomyelitis
DPTPM diphtheria, pertussis, tetanus, poliomyelitis, measles
DPW distal phalangeal width
DPX dextropropoxyphene

DQ deterioration quotient
developmental quotient
DR delivery room
diabetic retinopathy
diagnostic radiology
Diploma in Radiology
distribution ratio
dorsal raphe
dorsal root
D-related
drug receptor
reaction of degeneration
D.R. Diplomate in Radiology
Dr doctor (also d)
rare detail response
dr drachm
dram
dressing
unusual rare detail response
DRA dextran reactive antibody
disease-resistant antigen
DRAS Drug Regulatory Affairs Section
DRAT differential rheumatoid agglutination test
DRB daunorubicin (also DNR)
beta-D-ribofuranosylbenzimidazole
DRBC dog red blood cell
DRC damage risk criteria
dendritic reticulum cell
dog red blood cell
DRDS Division of Respiratory Disease Studies
DREF dose reduction effectiveness factor
DRF daily replacement factor
Deafness Research Foundation
Direct Relief Foundation
dose reduction factor
DRG diagnostic-related group
disease-related group
dorsal root ganglia
DRID double radioisotope derivative
DRMS drug reaction monitoring system
DRP digoxin reduction product
dorsal root potential
DRQ discomfort relief quotient
DRR Division of Research Resources
dorsal root reflex
DRS descending rectal septum
Diabetic Retinopathy Study
Dyskinesia Rating Scale
DRTC Diabetes Research and Training Centers
DS dead air space
deep sleep
dehydroepiandrosterone sulfate
delayed sensitivity
dendritic spine
deprivation syndrome
dermatan sulfate
dextran sulfate
dextrose-saline
diaphragm stimulation
difference spectroscopy
diffuse scleroderma
digit span (also DSp)
dihydrostreptomycin (also DHS, DHSM, DST)
dilute strength
dioptic strength
discrimination score
discriminative stimulus
donor's serum
doppler sonography
double stranded
double strength
double subordinance
Down's syndrome
driving signal
dry swallow
duration of systole
D.S. Diplomate in Surgery
Doctor of Science (also D.Sc.)
D-S Doerfler-Stewart
D/S dextrose in saline
D&S dermatology and syphilology
D5S 5% dextrose in saline
Ds associative detail response to white space
DSA digital substration angiography
disease-susceptible antigen
DSAP disseminated superficial actinic porokeratosis
Dsb single-breath diffusing capacity
DSBT donor specific blood transfusion
DSC differential scanning calorimeter
D.S.C.
Doctor of Surgical Chiropody
D.Sc. Doctor of Science (also D.S.)
DSCG disodium cromoglycate
DSCT dorsal spinocerebellar tract
DSD depressed spectrum disease
depression sine depression
dry sterile dressing
DSDB direct self-destruction behavior
DSDDT double sampling dye dilution technique
dsDNA double-stranded deoxyribonucleic acid
DSDS daughter sites of dimer strands
d seq on the following day (die sequente)
DSFI Derogatis Sexual Functioning Inventory
DSHEFS
Division of Surveillance Hazards Evaluation and Field Studies
DSHR delayed skin hypersensitivity reaction
DSIP delta sleep-inducing peptide
DSM dextrose solution mixture
dried skim milk
drink skim milk
DSM-III
Diagnostic and Statistical Manual of Mental Disorders, 3rd edition
D.S.N.
Doctor of Science in Nursing
DSO distal subungual onychomycosis
DSP dibasic sodium phosphate
DSp digit span (also DS)
DSPC disaturated phosphatidyl choline
distearoyl phosphatidyl choline
DSR distal splenorenal
double simultaneous recording
dynamic spacial reconstructor
dsRNA double-stranded ribonucleic acid
DSRS distal splenorenal shunt
DSS dengue shock syndrome
dioctyl sodium sulfosuccinate (also DOSS)
disability status scale
DST desensitization test
dexamethasone suppression test
dihydrostreptomycin (also DHS, DHSM, DS)
disproportionate septal thickening
donor-specific transfusion
DSU double setup
DSUH direct suggestion under hypnosis
DSVP downstream venous pressure
DSWI deep surgical wound infection

DSy digit symbol

DT delirium tremens
deuteron tritium
differently tested
diphtheria, tetanus
diphtheria toxoid
discharge tomorrow
distance test
doubling time
duration of tetany
dye test

dT thymidine (also dThd)

DTBP di-tert-butyl peroxide

DTC day treatment center
d-tubocurarine

dtd give such a dose (datur talis dosis)

dtd. no. V
give 5 such doses (dentur talis doses)

dTDP thymidine 5'-diphosphate

DTE desiccated thyroid extract

DTF Dean Thiel Foundation
9-dicyanomethylene-2,4,7-trinitrofluorene

DTGE des-tyrosine gamma-endorphin

DTH delayed-type hypersensitivity
Diploma in Tropical Hygiene

dThd thymidine (also dT)

DTIC dacarbazine (5-(dimethyltrazeno)imidazole-4-carboxamide) (also DIC)

DTICH delayed traumatic intracerebral hemorrhage

DTLA Detroit Test of Learning Aptitude

DTM dermatophyte test medium
Diploma in Tropical Medicine

DTMA deoxycorticosterone trimethylacetate

DTMC di(p-chlorophenyl)trichloromethylcarbinol

dTMP deoxythymidine-5'-monophosphate

DTN diphtheria toxin normal

DTNB 5'-5'-dithiobis-2-nitrobenzoic acid

DTP digital tingling on percussion
digital tingling on pressure
diphtheria, tetanus, pertussis
distal tingling on pressure

DTPA diethylenetriamine pentaacetic acid (also DPTA)

DTPT dithiopropylthiamine (also TPD)

DTR deep tendon reflex
detorubicin

DTRTT digital temperature recovery time test

DTS diphtheria toxin sensitivity
Division of Technical Services

D.T.S.
Diplomate in Thoracic Surgery

DTSP dithiobis (succinimidyl propionate)

DTT device for transverse traction
diagnostic and therapeutic team
diphtheria tetanus toxoid
dithiothreitol

dTTP thymidine 5'-triphosphate

DTVMI Developmental Test of Visual Motor Integration

DTVP Developmental Test of Visual Perception

DTX detoxification

DTZ diatrizoate

DU density unknown
deoxyuridine
dermal ulcer
diagnosis undetermined
diazouracil
dog unit
dose unit
duodenal ulcer

D.U. Diplomate in Urology

DUA dorsal uterine artery

DUB dysfunctional uterine bleeding

DUF Doppler ultrasonic flowmeter

DUL diffuse undifferentiated lymphoma

dulc sweet (dulcis)

dUMP deoxyuridylate

duod duodenum

DUR drug use review

dur hard (durus)

dur dolor
while the pain lasts (durante dolore)

DV Democratic Values
dependent variable
dilute volume
distemper virus
dorsoventral
double vibration

D&V diarrhea and vomiting

DVA desacetyl vinblastine amide
distant visual acuity
duration of voluntary apnea

DVC divanillalcyclohexanone

DVI digital vascular imaging

DVIS digital vascular imaging system

D.V.M.
Doctor of Veterinary Medicine (also V.D.M.)

D.V.M.S.
Doctor of Veterinary Medicine and Surgery

DVR Department (or Division) of Vocational Rehabilitation
double valve replacement

D.V.S.
Doctor of Veterinary Surgery

D.V.Sc.
Doctor of Veterinary Science

DVT deep vein thrombosis

DW distilled water
dry weight
whole response to detail

D/W dextrose in water
dry to wet

D5W 5% dextrose in water

DWDL diffuse, well-differentiated lymphocytic lymphoma

DWI driving while intoxicated

DWT deadweight ton

dwt denarius weight (pennyweight)

DX dextran
dicloxacillin (also DCL)

Dx diagnosis (also D, DG, Diag)

DXM dexamethasone

DXR deep x-ray
doxorubicin (also ADM--Adriamycin; DOX)

DXRT deep x-ray therapy (also DXT)

DXT deep x-ray therapy (also DXRT)

DY double Y

Dy dysprosium

^{165}Dy radioactive isotope of dysprosium

DYN dynorphin

dyn dynamometer
dyne

DZ diazepam (also DZP)
dizygous

Dz disease (also dis)

DZAPO daunorubicin, azacytidine, Ara-C, prednisone, vincristine (Oncovin)

DZC 5-diazoimidazole 4-carboxamide

DZP diazepam (also DZ)

E

E cortisone (compound E)
early
Echinococcus
Echinostoma
edema
Eikenella
Eimeria
einstein
einsteinium (also Es)
electromotive force
emmetropia (also EM)
endogenous
Endolimax
Endomyces
enema (also en, enem)
energy
Entamoeba
Enterobacter
Enterobius
enterococcus
Enteromonas
enzyme
eosinophil (also EOS)
epicondyle
Epidermophyton
epinephrine (also EPI)
error
Erwinia
Erysipelothrix
erythromycin (also EM, EMU)
Escherichia
esophoria, far viewing
ester
ethanal
ethanol
etiocholanolone
Eubacterium
examiner
exercise (also ex)
experimenter
expired gas
extraction ratio
eye

E^1 esophoria, near viewing

E_1 estrone

E_2 estradiol

17 E_2 17-alpha estradiol

E_3 estriol

E_4 estetrol

e electric charge
electron
erg
from (ex)

EA early antigen
educational age
elbow aspiration
electroacupuncture
enteral alimentation
enzymatic active
erythrocyte antibody
erythrocyte antisera
esterase activity

E&A evaluate and advise

ea each

EAA electroacupuncture analgesia
essential amino acid
extrinsic allergic alveolitis

EABV effective arterial blood volume

EAC Ehrlich ascites carcinoma
electroacupuncture
erythema action spectrum
erythema annulare centrifugum
erythrocyte antibody complement
external auditory canal

EACA epsilon-aminocaproic acid

EACD eczematous allergic contact dermatitis

EAD extracranial arterial disease

ead the same (eadem)

e-ADM 4'-epi-Adriamycin

EAE experimental allergic encephalitis
experimental allergic encephalomyelitis
experimental autoimmune encephalomyelitis

EAF emergency assistance to families

EAG electroantennogram

EAHF eczema, asthma, hay fever

EAHLG equine antihuman lymphoblast globuin

EAHLS equine antihuman lymphoblast serum

EAI Employment and Adaptation Index
erythrocyte antibody inhibition

EAM external auditory meatus

EAMG experimental autoimmune myasthenia gravis

EAN experimental allergic neuritis

EAO experimental allergic orchitis

EAP epiallopregnanolone

e-aq aqueous electron

EAR expired air resuscitation
reaction of degeneration (Entartungs-Reaktion)

EAT experimental autoimmune thyroiditis

EAV extra-alveolar vessel

EAVM extramedullary arteriovenous malformation

EB elbow bearing
elementary body
epidermolysis bullosa
Epstein-Barr
esophageal body
estradiol benzoate (also E_2B)
ethidium bromide
Evans blue

E_2B estradiol benzoate (also EB)

Eb See Er

EBA epidermolysis bullosa acquisita
extrahepatic biliary atresia

EBAA Eye Bank Association of America

EBAGGH epidermolysis bullosa atrophicans generalisata gravis Herlitz

EBAGMD epidermolysis bullosa atrophicans generalisata mitis Disentis

EBAIGA epidermolysis bullosa atrophicans inversa Gedde-Dahl/Anton Lamprecht

EBALSA epidermolysis bullosa atrophicans localisata Schnyder/Anton-Lamprecht

EBC esophageal balloon catheter

EBD epidermolysis bullosa dystrophica

EBDD epidermolysis bullosa dystrophica dominant

EBDGHS epidermolysis bullosa dystrophica generalisata Hallopeau-Siemens

EBDGP epidermolysis bullosa dystrophica generalisata Pasini
EBDIG epidermolysis bullosa dystrophica inversa Gedde-Dahl
EBDLCT epidermolysis bullosa dystrophica localisata Cockayne-Touraine
EBDR epidermolysis bullosa dystrophica recessive
EBF erythroblastosis fetalis
EBHDM epidermolysis bullosa herpetiformis Dowling-Meara
EBI emetine bismuth iodide
erythroblastic islands
estradiol-binding index
EBL erythroblastic leukemia
estimated blood loss
EBM expressed breast milk
EBNA Epstein-Barr nuclear antigen
EBP epidural blood patch
EBS elastic back strap
epidermolysis bullosa simplex
EBSK epidermolysis bullosa simplex Koebner
EBSMPFG epidermolysis bullosa simplex, mottled pigmentation, Fischer/Gedde-Dahl
EBSO epidermolysis bullosa simplex Ogna
EBSR Eye-Bank for Sight Restoration
EBSS Earle's balanced salt solution
EBSWC epidermolysis bullosa simplex Weber-Cockayne
EBV Epstein-Barr virus
estimated blood volume
EBZ epidermal basement zone
EC econazole
ejection click
electron capture
embryonal carcinoma
emetic center
endothelial cell
enteric coated
enterochromaffin cell
entorhinal cortex
entrance complaint
Enzyme Commission
enzyme-treated cell
epithelial cell
equalization-cancellation
Escherichia coli
esophageal carcinoma
excitation-contraction
Experienced Control
expiratory center
external carotid
extracellular
extracellular concentration
extracranial
extruded cell
Eye Care
eyes closed
See E (Echinococcus)
E/C estriol to creatine ratio
EC_{50} median effective concentration
ECA electrical control activity
enterobacterial common antigen
ethacrynic acid
external carotid artery
ECB electric cabinet bath
ECBO enteric cytopathic bovine orphan
ECBV effective circulating blood volume
ECC embryonal cell carcinoma
emergency cardiac care
endocervical curettage
estimated creatinine clearance
external cardiac compression
extracorporeal circulation
extrusion of cell cytoplasm
ECCE extracapsular cataract extraction
ECD electrochemical detection
electron capture detector
endocardial cushion defect
enzymatic cell dispersion
ECDB encourage to cough and deep breathe
ECDO enteric cytopathic dog orphan
ECE equine conjugated estrogen
ECF effective capillary flow
eosinophil chemotactic factor
Escherichia coli filtrate
extended care facility
extracellular fluid
ECF-A eosinophil chemotactic factor-anaphylaxis
ECF-C eosinophil chemotactic factor-complement
ECFMG Educational Commission for Foreign Medical Graduates
ECFMS Educational Council for Foreign Medical Students
ECFV extracellular fluid volume
ECG electrocardiogram (also EKG)
ECH epicholorohydrin
ECHO enteric cytopathogenic human orphan
ECI extracorporeal irradiation
ECIB extracorporeal irradiation of blood
ECIL extracorporeal irradiation of lymph
ECK extracellular potassium
ECL electrogenerated chemiluminescence
enterochromaffin-like
eclec eclectic
ECLT euglobulin clot lysis time
ECM erythema chronicum migrans
external cardiac massage
external chemical messenger
extracellular material
extracellular matrix
ECMO enteric cytopathic monkey orphan
extracorporeal membrane oxygenator
ECochG electrocochleography
ECOG Eastern Cooperative Oncology Group
Ecog See ECochG
ECP eosinophil cationic protein
erythroid committed precursor
external counterpulsation
ECR electrocardiographic response
ECRB extensor carpi radialis brevis
ECRI Emergency Care Research Institute
ECRL extensor carpi radialis longus
ECS electrocerebral silence
electroconvulsive shock
extracellular space
ECSO enteric cytopathic swine orphan
ECSP epidermal cell surface protein
ECT electroconvulsive therapy (or treatment)
emission computed tomography
enteric-coated tablet
extracellular tissue
ECTEOLA epichlorhydrin and triethanolamine
ECU environmental control unit
extensor carpi ulnaris
ECV extracellular volume
ECVD extracellular volume of distribution

ECVE extracellular fluid volume expansion

ECW extracellular water

ED ectodermal dysplasia
effective dose
Ehlers-Danlos
elbow disarticulation
elemental diet
embryonic death
emergency department
emotional disturbance
epileptiform discharge
equilibrium dialysis
erythema dose
ethylenediamine
ethynodiol
evidence of disease
exertional dyspnea (also DOE)
extensor digitorum
external diameter

ED_{50} median effective dose

EDA electrodermal audiometry
electrolyte-deficient agar

EDAX energy dispersive analysis of x-rays

EDB ethylene dibromide

EDBC ethylene bisdithiocarbamate

EDBP erect diastolic blood pressure

EDC end-diastolic count
estimated date of conception
estimated date of confinement
expected date of confinement
extensor digitorum communis

EDD effective drug duration
end-diastolic dimension
expected date of delivery

EDDHA ethylenediamine-di-o-hydroxyphenylacetic acid

EDF extradural fluid

EDH extradural hematoma

EDICP electron-dense iron containing particle

EDIM epidemic diarrhea of infant mice
epizootic diarrhea of infant mice

EDL end-diastolic load
end-diastolic segment length
extensor digitorum longus

EDM early diastolic murmur
extramucosal duodenal myotomy

EDMA ethylene glycol dimethacrylate

EDN electrodesiccation

EDNA Emergency Department Nurses' Association

EDP electronic data processing
end-diastolic pressure

EDPA2 ethyl-3,3-diphenyl-2-propenylamine

EDR early diastolic relaxation
effective direct radiation
electrodermal response

EDS Ehlers-Danlos syndrome
energy dispersive spectrometer
excessive daytime sleepiness
extradimensional shift

EDT end-diastolic cardiac wall thickness

EDTA ethylene diaminetetraacetic acid (or edetic acid, or ethylene dinitrilotetraacetic acid)
European Dialysis Transplant Association

educ education

EDV end-diastolic volume

EDVI end-diastolic volume index

EDWGT emergency drinking water germicidal tablet

EDx electrodiagnosis

EE embryo extract
end-expiration
end-to-end
energy expenditure
equine encephalitis
ethinylestradiol
expressed emotion
external ear
eye and ear

EEA electroencephalic audiometry
elemental enteral alimentation
end-to-end anastomosis

EEC ectrodactylia, ectodermal dysplasia, cleft lip and palate
enteropathogenic Escherichia coli

EEDQ 2-ethoxy-1(2H)-quinolinecarboxylic acid

EEE Eastern equine encephalitis

EEG electroencephalogram

EEME ethinylestradiol methyl ether

EENT eye, ear, nose, throat

EEP end-expiratory pressure

EEPI extraretinal eye position information

EER electroencephalographic response

EES erythromycin ethylsuccinate

EF ectopic focus
ejection factor
ejection fraction
elastic fibril (or fiber)
emotional factor
encephalitogenic factor
endothoracic fascia
endurance factor
equivalent focus
erythroblastosis fetalis
erythrocyte fragmentation
exposure factor
extended field
extra food
extrinsic factor

EFA Epilepsy Foundation of America
essential fatty acid
extrafamily adoptees

EFAD essential fatty acid deficiency

EFC elastin fragment concentration
endogenous fecal calcium

EFE endocardial fibroelastosis

eff effect
efferent

EF-G elongation factor G

EFL external fluid loss

EFM electronic fetal monitoring

EFP effective filtration pressure

EFPS epicardial fat pad sign

EFR effective filtration rate

EFS electric field stimulation
electric foot shock

EFT Embedded Figures Test

EFV extracellular fluid volume

EFVC expiratory flow volume curve

EFW estimated fetal weight

EG esophagogastrectomy

e.g. for example (exempli gratia)

EGA estimated gestational age

EGAM ethylene glycol acetate malonate

EGC early gastric cancer

EGD esophagogastroduodenoscopy (also OGD)

EGDA ethylene glycol diacetate

EGF epidermal growth factor

EGG electrogastrogram

EGL eosinophilic granuloma of the lung

EGLT euglobulin lysis time

EGM electogram

extracellular granular material
EGN experimental glomerulonephritis
EGOT erythrocyte glutamic oxaloacetic transaminase
EGT ethanol gelation test
EGTA esophageal gastric tube airway
ethylene glycol-bis (beta-aminoethyl ether)-N,N'-tetraacetic acid
EGW Economic and General Welfare
EH early healed
enlarged heart
enteral hyperalimentation
epidermolytic hyperkeratosis
essential hypertension
E&H environment and heredity
E_h oxidation-reduction potential (also E_o^+)
EHAA epidemic hepatitis-associated antigen
EHB elevate head of bed
EHBA extrahepatic biliary atresia
EHBF estimated hepatic blood flow
exercise hyperemia blood flow
extrahepatic blood flow
EHC enterohepatic circulation
enterohepatic clearance
essential hypercholesterolemia
extrahepatic cholestasis
EHD electrohemodynamics
EHDP etidronate (ethylene hydroxydiphosphonate)
EHF epidemic hemorrhagic fever
exophthalmos hyperthyroid factor
extremely high factor
extremely high frequency
E-HIDA
diethyl iminodiacetic acid
EHL effective half-life
endogenous hyperlipidemia
EHMS electrohydrodynamic ionization mass spectrometry
EHNA erythro-9-(2-hydroxy-3-nonyl)adenine
EHO extrahepatic obstruction
EHP excessive heat production
extra high potency
EHPH extrahepatic portal hypertension
EHR/HR
ethambutol-isoniazid-rifampicin/isoniazid-rifampicin
EHSDS experimental health services delivery system
EHT essential hypertension
EI electron impact
electron ionization
emotionally impaired
enzyme inhibitor
excretory index
external intervention
E/I expiration to inspiration ratio
EIA electroimmunoassay
enzyme immunoassay
equine infectious anemia
exercise-induced asthma
EIAB extracranial intracranial arterial bypass
EIB exercise-induced bronchoconstriction
exercise-induced bronchospasm
EIC elastase-inhibiting capacity
EID egg infective dose
electroimmunodiffusion
EIEC enteroinvasive Escherichia coli
EIF eukaryotic initiation factor
EIM excitability-inducing material
EINECS
European Inventory of Environmental Chemical Substances
EIP end-inspiratory pause
extensor indicis proprius
E_2IP estrogen-induced protein
EIS endoscopic injection sclerosis
EIT erythroid iron turnover
EIV external iliac vein
EJ elbow jerk
EJP excitatory junction potential
ejusd of the same (ejusdem)
EK enterokinase
erythrokinase
EKC epidemic keratoconjunctivitis
ethylketocyclazocine
EKG electrocardiogram (also ECG)
EKV erythrokeratodermia variabilis
EKY electrokymogram
EL early latent
egg lecithin
electroluminescence
erythroleukemia
external elastic
El elastase
elb elbow
ELBW extremely low birth weight
elec electric
elect electuary
elem elementary
ELH egg-laying hormone
ELIEDA
enzyme-linked immunoelectrodiffusion assay
ELISA enzyme-linked immunoabsorbent assay
elix elixir
ELK ear, nose, throat, lung, kidney
ELM external limiting membrane
ELP early labeled peak
elastase-like protein
ELS Eaton-Lambert syndrome
extralobar sequestration
ELT euglobulin lysis test
euglobulin lysis time
ELU extended length of utterance
EM early memory
ejection murmur
electromagnetic
electron microscope
emmetropia (also E)
emphysema
ergonovine maleate
erythema multiforme
erythrocyte mass
erythromycin (also E, EMU)
esophageal manometry
esophageal motility
e/m charge to mass ratio
EMA epithelial membrane antigen
EMAD equivalent mean age at death
EMB eosin-methylene blue
ethambutol
explosive motor behavior
emb embryology
EMBO European Molecular Biology Organization
EMC electron microscopy
encephalomyocarditis
essential mixed cryoglobulinemia
EMCRO Experimental Medical Care Review Organization
EMEM Eagle's minimum essential medium
EMF electromagnetic flowmeter

electromotive force
endomyocardial fibrosis
erythrocyte maturation factor
evaporated milk formula

EMG electromyogram
exophthalmos, macroglossia, gigantism

EMI electromagnetic interference

EMIC Emergency Maternal and Infant Care

EMIT enzyme-multiplied immunoassay technique
enzyme-multiplied immunoassay test

EMJH Ellinghausen, McCullough, Johnson, Harris

EML effective mandibular length

EMLD external muscle layer damaged

EMM erythema multiforme major

EMO Epstein, Macintosh, Oxford

EMP electromagnetic pulse
epimacular proliferation
external membrane protein
extramedullary plasmacytoma

emp as directed (ex modo prescripto)
plaster (emplastrum)

emp vesic
a blistering plaster (emplastrum vesicatorium)

EMR educable mentally retarded
electromagnetic radiation
ethanol metabolic rate
eye movement recording

EMRA Emergency Medicine Residents' Association

EMRC European Medical Research Council

EMS early morning stiffness
Emergency Medical Service
emergency medical system
ethyl methane sulfonate
extramedullary site

EMSA Electron Microscopy Society of America

EMSL Environmental Monitoring and Support Laboratory

EMT emergency medical team
Emergency Medical Technician

EMT-ALS
Emergency Medical Technician-Advanced Life Support

EMTDP
Environmental Mutagenesis Test Development Program

EMT-IV
Emergency Medical Technician-Intravenous

EMT-P Emergency Medical Technician-Paramedic

EMU early morning urine
electromagnetic unit
erythromycin (also E, EM)

emul emulsion

EMV eye opening, motor response, verbal response

EMVC early mitral valve closure

EN ecto-5'-nucleotidase
endocardial
enteral nutrition
erythema nodosum

en enema (also E, enem)

ENA extractable nuclear antigen

END elective node dissection

endo endocardial
endotracheal

endocrin
endocrinology

ENDP ethane-1-hydroxy-1,1-diphosphonate

ENE ethyl-norepinephrine

enem enema (also E, en)

ENG electronystagmography

ENK enkephalin

ENL erythema nodosum leprosum

ENN ethylnornicotine

Eno enolase

ENS enteric nervous system
ethyl-N-nitrososarcosinate
ethyl-norsuprarenin

ENT ear, nose, throat
extranodal tissue

entom entomology

ENU ethylnitrosourea

EO eosinophilia
ethylene oxide
eyes open

E_o^+ oxidation-reduction potential (also E_h)

EOA effective orifice area
erosive osteoarthritis
esophageal obturator airway
examination, opinion, advice

EOD electric organ discharge
every other day

EOG electro-oculogram
electro-olfactogram

EOJ extrahepatic obstructive jaundice

EOM equal ocular movements
error of measurement
extraocular movement
extraocular muscles

EOMI extraocular muscles intact

EORTC European Organization for Research on Treatment of Cancer

EOS eosinophil (also E)
ethanolamine-O-sulfate

EOT effective oxygen transport

EP ectopic pregnancy
Eder-Puestov
edible portion
electrophysiologic
emergency physician
endogenous pyrogen
endoperoxide
enteropeptidase
ependymal cell
epicardial
epicillin
erythrocyte protoporphyrin
erythropoietic porphoria
esophageal pressure
evoked potential

Ep erythropoietin

EPA eicosapentaenoic acid
Environmental Protection Agency
extrinsic plasminogen activator

EPAP expiratory airway pressure

EPAQ Extended Personal Attributes Questionnaire

EPB extensor pollicis brevis

EPC epilepsia partialis continua
external pneumatic compression

EPCA external pressure circulatory assistance

EPD effective pressor dose

EPEA expense per equivalent admission

EPEC enteropathogenic Escherichia coli

EPF early pregnancy factor
exophthalmos-producing factor

EPG eggs per gram

EPH edema proteinuria hypertension

EPI Emotions Profile Index
epileptic

epinephrine (also E)
epitympanic
extrapyramidal involvement
Eysenck Personality Inventory
epis episiotomy
epistom
a stopper (epistomium)
Epi-T epitestosterone
epith epithelium
EPL effective patient life
essential phospholipids
extensor pollicis longus
external plexiform layer
EPN O-ethyl-O-paranitrophenyl benzenethiophosphonate
EPO erythropoietin
expiratory port occlusion
EPP end-plate potential
erythropoietic protoporphyria
ethylphenylpropiolate
EPPS Edwards Personal Preference Schedule
N-hydroxyethylpiperazine propane sulfonic acid
EPQ Eysenenck Personallity Questionnaire
EPR electron paramagnetic resonance
electrophrenic respiration
estradiol production rate
extraparenchymal resistance
EPS enzymatic pancreatic secretion
exophthalmos-producing substance
expressed prostatic secretion
extrapyramidal side effect
extrapyramidal symptom
extrapyramidal syndrome
EPSDT early periodic screening, diagnosis, and treatment
EPSP excitatory postsynaptic potential
EPSS E-point septal separation
EPT endoscopic papillotomy
EPTE existed prior to enlistment
EPTS existed prior to service
EPVA Eastern Paralyzed Veterans Association
EQ educational quotient
equilibrium
Eq equation (also eqn)
eq equivalent (also equiv)
EQA external quality assessment
eqn equation (also Eq)
equip equipment
equiv equivalent (also eq)
ER early reticulocyte
efficacy ratio
ejection rate
emergency room
endoplasmic reticulum
equivalent roentgen
erythrocyte receptor
esophageal rupture
estrogen receptor
evoked response
expiratory reserve
external resistance
extraction ratio
Eye Research
Er erbium
^{169}Er radioactive isotope of erbium
^{171}Er radioactive isotope of erbium
er erythrocyte (also Ery)
ERA electrical response activity
electrical response audiometry
Electroshock Research Association
estradiol receptor assay
evoked response audiometry
ERB ethnic relational behavior
ERBF effective renal blood flow
ERC erythropoietin-responsive cell
ERCP endoscopic retrograde cannulation of the pancreatic duct
endoscopic retrograde cholangiopancreatography
endoscopic retrograde choledochopancreatography
ERD evoked response detector
ERF Education and Research Foundation
ERFC erythrocyte rosette-forming cells
ERG electroretinogram
ERH egg-laying release hormone
ERHD exposure-related hypothermia death
ERI Ear Research Institute
E rosette inhibitor
ERM extended radical mastectomy
ERP early receptor potential
effective refractory period
endoscopic retrograde pancreatography
equine rhinopneumonitis
estrogen receptor protein
event-related potential
ERPF effective renal plasma flow
ERPLV effective refractory period of the left ventricle
ERS endoscopic retrograde sphincterotomy
ERT esophageal radionuclide transit
estrogen replacement therapy
external radiation therapy
ERV expiratory reserve volume
Ery erythrocyte (also er)
ES ejection sound
electrical stimulation
emergency service
Endocrine Society
endoscopic sclerosis
endoscopic sphinterotomy
end-to-side
enzyme substrate
esophageal scintigraphy
esophagus (also eso, esoph)
experimental study
exsmoker
exterior surface
Es einsteinium (also E)
ESA Entomological Society of America
ESAO European Society for Artificial Organs
ESB electrical stimulation of the brain
ESC end-systolic count
European Society of Cardiology
ESCA electron spectroscopy for chemical analysis
ESCC epidural spinal cord compression
Esch See E (Escherichia)
ESCS Early Social Communication Scale
ESD electronic summation device
electron-stimulated desorption
end-systolic dimension
exoskeletal device
EsD esterase D
ESEP elbow sensory potential
ESF electrosurgical filter
erythropoietic-stimulating factor
European Science Foundation
ESI enzyme substrate inhibitor
epidural steroid injection
extent of skin involvement
ESL end-systolic segment length
English as a second language

ESM ejection systolic murmur
endothelial specular microscope
ethosuximide (also ETX)
ESN educationally subnormal
estrogen-stimulated neurophysin
eso esophagus (also, ES, esoph)
esoph esophagus (also, ES, eso)
ESP early systolic paradox
end-systolic pressure
eosinophil stimulation promoter
epidermal soluble protein
extrasensory perception
esp especially
ESR electron spin resonance
erythrocyte sedimentation rate
ESRD end-stage renal disease
ESRF end-stage renal failure
ESRS Extrapyramidal Symptom Rating Scale
ESS erythrocyte-sensitizing substance
excited skin syndrome
ess essence
essential
EST electroshock therapy
endodermal sinus tumor
exercise stress test
est estimated
ESU electrostatic unit
ESV end-systolic volume
ESVI end-systolic volume index
ESVS epiurethral suprapubic vaginal suspension
ESWS end-systolic wall stress
ESWL extracorporeal shock-wave lithotripsy
ET constant esotropia
edge thickness
educational therapy
effective temperature
ejection time
embryo transfer
endotracheal
endurance time
enterostomal therapist
epithelial tumor
essential thrombocythemia
essential tremor
ethanol (also ETOH)
etiology
eustachian tube
exchange transfusion
exercise treadmill
expiration time
extracellular tachyzoite
E(T) intermittent esotropia
E.T. Enterostomal Therapist
E/T effector to target ratio
Et ethyl
ETA eicosatetraynoic acid
endotracheal airway
ethionamide
et al and elsewhere (et alibi)
and others (et alii)
ETB Education and Training Board
E_2TBG estradiol-testosterone-binding globulin
ETD eustachian tube dysfunction
ETDRS Early Treatment Diabetic Retinopathy Study
ETEC enterotoxigenic Escherichia coli
ETH elixir of terpin hydrate
ethionamide
ethmoid
ETH/C elixir of terpin hydrate with codeine
etiol etiology
ETIP Experimental Technology Incentives Program
ETKM every test known to man
ETL expiratory threshold load
Et_3N triethylamine
EtO ethylene oxide
ETOH ethanol (or ethyl alcohol) (also ET)
ETOX See EtO
ETP electron transfer particle
electron transport particle
entire treatment period
ephedrine, theophylline, phenobarbital
eustachian tube pressure
ETPBBR European Training Programme in Brain and Behavior Research
ETR effective thyroxine ratio
ETS electrical transcranial stimulation
et seq and the following (et sequentia)
ETT endotracheal tube
ethylenethiourea
extrathyroidal thyroxine
ETU emergency treatment unit
ETV educational television
ETX ethosuximide (also ESM)
ETYA eicosatetraynoic acid
EU Ehrlich unit
enzyme unit
esophageal ulcer
esterase unit
Eu europium
^{152}Eu radioactive isotope of europium
^{154}Eu radioactive isotope of europium
^{155}Eu radioactive isotope of europium
EUA examination under anesthesia
EUCD emotionally unstable character disorder
EULAR European League Against Rheumatism
EUM external urethral meatus
EUP extrauterine pregnancy
EUS external urethral sphincter
EV enterovirus
evoked response
excessive ventilation
extravascular
eV electron volt
ev eversion
evac evacuated
eval evaluation
evap evaporated
EVD external ventricular drainage
ever eversion
EVF ethanol volume fraction
EVI endocardial, vascular, interstitial
endocardial, vascular, intestinal
EVLW extravascular lung water
EVM extravascular mass
evol evolution
EVR endocardial viability ratio
EVS endoscopic variceal sclerosis
EVSD Eisenmenger ventricular septal defect
EVTV extravascular thermal volume
EW emergency ward
EWL egg white lysozyme
evaporative water loss
EWPHE European Working Party High Blood Pressure in the Elderly
Ex exacerbation
exposure
extraction
ex exaggerated (also exag)
examined

example
excision (also exc)
exercise (also E)
exophthalmos
exposure

ex aff of affinity (ex affinis)

EXAFS x-ray absorption fine structure

exag exaggerated (also ex)

exam examination

ex aq in water (ex aqua)

EXBF exercise hyperemia blood flow

exc except
excision (also ex)

EXD ethylxanthic disulfide

ex gr of the group of (ex grupa)

exhib let it be given (exhibeatur)

EXO exonuclease

exp expected
expectorant (also expec)
expired
exposed

expec expectorant (also exp)

expir expiration

EXS externally supported
extrinsically supported

ext extension
exterior
external
extract
extremity
spread (extende)

ext fl fluid extract

EXU excretory urogram

EY epidemiology year

EYA egg yolk agar

F

F cortisol (compound F)
facies
factor
Fahrenheit
failed
fair
false
farad
faraday
fascia
father
feces
fellow
female (also fem)
fermentative
Fermi
fibrous
Ficoll
field of vision
Filaria
Fischer
flexed
fluorine
fontanelle
foramen
force
form response
formula
fossa
fractional
fradiomycin
Francisella
free
French (also Fr)
frequency (also freq)
frontal
Fusarium
Fusiformis
gilbert
luminous flux
variance ratio

^{18}F radioactive isotope of fluorine

F_1 first filial generation

F_2 second filial generation

F+ good form response

F- poor form response

f breaths per unit time
fission
following
make (fiat) (also ft)

FA Fanconi's anemia
far advanced
fatty acid
femoral artery
fibrinolytic activity
fibroadenoma
field ambulance
filterable agent
filterable air
first aid
fluorescent antibody
fluoroalanine
folic acid
forearm
fortified aqueous
free acid
Friedreich ataxia
functional activity
fusaric acid
fusidic acid

FAA N-2-fluorenyl-acetamide (also AAF)

FAAN Fellow of the American Academy of Nursing

FAAO Fellow of the American Association of Optometrists

FAAP Fellow of the American Academy of Pediatrics

FAB fast atom bombardment
French-American-British
functional arm brace

Fab fraction antigen binding

FABF femoral artery blood flow

FAB/MS fast atom bombardment mass spectrometry

FABP fatty acid binding protein
folic acid binding protein

FAC 5-fluorouracil, doxorubicin (Adriamycin), cyclophosphamide
fractional area change

FACA Fellow of the American College of Anesthetics
Fellow of the American College of Angiology

FACAL Fellow of the American College of Allergists

FACC Fellow of the American College of Cardiologists

FACCP Fellow of the American College of Chest Physicians

FACD Fellow of the American College of Dentists
FACG Fellow of the American College of Gastroenterology
FACNHA
Foundation of American College of Nursing Home Administrators
FACOG Fellow of the American College of Obstetricians and Gynecologists
FACP Fellow of the American College of Physicians
FACPM Fellow of the American College of Preventive Medicine
FACR Fellow of the American College of Radiology
FACS Fellow of the American College of Surgeons
fluorescence-activated cell sorter
FACSM Fellow of the American College of Sports Medicine
FAD fetal activity determination
flavin-adenine dinucleotide
FADF fluorescent antibody dark field
$FADH_2$ flavin-adenine dinucleotide, reduced
FADU fluorometric analysis of DNA unwinding
FAF fibroblast-activating factor
FAGA Friedreich's Ataxia Group in America
FAH Federation of American Hospitals
Fahr See F (Fahrenheit)
FAHRB Federation of Associations of Health Regulatory Boards
FAJ fused apophyseal joints
FAM Faschingbauer Abbreviated Minnesota Multiphasic Personality Inventory
5-fluorouracil, doxorubicin (Adriamycin), mitomycin C
fam family
FAMA Fellow of the American Medical Association
fluorescent antibody to membrane antigen
FAME fatty acid methyl ester
FAMMM familial atypical mole malignant melanoma
familial atypical multiple mole melanoma
FANA fluorescent antinuclear antibody
FANCAP
fluids, aeration, nutrition, communication, activity, pain
FANCAS
fluids, aeration, nutrition, communication, activity, stimulation
FANFT N-(4-nitro-2-furyl)-2-thiazolyl formamide
FAO Food and Agricultural Organization
FAOTA Fellow of the American Occupational Therapy Association
FAP familial amyloid polyneuropathy
fatty acid poor
femoral artery pressure
fixed action pattern
FAPA Fellow of the American Psychiatric Association
FAPHA Fellow of the American Public Health Association
FAQ Family Attitudes Questionnaire
FAR fractional albuminuria rate
far faradic
FARE Federation of Alcohol Rehabilitation Establishments
FARS Fatal Accident Reporting System
FAS Federation of American Scientists
fetal alcohol syndrome
FASC free-standing ambulatory surgical center
fasc fasciculus
FASEB Federation of American Societies for Experimental Biology
FASF Factor Analyzed Short Form
FAST Filtered Audiometer Speech Test
FASRT Fellow of the Association of Radiological Technologists
FASXT Fellow of the American Society of X-Ray Technicians
FAT fast axoplasmic transport
fluorescent antibody test
FAUS Feingold Association of the United States
FAV feline ataxia virus
FAZ foveal avascular zone
FB factor B
fiberoptic bronchoscopy (see also FOB)
fingerbreath
foreign body
FBA fecal bile acid
Fellow of the British Academy
FBD functional bowel disorder
FBE full blood examination
FBF forearm blood flow
FBG fasting blood glucose
FBH familial benign hypercalcemia
FBL Foundation for Better Living
FBM fetal breathing movement
FBN Federal Bureau of Narcotics
FBP femoral blood pressure
fibrinogen breakdown product
FBPsS Fellow of the British Psychological Society
FBS fasting bile reflux
fasting blood sugar
fetal bovine serum
FC fasciculus cuneatur
febrile convulsions
fibrocyte
finger clubbing
finger counting
flucytosine
Foley catheter
form response determined by color
foster care
free cholesterol
nitrofural
5-FC 5-fluorocytosine
Fc fragment, crystallizable
shade response to black areas
Fc' fragment crystallized in minute quantities
shade response to light gray area
fc foot candle
FCA ferritin-conjugated antibody
Freund's complete adjuvant
FCAL familial combined hyperlipidemia
FCAP Fellow of the College of American Pathologists
fluorchrome arsenate phenol
FCC follicular center cell
FCCP flurocarbonyl-cyamidephenylhydrazone
FCD fibrocystic dysplasia
focal cytoplasmic degradation
FCER Foundation for Chiropractic Education and Research
FCF fibroblast chemotactic factor
FCFC fibroblast colony forming cells

FCGP Fellow of the College of General Practitioners
FCI fixed cell immunofluorescence
food-chemical intolerance
FCLM Fellow of the College of Legal Medicine
fcly face lying
FCM flow cytometric
FCMW Foundation for Child Mental Welfare
FCP final common pathway
5-fluorouracil, cyclophosphamide, prednisone
Functional Communication Profile
FCPS Fellow of the College of Physicians and Surgeons
FCR flexor carpi radialis
fractional catabolic rate
FcR Fc receptor
FCRA Fellow of the College of Radiologists, Australia
FCS Fellow of the Chemical Society
fetal calf serum
FCU flexor carpi ulnaris
fraud control unit
FCV forced vital capacity
FCVDS Framingham Cardiovascular Disease Survey
FCx frontal cortex
FD familial dysautonomia
fan douche
fatal dose
fibrinogen derivative
field desorption
fluorescence depolarization
fluphenazine decanoate
focal distance
foot drape
forceps delivery
freedom from distractability
freeze dried
frequency deviation
FD_{50} median fatal dose
Fd ferredoxin
FDA fluorescein diacetate
Flying Dentists Association
Food and Drug Administration
frontodextra anterior
FDBL fecal daily blood loss
FDC frequency dependence of compliance
FDDQ Freedom from Distractibility Deviation Quotient
FDDS Family Drawing Depression Scale
Federation of Dental Diagnostic Sciences
Federation of Digestive Disease Societies
FDE final drug evaluation
FDG ^{18}F-2-deoxy-2-fluoro-D-glucose
F-labeled deoxyglucose
FDH familial dysalbuminemic hyperthyroxinemia
FDI first dorsal interosseus
International Dental Federation (Federation Dentaire Internationale)
FDL flexor digitorum longus
FDM fetus of a diabetic mother
FDMD Foundation for Depression and Manic Depression
FDNB fluorodinitrobenzene (see also DNFB)
FDP fibrin degradation product
fibrinogen degradation product
flexor digitorum profundus
frontodextra posterior
fructose 1,6-diphosphate
FDPase
fructose-1,6-diphosphatase
FDR fractional disappearance rate
frequency dependence of resistance
FDS Fellow in Dental Surgery
flexor digitorum superficialis
FDT frontodextra transversa
5-FdUMP
5-fluorodeoxyuridine monophosphate
FE fatty ester
fetal erythrocyte
fluorescing erythrocyte
formalin and ethanol
freely eating
Fe iron
^{52}Fe radioactive isotope of iron
^{55}Fe radioactive isotope of iron
^{59}Fe radioactive isotope of iron
feb fever (febris)
feb dur
while the fever lasts (febre durante)
FEBS Federation of European Biochemical Societies
FEC forced expiratory capacity
free erythrocyte coproporphyrin (also FECP)
FECG fetal electrocardiogram
$FECO_2$ fractional expired carbon dioxide
FECP free erythrocyte coproporphyrin (also FEC)
FEF Family Evaluation Form
forced expiratory flow
FEFV forced expiratory flow volume
FEIBA Factor VIII inhibitor bypassing activity
FEKG See FECG
FELC Friend erythroleukemia cell
FeLV feline leukemia virus
FEM finite element method
fluid-electrolyte malnutrition
fem female (also F)
femur
FEMA Federal Emergency Management Agency
Flavor and Extracts Manufacturer's Association
fem intern
at the inner side of the thighs (femoribus internus)
FENa excreted fraction of filtered sodium
FENF fenfluramine
FeNTA ferric nitrilotriacetate
FEP free erythrocyte porphyrin
free erythrocyte protoporphyrin (also FEPP)
FEPP free erythrocyte protoporphyrin (also FEP)
FER fractional esterification rate
Friends of Eye Research
FERV Foundation for Education and Research in Vision
ferv boiling (fervens)
FES Family Environment Scale
fat embolism syndrome
forced expiratory spirogram
functional electrical stimulation
FESA finite element stress analysis
FeSV feline sarcoma virus
FET Fisher exact test
forced expiratory time
FEV forced expiratory volume
FEV_1 forced expiratory volume in one second

FEXE formalin, ethanol, xylol, ethanol
FeZ iron zone
FF fat free
fear of failure
fecal frequency
filtration factor
filtration fraction
fine fiber
fine fraction
finger to finger
fixing fluid
flat feet
force fluids
forearm flow
foster father
free fraction
fF ultrafine fiber
ultrafine fraction
ff following
FFA free fatty acid
FFARCS
Fellow of the Faculty of Anaesthetists, Royal College of Surgeons
FFB fast feedback
flexible fiberoptic bronchoscopy
FFBI Foundation for Blood Irradiation
FFC Federal Funding Criteria
Foundation for Cure
free from chlorine
FFD focal film distance
FFDW fat-free dry weight
FFE fecal fat excretion
FFEM freeze fracture electron microscopy
FFF field flow fractionation
FFI free from infection
FFM fat-free mass
FFMTP fatigue fracture of the medial tibial plateau
FFP fresh-frozen plasma
FFPS Fellow of the Faculty of Physicians and Surgeons
FFR Fellow of the Faculty of Radiology
frequency-following response
FFS failure of fixation suppression
fat-free solid
fee for service
FFT fast Fourier transform
flicker fusion test
flicker fusion threshold
FFU focus-forming unit
FFW fat-free weight
FFWC fractional free water clearance
FFWW fat-free wet weight
FG fasciculus gracilis
fast glycolytic
Fast Green
Feeley-Gorman (also F-G)
fibrinogen (also fib)
field gain
French gauge
F-G Feeley-Gorman (also FG)
fg femtogram
FGAM formylglycinamidine ribonucleotide
FGAR formylglycinamide ribonucleotide
FGC fibrinogen gel chromatography
FGD fatal granulomatous disease
FGF father's grandfather
fibroblast growth factor
fresh gas flow
FGG focal global glomerulosclerosis
fowl gamma globulin
FGL fasting gastrin level
FGM father's grandmother
FGN focal glomerulonephritis
FGP Federation of General Practitioners
FGS focal glomerulosclerosis
FGT female genital tract
FGU French gauge, urodynamic
FH familial hypercholesterolemia
family history
fasting hyperbilirubinemia
favorable histology
fetal head
fetal heart
Ficoll-Hypaque
Floating Hospital
follicular hyperplasia
fh let a draught be made (fiat haustus)
FHA filamentous hemagglutinin
filterable hemolytic anemia
fimbrial hemagglutinin
FHC family health center
FHCH fortified hexachlorocyclohexane
FHD family history of diabetes
FHF fulminant hepatic failure
FHH familial hypocalciuric hypercalcemia
family history of hirsutism
FHL flexor hallicus longus
functional hearing loss
FHLDL familial hypercholesterolemia (low density lipoprotein)
FH-M fumarate hydratase, mitochondrial
FHN family history negative
FHP family history positive
Friends of Historical Pharmacy
FHR fetal heart rate
fetal heart rhythm
Foundation for Hand Research
FHRDC family history, research diagnostic criteria
FHR-NST
fetal heart rate nonstress test
FHS fetal heart sound
fetal hydantoin syndrome
FH-S fumarate hydratase, soluble
FHT fetal heart tone
FHTG familial hypertriglyceridemia
FI fasciculus interfascicularis
fever from infection
fixed interval
FIA Freund's incomplete adjuvant
FIAC fluoroiodoarabinosylcytosine
FIAMC International Federation of Catholic Medical Associations
fib fiber
fibrillation
fibrinogen (also FG)
FIBER Fund for Integrative Biomedical Research
FIC Fellow of the Institute of Chemistry
FICD Fellow of the International College of Dentists
$FICO_2$ fraction of inspired carbon dioxide
FICS Fellow of the International College of Surgeons
FID flame ionization detector
free induction decay
fungal immunodiffusion
FIDE Foundation for International Dermatologic Education
FIF forced inspiratory flow
formaldehyde-induced fluorescence
fig figure
FIGLU formiminoglutamic acid

FIGO International Federation of Gynecology and Obstetrics
filt filter
FIMS International Federation of Sports Medicine
FIO_2 forced inspiratory oxygen
FiO_2 fractional inspired oxygen
FIQ full-scale intellegence quotient
FIRO-B Fundamental Interpersonal Relations Orientation Behavior Inventory
fist fistula
FIT fusion inferred threshold
FITC fluorescein isothiocyanate
FJN familial juvenile nephrophthisis
FJROM full joint range of motion
FJS finger joint size
FK functioning kasai
FL factor level
fatty liver
fibers of Luschka
fibroblast-like
filtration leukapheresis
flavomycin
fluorescein
focal length
full liquids
functional length
Fl florentium
fl femtoliter
flexion
fluid
FLA fluorescent-labeled antibody
frontolaeva anterior
fla according to rule (fiat lege artis)
flac flaccid
flav yellow (flavus)
FLC fatty liver cell
fetal liver cell
Friend leukemia cell
FLD fibrotic lung disease
fld See fl (fluid)
fl dr fluid dram
FLEP Family Life Education Program
FLEX Federation Licensing Examination
FLG Finnish Leukemia Group
FLK funny looking kid
FLKS fatty liver and kidney syndrome
flocc flocculation
flor flowers (flores)
fl oz fluid ounce
FLP frontolaeva posterior
FLPR flurbiprofen
FLS Fellow of the Linnean Society
fibrous long-spacing
flow limiting segment
Functional Life Scale
FLSA follicular lymphosarcoma
FLT frontolaeva transversa
FLU fluphenazine
FLUO fluothane
fluor fluorescent
FLV Friend leukemia virus
FM fathom
fetal movement
fibromuscular
filtered mass
flowmeter
fluid movement
foster mother
frequency modulation
functional movement
Fm fermium
fm from (also fr)
make a mixture (fiat mistura)
FMA Forum for Medical Affairs
FMAC fetal movement acceleration test
FMAU 2'-fluoro-5-methyl-1-beta-D-arabinosyl-uracil
FMB full maternal behavior
FMD fibromuscular dysplasia
foot and mouth disease
FMDV foot and mouth disease virus
FME full-mouth extraction
FMEN familial multiple endocrine neoplasia
fMet formylmethionine
FMF familial Mediterranean fever
flow microfluorometry
FMFD1 familial multiple factor deficiency 1
FMG foreign medical graduate
FMH fetomaternal hemorrhage
FML fluorometholone
FMLP N-formyl-methionyl-leucyl-phenylalanine
FMN first malignant neoplasm
flavin mononucleotide
$FMNH_2$ flavin mononucleotide, reduced
fmol femtomole
FMS fat-mobilizing substance
full-mouth series
FMT Foundation for Medical Technology
FN false negative
fastigial nucleus
fibronectin
final nitrogen
finger to nose
FNA fine needle aspiration
FNAB fine needle aspiration biopsy
FNB Food and Nutrition Board
FNF false negative fraction
femoral neck fracture
FNH focal nodular hyperplasia
FNIF Florence Nightingale International Foundation
FNM flunitrazepam (also FNZP)
FNP family nurse practitioner
FNS Frontier Nursing Service
functional neuromuscular stimulation
FNT 2-(2-formylhydrazino)-4-(5-nitro-2-furyl)thiazole
FNZP flunitrazepam (also FNM)
FO fast oxidative
foot orthosis
foramen ovale
forced oscillation
fronto-occipital
FOA Federation of Orthodontic Association
FOB fecal occult blood
feet out of bed
fiberoptic bronchoscope (see also FB)
foot of bed
FOC Frequency of contact scale
fronto-occipital circumference
FOCMA feline oncornavirus cell membrane antigen
FOD free of disease
FOG fast oxidative, glycolytic
fol leaves (folia)
for foreign
fort strong (fortis)
FOS fractional osteoid surface
FOX cefoxitin
fosfomycin
FP false positive
family physician

family planning
family practice
family practitioner
fibrinolytic potential
filling pressure
first pass
flat plate
flavin phosphate
flavoprotein
flexor profundus
fluorescence polarization
forearm pronated
foreperiod
freezing point
full period
See AFP (alpha-fetoprotein)

F/P fluorescein to protein ratio
fp foot pound
let a potion be made (fiat potio)
FPA fibrinopeptide A
Flying Physicians Association
FPB flexor pollicis brevis
FPC familial polyposis coli
fish protein concentrate
Future Physicians Clubs
FPCL fibroblast populated collagen lattice
FPDD familial pure depressive disease
FPF false positive fraction
fibroblast pneumocyte factor
FPG fasting plasma glucose
FPGN focal proliferative glomerulonephritis
FPHA family planning health assistant
FPI femoral pulsatility index
f pil let pills be made (fiant pilulae)
FPL fasting plasma lipid
flexor pollicis longus
FPLA fibrin plate lysis area
FPM filter paper microscopic
fpm feet per minute
FPN ferric chloride, perchloric acid, nitric acid
FPO Federation of Prosthodontic Organizations
FPP free portal pressure
FPPH familial primary pulmonary hypertension
FPR Federal Procurement Regulations
FPS Fellow of the Pharmaceutical Society
footpad swelling
fps feet per second
foot pound second
frames per second
FPU Family Participation Unit
FR Federal Register
fibrinogen related
fixed ratio
flocculation reaction
flow rate
fluid restriction
fluid retention
F&R force and rhythm
Fr francium
French (also F)
fr fried
from (also fm)
FRA fibrinogen-related antigen
fluorescent rabies antibody
FRACON
framycetin, colistin, nystatin
FRACPS
Fellow of the Royal Australian Colleges of Physicians and Surgeons
fract fracture
fract dos
in divided doses (fracta dosi)
frag fragility
FRAI Fellow of the Royal Anthropological Institute
FRAT free radical assay technique
FRBB fracture of both bones
FRBS fast red B salt
FRC Federal Radiation Council
frozen red cell
functional reserve capacity
functional residual capacity
FRCA Fellow of the Royal College of Anesthesiologists
FRCOG Fellow of the Royal College of Obstetricians and Gynecologists
FRCP Fellow of the Royal College of Physicians
FRCPath
Fellow of the Royal College of Pathologists
FRCPC Fellow of the Royal College of Physicians of Canada
FRCPE Fellow of the Royal College of Physicians of Edinburgh
FRCPI Fellow of the Royal College of Physicians of Ireland
FRCS Fellow of the Royal College of Surgeons
FRCSC Fellow of the Royal College of Surgeons of Canada
FRCSE Fellow of the Royal College of Surgeons of Edinburgh
FRCSI Fellow of the Royal College of Surgeons of Ireland
FRCVS Fellow of the Royal College of Veterinary Surgeons
FRD flexion-rotation-drawer
freq frequency (also F)
FRES Fellow of the Royal Entomological Society
FRF fasciculus retroflexus
follicle-releasing factor
FRFPS Fellow of the Royal Faculty of Physicians and Surgeons
FRFPSG
Fellow of the Royal Faculty of Physicians and Surgeons of Glasgow
FRH follicle-releasing hormone
FRIC Fellow of the Royal Institute of Chemistry
FRIPHH
Fellow of the Royal Institute of Public Health and Hygiene
FRJM full-range joint movement
FRMS Fellow of the Royal Microscopical Society
FRN fully resonant nucleus
FRNS frequently relapsing nephrotic syndrome
FROM full range of motion
full range of movement
FROS front routing of signal
FRP functional refractory period
FRPS functional resting position splint
FRS Fellow of the Royal Society
ferredoxin-reducing substance
first rank symptom
Frs furosemide
FRSC Fellow of the Royal Society of Canada
FRSE Fellow of the Royal Society of Edinburgh
FRSPH Fellow of the Royal Society for the Promotion of Health

Fru fructose
FS dihydroxymethylfuralazine
field stimulation
Fight for Sight
fine structure
fire setter
Fleischner Society
forearm suppinated
for skin
Fourier series
frozen section
full and soft
full scale
full strength
FSA fetal sulfoglycoprotein antigen
fsa let it be made skillfully (fiat secundum artem)
FSB Family Service Bureau
fetal scalp blood
FSC free secretory component
FSD focal skin distance
full-scale deflection
FSE filtered smoke exposure
FSEB Federation of Societies for Experimental Biology
FSF fibrin-stabilizing factor
FSG fasting serum glucose
focal sclerosing glomerulonephritis
focal segmental glomerulosclerosis
FSGO floating spherical Gaussian orbitals
FSGS focal segmental glomerulosclerosis
FSH facioscapulohumeral
follicle-stimulating hormone
FSHRF follicle-stimulating hormone-releasing factor
FSI Foam Stability Index
Function Status Index
FSIA foot shock-induced analgesia
FSID Fellow of the Society for Investigative Dermatology
FSIMT Foundation for the Support of International Medical Training
FSIQ Full Scale Intelligence Quotient
FSL fasting serun level
fixed slit light
FSMB Federation of State Medical Boards of the United States
FSP fibrinogen split products
fibrin split products
fine suspended particulate
free secretory piece
FSR Fellow of the Society of Radiographers
film screen radiography
FSS Fear Survey Schedule
French steel sound
front support strap
functional systems scale
FSST Full Scale Score Total
FST foam stability test
FSV feline sarcoma virus
FT family therapy
ferritin
ferromagnetic tamponade
fetal tonsil
fibrous tissue
finger tapping
Fourier transform
full term
nitrofurantoin
FT_3 free triiodothyromine
FT_4 free thyroxine
ft foot
make (fiat) (also f)
FTA fluorescent treponemal antibody
FTA-ABS
fluorescent titer antibody absorption
fluorescent treponemal antibody absorption
FTB fingertip blood
FTC frequency threshold curve
ft c foot-candle
FTE full-time equivalent
ft garg
make a gargle (fiat gargarisma)
FTI free thyroxine index (also FT_4I)
FT_4I free thyroxine index (also FTI)
ft infus
make an infusion (fiat infusum)
FTLB full-term living birth
ft lb foot-pound
ft mas div in pil
make a mass and divide into pills (fiat massa dividenda in pilulae)
ft mist
make a mixture (fiat mistura)
FTNB full-term newborn
FTND full-term normal delivery
FTNS functional transcutaneous nerve stimulation
ft pulv
make a powder (fiat pulvis)
FTR fractional turnover rate
FTS Family Tracking System
serum thymic factor (facteur thymique serique)
FTSG full-thickness skin graft
FTT failure to thrive
fat tolerance test
fraternal twins raised together
FTTPP Federation of Trainers and Training Programs in Psychodrama
ft troch
make lozenges (fiat trochisci)
ft ung
make an ointment (fiat unguentum)
FTX field training exercise
FU fecal urobilinogen
flucloxacillin
follow-up (also F/U)
F/U follow-up (also FU)
5-FU 5-fluorouracil
FUB functional uterine bleeding
FUC fucosidase
Fuc fucose
FUDR fluorodeoxyuridine
FUM 5-fluorouracil, methrotrexate
5-FUMP
5-fluorouridine monophasphate
funct functional
FUO fever of undetermined origin
fever of unknown origin
FUR fluorouracil riboside
furasemide
FV femoral vein
flow volume
fluid volume
formaldehyde vapors
Friend virus
FVC false vocal cord
forced vital capacity
FVD fibrovascular tissue on disk
FVE fibrovascular tissue elsewhere
FVFR filled voiding flow rate
FVL femoral vein ligation

force, velocity, length
FVM familial visceral myopathy
f vs let the patient be bled (fiat venaesectio)
FW Felix-Weil
Folin and Wu
fracturing wall
fw fresh water
FWB full weight bearing
FWHF Federation of World Health Foundations
FWR Felix-Weil reaction
FWW Family Welfare Worker
FX fornix
frozen section
fx fracture
fx-dis fracture-dislocation
FY fiber year
fiscal year
framycetin
FYI for your information
FZ frazolidine
FZS Fellow of the Zoological Society

G

G free energy
gallop
Gasterophilus
Gastrodiscoides
Gemella
Giardia
giga
gingival
Glossina
glucose (also Glc, Glu)
Gnathostoma
gonidial
good
Gordius
grade (also gr)
gravida
gravitational constant
guanine
guanosine
See B (gauss)
G1 gap 1
G_1 period between cell division and DNA replication
G_2 period between DNA replication and onset of mitosis
g gauge
grain (also gr)
gram (also gm)
gravity (also gr)
GA airway conductance
Gamblers Anonymous
gastric analysis
gastric antrum
general anesthesia
gestational age
gingivoaxial
glucuronic acid
Golgi appartus
gramicidin
granuloma annulare
Ga gallium
^{66}Ga radioactive isotope of gallium
^{67}Ga radioactive isotope of gallium
^{72}Ga radioactive isotope of gallium
GABA gamma-aminobutyric acid (also GAMA)
GABA-T gamma-aminobutyric acid transaminase
GABHS group A beta-hemolytic streptococci (also GABS)
GABOB gamma-amino-beta-hydroxybutyric acid
GABS group A beta-hemolytic streptococci (also GABHS)
GAD generalized anxiety disorder
glutamic acid decarboxylase
GAF giant axon formation
GAG gamma-acetylenic gamma-aminobutyric acid
glycosaminoglycan
GAHS galactorrhea-amenorrhea hyperprolactinemia syndrome
GAI guided affective imagery
GAL gallus adenolike
Gal galactose
gal gallon (also C, cong)
GalC galactocerebroside
GalN galactosamine
GalNAc n-acetylgalactosamine
GALT gut-associated lymphoid tissue
GALV gibbon ape leukemia virus
galv galvanic
GAMA gamma-aminobutyric acid (also GABA)
GAMG goat antimouse immunoglobulin G
GAN giant axonal neuropathy
gang ganglion
GAP Glaucoma Alert Program
glucopyranosyl adenine 6'-phosphate
Group for the Advancement of Psychiatry (also GAPsy)
GAPD glyceraldehyde phosphate dehydrogenase
GAPDH glyceraldehyde-3-phosphate dehydrogenase
GAPsy Group for the Advancement of Psychiatry (also GAP)
GAR glycinamide ribonucleotide
goat antirabbit
garg gargle
GARGG goat antirabbit gamma globulin
GAS gastric acid secretion
general adaptation syndrome
generalized arteriosclerosis
Global Assessment Scale
group A Streptococcus
GASA growth-adjusted sonographic age
GASP Global Atomospheric Sampling Program
Group Against Smoking Pollution
GAST gastrocnemius
GAT gas antitoxin
gelatin agglutination test
l-glutamic acid-l-alanine-l-tyrosine
group adjustment therapy
GATLA Argentinean Group for the Treatment of Acute Leukemia
GB gallbladder
glass bead
Guillain-Barre
GBA ganglionic-blocking agent
gingivobuccoaxial
GBD granulomatous bowel disease
GBG glycine-rich beta-glycoprotein
GBH gamma benzene hexachloride
GBI globulin-bound insulin
GBL gamma butyrolactone

GBM glomerular basement membrane
GBPS gallbladder pigment stones
GBq gigabequerel
GBS gallbladder series
gastric bypass surgery
glycine-buffered saline
group B Streptococcus
Guillain-Barre syndrome
GC ganglion cell
gas chromatography
gel chromatography
glucocorticoid
glycocholate
goblet cell
Golgi cell
Golgi complex
gonococcus
good condition
granular cast
granule cell
guanine cytosine
Gc gigacycle
GCA gastric cancerous area
giant cell arteritis
g-cal gram-calorie
GCDC glycochenodeoxycholate
GCDFP gross cystic disease fluid protein
GCFT gonococcal complement-fixation test
GCII glucose-controlled insulin infusion
GCIIS glucose-controlled insulin infusion system
GCMS gas chromatography-mass spectrometry
GCN giant cerebral neuron
GCR glucocorticoid receptor
GCRC General Clinical Research Centers
GCS general clinical service
Generalized Contentment Scale
Glasgow Coma Scale
glucocorticosteroid
GCSA Gross cell surface antigen
GCU gonococcal urethritis
GCV great cardiac vein
GD general duties
Gianotti disease
Gd gadolinium
^{153}Gd radioactive isotope of gadolinium
^{159}Gd radioactive isotope of gadolinium
GDA germine diacetate
GDB Guide Dogs for the Blind
GDFB Guide Dog Foundation for the Blind
GDH glucose dehydrogenase
glutamate dehydrogenase
glycerophosphate dehydrogenase
growth and development hormone
GDID genetically determined immunodeficiency disease
GDM gestational diabetes mellitus
GDP gastroduodenal pylorus
gel diffusion precipitin
guanosine diphosphate
GDU Guide Dog Users
GE gastric emptying
gastroenterology
gastroenterostomy
gastroesophageal
gastrointestinal endoscopy
generalized epilepsy
glandular epithelium
Ge germanium
^{68}Ge radioactive isotope of germanium
^{71}Ge radioactive isotope of germanium
^{77}Ge radioactive isotope of germanium
GEB Guiding Eyes for the Blind
GEC galactose elimination capacity
GEF glossoepiglottic fold
gonadotropin-enhancing factor
gel gelatin
gel quav
any kind of jelly (gelatina quavis)
GEMS Good Emergency Mother Substitute
gen general
genus
GEP gastro-entero-pancreatic
GEPG gastroesophageal pressure gradient
GER gastroesophageal reflux
granular endoplasmic reticulum
Ger geriatrics
GERD gastroesophageal reflux disease
GET gastric emptying time
graded exercise test
GeV giga electron volt
GF gastric fistula
germ free
glomerular filtrate
grandfather
griseofulvin
growth factor
growth failure
growth fraction
gf gram force
GFA global force applicator
GFAP glial fibrillary acidic protein
GFD gluten-free diet
GFP glomerular filtered phosphate
GFR glomerular filtration rate
GG gamma globulin
genioglossus
guar gum
GGA general gonadotropic activity
GGE generalized glandular enlargement
gradient gel electrophoresis
GGFC gamma globulin-free calf serum
GGG gamboge (gummi guttae gambiae)
GGM glucose-galactose malabsorption
GGS glands, goiter, or stiffness
GGT galactosylhydroxylysyl glucosyltransferase
gamma glutamyl transferase
GGTP gamma glutamyl transpeptidase
GH galactosylhydroxylysine
geniohyoid
glucoheptonate (also GHA)
growth hormone
GHA glucoheptonate (also GH)
GHAA Group Health Association of America
GHAQ general high altitude questionnaire
GHB gamma hydroxybutyric acid
GHD growth hormone deficiency
GHK Goldman-Hodgkin-Katz
GHQ General Health Questionnaire
GHRF growth hormone-releasing factor
GHRH growth hormone-releasing hormone
GHRIH somatostatin (growth hormone release-inhibiting hormone)
GHz gigahertz
GI gastrointestinal
Gingival Index
globin insulin
glomerular index
glucose intolerance
granuloma inguinal
growth inhibiting
GIA gastrointestinal anastomosis
GIC gastric interdigestive contraction

GICA gastrointestinal cancer
gastrointestinal cancer antigen

GIFT granulocyte immunofluorescence test

GIG Gluten Intolerance Group

GIH gastrointestinal hemorrhage

GIK glucose-insulin-potassium

GILCU gradual increase in length and complexity of utterance

GIM gonadotropin-inhibitory material

GIMS Graduates of Italian Medical Schools

GIP gastric inhibitory peptide
gastric inhibitory polypeptide
giant cell interstitial pneumonia
glucose-dependent insulin-releasing peptide

GIR global improvement rating

GIRF Gastro-Intestinal Research Foundation

GIRSO International Group for Scientific Research in Stomatology and Odontology

GIS gas in stomach
gastrointestinal symptom
gastrointestinal system
Gender Identity Service

GIT gastrointestinal tract
glutathione insulin transhydrogenase

GITS gastrointestinal therapeutic system

GITSG Gastrointestinal Tumor Study Group

GITT gastrointestinal transit time
glucose-insulin tolerance test

GIX See DFDT

GJ gap junction
gastrojejunostomy

GK galactokinase
glycerol kinase

GKA guinea pig keratocyte

GKN glucose-potassium-sodium

GL glomerular layer
granular layer (also GRL)
greatest length

Gl glucinium

gl gland

GLA D-glucaric acid
gingivolinguoaxial

GLAT glutamic acid, lysine, alanine, tyrosine

glau glaucoma

GLC gas-liquid chromatography

Glc glucose (also G, Glu)

GlcA gluconic acid

GLC/MS
gas-liquid chromatography/mass spectrometry

GlcN glucosamine

GlcNAc
N-acetylglucosamine (also NAG)

GlcUA glucuronic acid

GLD globoid leukodystrophy

GLDH glutamate dehydrogenase

GLH germinal layer hemorrhage

GLI glucagon-like immunoreactivity

GLM general linear model

Gln glutamine (also Glx)

GLO glyoxalase

glob globulin

GLS guinea pig lung strip

GLTT glucose-lactate tolerance test

Glu glucose (also G, Glc)
glutamic acid (also Glx)

GLV Gross leukemia virus

Glx glutamic acid (also Glu)
glutamine (also Gln)

Gly glycine

GM gastric mucosa
general medical
gentamicin
geometric mean
grand mal
grandmother
granulocyte-macrophage

Gm gamma

gm gram (also g)

GMA glyceryl methacrylate
glycol methacrylate
gross motor activity

GMB gastric mucosal barrier

GMBF gastric mucosal blood flow

GMC General Medical Council

GM-CFU
granulocyte-macrophage colony-forming unit

GM-CSF
granulocyte-macrophage colony-stimulating factor

GMCU gracillis myocutaneous unit

GME graduate medical education

GMENAC
Graduate Medical Education National Advisory Committee

GMEPP giant miniature end-plate potential

GMH germinal matrix hemorrhage

GMK green monkey kidney

GML gut mucosal lymphocyte

GMO general medical officer

GMP guanosine monophosphate

GMR gallops, murmurs, or rubs

GMS Gomori's methenamine silver

GM&S general medicine and surgery

GMT geometric mean titer

GMW gram molecular weight

GN gaze nystagmus
glomerulonephritis
glucagon
gram negative

GNB gram-negative bacillus

GNBM gram-negative bacillus meningitis

GNC General Nursing Council
glandular neck cell

GNCA gastric noncancerous area

GNID gram-negative intracellular diplococcus

GnRF gonadotropin-releasing factor (also GRF)

GnRH gonadotropin-releasing hormone (also GRH)

GO glucose oxidase

Go Golgi

GOD generation of diversity
glucose oxidase

GOE gas, oxygen, and ether

GOG Gynecologic Oncology Group

GON gonococcal ophthalmia neonatorum

GOR gastroesophageal reflux
general operating room

GOT glutamic oxaloacetic transaminase
goals of treatment

GOT-M glutamic oxaloacetic transaminase, mitochondrial

GOT-S glutamic oxaloacetic transaminase, soluble

GP gastroplasty
general paralysis
general paresis
general practice
general practitioner
general proprioception

general purpose
geometric progression
globus pallidus
glucose production
glutathione peroxidase (also GPx)
glycoprotein
gram positive
guinea pig
gutta-percha

G3P glyceraldehyde 3-phosphate
G6P glucose 6-phosphate
gp group
GPA glutaraldehyde, picric acid, acetic acid
grade point average
GPAIS guinea pig anti-insulin serum
GPB glossopharyngeal breathing
GPC gel permeation chromatography
giant papillary conjunctivitis
glycerol-3-phosphorylcholine
granular progenitor cell
GPD glucose phosphate dehydrogenase
glycerophosphate dehydrogenase
guinea pig dander
G6PD glucose-6-phosphate dehydrogenase
GPDH glycerol phosphate dehydrogenase
GPE glycerol-3-phosphoryethanolamine
guinea pig embryo
GPF glomerular plasma flow
GPHN giant pigmented hairy nevus
GPHV guinea pig herpes virus
GPI general paralysis of the insane
general paresis of the insane
gingival periodontal index
glucose phosphate isomerase
guinea pig ileum
GPIPID
guinea pig intraperitoneal infectious dose
GPK guinea pig kidney
GPKA guinea pig kidney absoprtion
GPLV guinea pig leukemia virus
GPM general preventive medicine
GPR good partial response
GPS Goodpasture's syndrome
guinea pig serum
guinea pig spleen
GPT glutamic pyruvic transaminase
GpTh group therapy (also GT)
GPTSM guinea pig tracheal smooth muscle
GPUT galactose phosphate uridyl transferase
GPx glutathione peroxidase (also GP)
GR gastric resection
generalized rash
glucose response
glutathione reductase
good recovery
granulocyte
gr gamma roentgen
grade (also G)
grain (also g)
gravid
gravity (also g)
gross
GRA gonadotropin-releasing agent
grad by degrees (gradatim)
gradient
gradually
GRAE generally recognized as effective
GRAS generally recognized as safe
GRD Gender Role Definition
GRE Graduate Record Examination
GRF gonadotropin-releasing factor (also GnRF)
growth hormone releasing factor
GRG Gastroenterology Research Group
GRH gonadotropin-releasing hormone (also GnRH)
growth hormone-releasing hormone
GRID gay-related immunodeficiency
GRIF growth hormone release-inhibiting factor
GRL granular layer (also GL)
Grn glycerone
GRP gastrin-releasing peptide
GS Gardner syndrome
general surgery
Gerontological Society
Gilbert's syndrome
glomerulosclerosis
glucagon secretion
glutamine synthetase
graft survival
group specific
G/S glucose and saline
GSA general somatic afferent
Genetics Society of America
GSB graduated spinal block
G-SC guanosine-coupled spleen cell
GSD glycogen storage disease
GSE general somatic efferent
gluten-sensitive enteropathy
GSH reduced glutathione
GSHP reduced glutathione peroxidase
GSK glycogen synthetase kinase
GSoA Gerontological Society of America
GSP glycogen synthetase phosphatase
glycosylated serum protein
GSR galvanic skin response
GSS glutamate-gamma-semialdehyde synthetase
GSSG oxidized glutathione
GSSI Global Sexual Satisfaction Index
GST aurothiomalate (gold sodium thiomalate) (also GTM)
gold salt therapy
graphic stress thermography
GSW gunshot wound
GT gait training
galactosyl transferase
Gamow-Teller
gastrostomy
gingiva treatment
glucagon test
glucose tolerance
glucose transport
glucuronyl transferase
group therapy (also GpTh)
gt drop (gutta)
GTF glucose tolerance factor
GTG gold thioglucose
GTH gonadotropic hormone
GTM aurothiomalate (gold sodium thiomalate) (also GST)
GTN gestational trophoblastic neoplasm
GTO Golgi tendon organ
GTP guanosine triphosphate
GTR galvanic tetanus ratio
generalized time reflex
GTS glucose transport system
GTT glucose tolerance test
gtt drops (guttae)
GU gastric ulcer
genitourinary
glucose uptake

gonococcal urethritis
Gua guanine
GUK guanylate kinase
Guo guanosine
GUS genitourinary system
guttat
drop by drop (guttatum)
GV gastric volume
gentian violet
granulosis virus
griseoviridin
GVA general visceral afferent
GVB gelatin-veronal buffer
GVBE gelatin-veronal buffer, ethylene diaminetetraacetate
GVE general visceral efferent
GvH graft versus host
GvHR graft versus host reaction
GVL graft versus leukemia
GW Gray-Wheelwright
group work
GWG generalized Wegener's granulomatosis
GX glycinexylidide
GXT graded exercise testing
Gy gray
Gyn gynecology
GYS guaranteed yield strength
GZTS Guilford-Zimmerman Temperament Survey

H

H Haemaphysalis
Haemophilus (or Hemophilus)
Hancock
Hauch
height (also ht)
henry
heparin
hetacillin
Heterophyes
high
Hippelates
Histoplasma
Holzknecht
horizontal
hormone
hot
Hounsfield
human
hydrogen
Hymenolepis
hyperopia
hyperplasia
hypodermic (also Hypo)
oersted
^{1}H protium (also H1, H^{1})
^{2}H deuterium (also H2, H^{2})
^{3}H tritium (also H3, H^{3})
H^{+} hydrogen ion
(H^{+}) hydrogen ion concentration
h at bedtime (hora decubitus) (also hd, hor decub)
draft (haustas)
hour (also hr)
human response
hundred
Planck's constant
HA halothane anesthesia
headache
Healthy America
hearing aid
height age
hemadsorbent
hemagglutination
hemagglutinin
hemolytic anemia
hepatic adenoma
hepatic artery
hepatitis A
herpangina
high anxiety
hippuric acid
histamine
histidine ammonialyase
Horton's arteritis
hospital acquired
hospital admission
household activity
hyaluronic acid
hydroxyanisole
hydroxyapatite
hyperalimentation
hyperopia, absolute
H/A head to abdomen ratio
HA1 hemeabsorption virus, type 1
HA2 hemeabsorption virus, type 2
Ha hahnium
HAA hepatitis-associated antigen
hospital activity analysis
HABA hydroxybenzeneazobenzoic acid
HABF hepatic artery blood flow
HACS hyperactive child syndrome
HAD hemadsorption
hexamethylmelamine, doxorubicin (Adriamycin), cisplatin (DDP)
HAd hospital administration
HADH hydroxyacyl dehydrogenase
HAE health appraised examination
hearing aid evaluation
hereditary angioedema
HAF hepatic arterial flow
HaF Hageman factor (also HF)
HAFP human alpha-fetoprotein
HAHTG horse antihuman thymus globulin
HAI hemagglutination inhibition (also HI)
HAL haloperidol
Hal halogen
halothane
HALO hemorrhage, abruption, labor, placental previa with mild bleeding
HALT Heroin Antagonist and Learning Therapy
HAM helical axis of motion
human albumin microsphere
human alveolar macrophage
HAMM human albumin minimicrosphere
HANA hemagglutinin neuraminidase (also HN)
HANE hereditary angioneurotic edema
HANES Health and Nutrition Examination Survey
HAOX L-alpha-hydroxyacid oxidase
HAP held after positioning
heredopathia atactia polyneuritiformis
high amplitude peristalsis
histamine acid phosphate
HAPE high altitude pulmonary edema
4HAQO 4-hydroxyaminoquinoline 1-oxide
HAR high altitude retinopathy
HARH high altitude retinal hemorrhage
HARS Hamilton Anxiety Rating Scale
HAS highest asymptomatic

hyperalimentation solution
HASCHD
hypertensive arteriosclerotic heart disease
HAT head, arms, trunk
hospital arrival time
hypoxanthine, aminopterin, thymidine
HATG See HAHTG
HAU hemagglutination unit
haust a drink (haustus)
HAV hepatitis A virus
HB heart block
held backward
hemolysis blocking
hepatitis B
His bundle
housebound
hyoid body
Hb hemoglobin (also Hg, Hgb)
HbA hemoglobin A
HBABA 2-(4-hydroxybenzene)azobenzoic acid
HBAg hepatitis B antigen
Hb AS heterozygosity for hemoglobins A and S
HB_c hepatitis B core
HbC hemoglobin C
HB_cAb hepatitis B core antibody
HB_cAg hepatitis B core antigen
HbCO carboxyhemoglobin
HBD hydroxybutric dehydrogenase
HBDH See HBD
HBDT human basophil degranulation test
HBE His bundle electrogram
HBE_1 His bundle electrogram, distal
HBE_2 His bundle electrogram, proximal
HB_eAg hepatitis B "e" antigen
HBF hand blood flow
hepatic blood flow
hypothalamic blood flow
HbF fetal hemoglobin
HBGM home blood glucose monitoring
HBI high serum-bound iron
Hospital Bureau, Inc.
HBIG hepatitis B immune globulin
HBM hypertonic buffered medium
HBO hyperbaric oxygen
HbO_2 oxyhemoglobin
HBOT hyperbaric oxygen treatment
HBP high blood pressure
HBRI Hospital Bureau Research Institute
HB_s hepatitis B surface
HbS sickle cell hemoglobin
HB_sA hepatitis B surface associated
HB_sAg hepatitis B surface antigen
HBSC hemopoietic blood stem cell
HbSC sickle cell hemoglobin C
HBSS Hanks' balanced salt solution
HbSS homozygosity for hemoglobin S
HBSSG Hanks' balanced salt solution plus glucose
HBV hepatitis B virus (or virions)
HBW high birth weight
H/BW heart to body weight ratio
HC hair cell
head circumference
head compression
heart cycle
heat conservation
heavy chain
heparin cofactor
hepatocellular cancer
histamine challenge
Histamine Club
histochemistry
home care
hospital corps
hospitalized controls
house call
Huntington's chorea
hyaline cast
hydrocortisone
hyoid cornu
hypertrophic cardiomyopathy (also HCM)
HCA homocysteic acid
HCB hexachlorobenzene
HCC hepatocellular carcinoma
25-HCC
25-hydroxycholecalciferol
HCD health care delivery
heavy chain disease
high caloric density
homologous canine distemper
HCDD hexachlorodibenzo-p-dioxin
HCF high carbohydrate, high fiber
HCFA Health Care Financing Administration
HCFSH human chorionic follicle-stimulating hormone
hCG human chorionic gonadotropin
HCH hexachlorocyclohexane
Hch hemochromatosis
HCL hairy cell leukemia
HCM hypertrophic cardiomyopathy (also HC)
HCMV human cyclomegalovirus
HCP hereditary coproporphyria
hexachlorophene
HCQ hydroxychloroquine
HCR human controlled repressor
hysterical conversion reaction
HCS Histochemical Society
human chorionic somatomammotropin
HCT Health Check Test
homocytotrophic
human calcitonin
human chorionic thyrotropin
hydrochlorothiazide (also HCTZ)
Hct hematocrit
HCTD hepatic computed tomography density
high cholesterol and tocopherol deficient
HCTS high cholesterol and tocopherol supplemented
HCTZ hydrochlorothiazide (also HCT)
HCU homocystinuria
HCVD hypertensive cardiovascular disease
HCVR hypercapnic ventilatory response
Hcy hemocyanin
HD Hanganutziu-Deicher
Hansen's disease
hearing distance
heart disease
helium dilution
hemidiaphragm
hemodialysis
hemolytic disease
2,5-hexanedione
high density
high dosage
hip disarticulation
histidine decarboxylase (also HDC)
Hodgkin's disease
house dust
Huntington's disease
hydatid disease
HD_{50} 50 percent hemolyzing dose of complement

Hd response to parts of the human figure
hd at bedtime (hora decubitus) (also h, hor decub)
head
HDC heptadecylcatechol
histidine decarboxylase (also HD)
human diploid cell
hypodermoclysis
HDCS human diploid cell system
HDCV human diploid cell vaccine
HDD half-dose depth
HDF high dry field
HDFL human development and family life
HDFP Hypertension Detection and Follow-up Program
HDG high-dose group
HDH heart disease history
HDHQ Hostility and Direction of Hostility Questionnnaire
HDI hexamethylene diisocyanate
HDL high-density lipoprotein
HDLC high-density lipoprotein cholesterol
HDLW distance at which a watch is heard by the left ear
HDM hexadimethrine
HDMP high-dose methylprednisolone
HDMTX high-dose methotrexate
HDMTX-CF
high-dose methotrexate-citrovorum factor
HDN hemolytic disease of the newborn
HDP high density polyethylene
HDRF Heart Disease Research Foundation
HDRS Hamilton Depression Rating Scale
HDRV human diploid rabies vaccine
HDRW distance at which a watch is heard by the right ear
HDS health delivery system
herniated disk syndrome
HDU hemodialysis unit
HDZ hydralazine
HE hard exudate
hepatic encephalopathy
human enteric
hypoxemic episode
H&E hematoxylin and eosin
hemorrhage and exudate
heredity and environment
He helium
^{4}He radioactive isotope of helium
HEA hexone extracted acetone
2-hydroxyethyl acrylate
HEART Health Evaluation and Risk Tabulation
HEAT human erythrocyte agglutination test
hebdom
a week (hebdomada)
HEC hamster embryo cell
hydroxyergocalciferol
HED Haut-Einheits-Dosis
HeD helper determinant
HEDP 1-hydroxyethylidene diphosphonate
HEENT head, eyes, ears, nose, throat
HEI homogeneous enzyme immunoassay
HEIR high energy ionizing radiation
HEK human embryonic kidney
HEL human embryonic lung
human erythroleukemia line
HELF human embryonic lung fibroblast
HELP Hawaii Early Learning Profile
Herpetics Engaged in Living Productively
HELT Hypertension Education Level Test
Hem hematology
HEMA Health Education Media Association
hydroxyethylmethacrylate
HEMPAS
hereditary erythroblastic multinuclearity associated with positive acidified serum
HEOD dieldrin (hexachloro-octahydro-dimethanonaphth-oxirene
HEP hemolysis end point
hepatic
hepatoerythropoietic porphyria
high egg passage
high energy phosphate
HEPA high-efficiency particulate air
HEPES N-2-hydroxyethyl-piperazine-N'-2-ethanesulfonic acid
herb recent
of fresh herbs (herbarium recentium)
HES hemotoxylin-eosin stain
hydroxyeicosatetraenoic acid
hydroxyethyl starch
hypereosinophilic syndrome
HeSCA Health Sciences Communications Association
HETE 12-hydroxyeicosatetraenoic acid
HETP hexethyltetraphosphate
HEW see DHEW
Hex A hexosaminidase A
Hex B hexosaminidase B
HF Hageman factor (also HaF)
haplotype frequency
hard feces
hard filled
hay fever
head forward
heart failure
helper factor
hemofiltration
hemorrhagic factor
hemorrhagic fever
hepatocyte function
high fat
high flow
high frequency
human fibroblast
Hf hafnium
^{175}Hf radioactive isotope of hafnium
^{181}Hf radioactive isotope of hafnium
hf half
HFB heptafluorobutyryl
HFBA heptafluorobutyric acid
heptafluorobutyric anhydride
HFC hard-filled capsule
histamine-forming capacity
HFCS high-fructose corn syrup
HFCWC high-frequency chest wall compression
HFD high-fiber diet
Human Figure Drawing
HFDA Hospital Food Directors Association
HFDK human fetal diploid kidney
HFDL human fetal diploid lung
HFEC human foreskin epithelial cell
HFI hereditary fructose intolerance
human fibroblast interferon
HFJV high-frequency jet ventilation
HFM hemifacial microsomia
HFO hard food orientation
high-frequency oscillation
HFOV high-frequency oscillatory ventilation
HFPPV high-frequency positive pressure ventilation

HFR high-frequency recombination
HFRS hemorrhagic fever with renal syndrome
HFS hemifacial spasm
hFSH human follicle-stimulating hormone
HFST hearing-for-speech test
HFUPR hourly fetal urine production rate
HFV high-frequency ventilation
HG heptadecapeptide gastrin
herpes gestationes
high glucose
hypoglycemia
Hg hemoglobin (also Hb, Hgb)
mercury (hydrargyrum)
^{197}Hg radioactive isotope of mercury
^{203}Hg radioactive isotope of mercury
hg hectogram
Hgb hemoglobin (also Hb, Hg)
HGF Human Growth Foundation
hyperglycemic-glycogenolytic factor
Hg-F fetal hemoglobin
HGG human gamma globulin
HGH high growth hormone
hGH human growth hormone
HGM hog gastric mucin
human glucose monitoring
HGO hepatic glucose output
HGP hepatic glucose production
HGPRT hypoxanthine guanine phosphoribosyl-transferase
HH halothane hepatitis
hard of hearing
hiatus hernia
hydroxyhexamide
hyporeninemic hypoaldosteronism
H&H hematocrit and hemoglobin
HHA hereditary hemolytic anemia
home health agency
home health aide
HHAA hypothalamo-hypophyseal-adrenal axis
HHb reduced hemoglobin
HHC home health care
HHD hypertensive heart disease
HHE health hazard evaluation
hemiplegia, hemiconvulsions, epilepsy
HHHO hypotonia, hypomentia, hypogonadism, obesity
HHL hippuryl-L-histidyl-L-leucine
H+Hm hyperopia plus astigmatism
HHNKS hyperglycemic hyperosmolar nonketotic syndrome
HHPC hyperoxic-hypercapnic
HHS Hearing Handicap Scale
See DHHS
HHSSA Home Health Services and Staffing Association
HHT heptadecatrienoic acid (12L-hydroxyl-5, 8,10-hepadecatrienoic)
hereditary hemolytic telangiectasia
heterotopic heart transplantation
HHTA hypothalamo-hypophyseal thyroidal axis
HI hearing impaired
heart infusion
heat inactivated
heat input
hemagglutination inhibition (also HAI)
high impulsiveness
hormone insensitive
hospital induced
humoral immunity
hyperglycemic index
HIA hemagglutination-inhibition antibody
HIAA Health Insurance Association of America
5-HIAA
5-hydroxyindoleacetic acid
HIB Haemophilus influenzae, type B
H-ICDA
International Classification of Disease Adopted Code for Hospitals
HIDA dimethyl iminodiacetic acid
Health Industry Distributers Association
HIE hyperimmunoglobulin E
HIEFSS
Hospital, Institution and Educational Food Service Society
HIF higher intellectual function
Historical Information Form
HIg human immunoglobulin
HIHA high impulsiveness, high anxiety
HILA high impulsiveness, low anxiety
HIM hemopoietic inductive microenvironment
HIMA Health Industry Manufacturers Association
HIMP high-dose intravenous methylprednisolone
HIOMT hydroxyindole-O-methyltransferase
HIP Health Insurance Plan of Greater New York
HIR high irradiance response
HIS Health Interview Survey
hospital information systems
hyperimmunized suppressed
His histidine
HISG human immune serum globulin
HISSG Hospital Information Systems Sharing Group
HIT hemagglutination inhibition test
histamine inhalation test
Holtzman Inkblot Technique
hypertrophic infiltrative tendinitis
HITES hydrocortisone, insulin, transferrin, estradiol, selenium
HJB Howell-Jolly bodies
HJR hepatojugular reflux
HK hand to knee
heat killed
heel to knee
hexokinase
human kidney
HKI Helen Keller International
HL hairline
half-life
hearing level
hearing loss
hemolysis
histocompatibility locus
human leukocyte
human lymphocyte
hyperlipidemia
latent hyperopia
H&L heart and lungs
hl hectoliter
HLA histocompatibility locus antigen
homologous leukocyte antibody
human leukocyte antigen
human lymphocyte antigen
HLA-A human leukocyte antigen A
HLA-B human leukocyte antigen B
HLA-D human leukocyte antigen D
HLA-L human leukocyte antigen L
HLC Health Locus of Control
heat loss center
HLD hepatolenticular degeneration
HLE human leukocyte elastase

HLF Holistic Life Foundation
human lung fluid
HLFCB horizontal laminar flow clean benches
HLH human luteinizing hormone
hypoplastic left heart
HLK heart, liver, kidney
HLI hemolysis inhibition
human leukocyte interferon
human lymphocyte interferon
HLN hilar lymph node
HLP hyperlipoproteinemia
HLR heart-lung resuscitation
HLV herpeslike virus
HM hand motion
hand movement
harmonic mean
health maintenance
heart murmur
hepatic metabolism
hexamethylmelamine (also HMM)
human milk
hydatidiform mole
hypoxic-metabolic
manifest hyperopia
hm hectometer
HMA 4-hydroxy-3-methoxy mandelic acid
HMB hydroxymethylbilane
HMBA hexamethylenebisacetamide
HMC hand mirror cell
health maintenance cooperative
3-HMC 3-hydroxymethyl-beta-carboline
HMD dihydroxybenzyl-alpha-hydrazinopropionic acid monohydrate
hyaline membrane disease
HMDS hexamethyldisilazane
HME Health Media Education
heat and moisture exchanger
HMF hydroxymethylfurfural
HMG high mobility group
human menopausal gonadotropin
hydroxymethylglutarate
HMGCoA
hydroxymethylglutaryl coenzyme A
HMGCoAR
hydroxymethylglutaryl coenzyme A reductase
HMK high molecular weight kininogen
HML human milk lysozyme
HMM heavy meromyosin
hexamethylmelamine (also HM)
HMO Health Maintenance Organization
HMP hexose monophosphate
hot moist pack
human menopausal
hydromotive pressure
HMPA hexamethylphosphoramide (also HMPT)
HMPG hydroxymethoxyphenylglycol
HMPS hexose monophosphate shunt
HMPT hexamethylphosphoric triamide (also HMPA)
HMR histiocytic medullary reticulosis
HMRA Hadassah Medical Relief Association
HMS hexose monophosphate shunt
high methacholine sensitivity
hypermobility score
hypermobility syndrome
hypothetical mean strain
HMSAS hypertrophic muscular subaortic stenosis
HMSN hereditary motor and sensory neuropathy
HMSS Hospital Management Systems Society
HMT hexamethylenetetramine
hydromethyltrioxsalen
See Hct
HMW high molecular weight
HMWK high molecular weight kininogen
HN head and neck
head nurse
hemagglutinin neuraminidase (also HANA)
hereditary nephritis
hilar node
HN_2 nitrogen mustard (also MBA)
hn tonight (hac nocte)
HNC hyperosmolar nonketotic coma
hyperoxic normocapnic
HNKDS hyperosmolar nonketotic diabetic state
HNMT histamine-N-methyltransferase
HNP herniated nucleus pulposus
hnRNA heterogeneous nuclear ribonucleic acid
HNS head and neck surgery
HNSHA hereditary nonspherocytic hemolytic anemia
HNTD highest nontoxic dose
HNV has not voided
HO hand orthosis
heterotopic ossification
high oxygen
house officer
hyperbaric oxygen
H/O history of
Ho holmium
^{166}Ho radioactive isotope of holmium
Ho null hypothesis
HOA hip osteoarthritis
hypertrophic osteoarthritis
HOAM Home Observation Assessment Method
HOB head of bed
HOC hydroxycorticoid
HOCM hypertrophic obstructive cardiomyopathy
hoc vesp
this evening (hoc vespere)
HOD hereditary opalescent dentin
Hoffer-Osmond Diagnostic
HOF hepatic outflow
HOG See HGO
See PCP (phencyclidine)
HOI hospital onset of infection
hypoiodous acid
HOME Home Observation for Measurement of the Environment
Home Oriented Maternity Experience
HOMO highest occupied molecular orbital
HON delta-hydroxy-gamma-oxo-L-norvaline
HOOD hereditary osteo-onychodysplasia
HOP high oxygen pressure
hydroxydaunorubicin, vincristine (Oncovin), prednisone
HOPE Healthcare Options Plan Entitlement
health-oriented physician education
HOPP hepatic occluded portal pressure
hor decub
at bedtime (hora decubitus) (also h, hd)
hor interm
at intermediate hours (horis intermediis)
hor som
at bedtime (hora somni) (also hs)
hor un spatio
at the end of an hour (horae unius spatio)
hosp hospital
HOST hypo-osmotic shock treatment
HOT human old tuberculin

HP Harding Passey
hard palate
hastening phenomenon
health professional
heater probe
high potency
high power
high pressure
high protein
horsepower (also hp)
hot pack
hot pad
house physician
human pituitary
hybridoma product
hydrophobic protein
hydrostatic pressure
hydroxyproline
hyperphoria
hypersensitivity pneumonitis
hypoparathyroid
H&P history and physical (see also HPE)
Hp haptoglobin
hp horsepower (also HP)
HPA Hereford Parental Attitude Survey
2-hydroxypropyl acrylate
hypothalmic-pituitary-adrenal axis
hypothalmic-pituitary-adrenocortical axis
15-HPAA
15-hydroperoxy-arachidonic acid
HPBL human peripheral blood leukocyte
HPC 3-hydroxy-2-phenykcinchoninic acid
HPD hematoporphyrin derivative
HPE hepatic portoenterostomy
high permeability edema
history and physical examination (see also H&P)
hydrostatic pulmonary edema
HPETE hydroperoxyeicosatetraenoic acid
HPF heparin-precipitable fraction
high-pass filter
high-power field
HPFH hereditary persistence of fetal hemoglobin
HPFSH human pituitary follicle-stimulating hormone
HPG human pituitary gonadotropin
hypothalamic-pituitary-gonodal
HPH halothane-percent-hour
HPI hepatic perfusion index
history of present illness
HPL human placental lactogen
HPLC high performance liquid chromatography
high pressure liquid chromatography
HPLE hereditary polymorphic light eruption
HPMA 2-hydroxypropyl methyl acrylate
HPMC human peripheral mononuclear cell
HPMIS Hospital Pharmacy Management Information System
HPN home parenteral nutrition
hypertension
hpn our own purgative draft (haustus purgans noster)
HPO high pressure oxygen
hypertrophic pulmonary osteoarthropathy
HPP human pancreatic polypeptide
hydroxypyrazolo-pyrimidine
HPPH hydroxyphenyl-5-phenylhydantoin
hPRL human prolactin
HPRP human platelet-rich plasma
HPRT hot plate reaction time
hypoxanthine phosphoribosyltransferase
HPS Health Physics Society
high protein supplement
His-Purkinje system
human platelet suspension
hypertrophic pyloric stenosis
HPT hyperparathyroidism
hypothalmic-pituitary-thyroid
HPV Hemophilus pertussis vaccine
human papilloma virus
hypoxic pulmonary vasoconstriction
HPVD hypertensive pulmonary vascular disease
HPX hypophysectomized
HPZ high-pressure zone
HQ hydroquinone
HR heart rate
Hemophilia Research
hospital record
hospital report
hypoxic responder
hr hour (also h)
HRA Health Resources Administration
high right atrium
histamine-releasing activity
HRAE high right atrium electrogram
HRB Halstead-Reitan Battery
histamine release from basophils
HRBC horse red blood cell
HRC help-rejecting complainer
HRE high-resolution electrocardiography
HREC hepatic reticuloendothelial cell
HREH high-renin essential hypertension
HRG Health Research Group
HRIG human rabies immune globulin
HRL head rotated left
hRNA heterogeneous ribonucleic acid
HRP high-risk pregnancy
horseradish peroxidase
horseradish peroxide
HRPO See HPR (horseradish peroxidase)
HRR head rotated right
heart rate range
HRS Hamilton Rating Scale
hepatorenal syndrome
Hunza Research Society
HRT half relaxation time
hormone replacement therapy
HRVL human reovirus-like
HS half-strength
hand surgery
Harvey Society
head sling
healthy subject
heart sounds
heat stable
heavy smoker
heme synthetase
heparin sulfate
hereditary spherocytosis
herpes simplex
hidradenitis suppurativa
homologous serum
Hopelessness Scale
horse serum
hospital stay
hours of sleep
house surgeon
human serum
Hurler's syndrome
hypersensitivity
hypertonic saline
H/S helper/suppressor

Hs hypochondriasis
hs at bedtime (hora somni) (also hor som)
HSA health service area
Health Services Administration
health systems agency
human serum albumin
HSAEP Hypertension Screening, Awareness, and Education Program
HSAG HEPES-saline-albumin-gelatin
HSAP heat-stable alkaline phosphotase
HSC health sciences center
health screening center
hemopoietic stem cell
horizontal semicircular canal
HSCD Hand-Schuller-Christian disease
HSCL Hopkins Symptom Check List
HSD Honest Significance Difference
See HDRS
HSDA high single dose alternate day
HSE herpes simplex encephalitis (see also HSVE)
human serum esterase
HSF heated soybean flower
histamine-induced suppressor factor
HSFR Health Services Funding Regulations
HSG hysterosalpingography
hSGF human skeletal growth factor
HSI heat stress index
HSL herpes simplex labialis
HSMHA Health Services and Mental Health Administration
HSP Henoch-Schoenlein purpura
HSPM hippocampal synaptic plasma membrane
HSPQ High School Personality Questionnaire
HSR homogeneously staining region
HSRS Health-Sickness Rating Scale
HSS Hallevorden-Spatz syndrome
hepatic stimulator substance
HSV herpes simplex virus
highly selective vagotomy
hyperviscosity syndrome
HSV-1 herpes simplex virus type 1
HSV-2 herpes simplex virus type 2
HSVE herpes simplex virus encephalitis (see also HSE)
HT Hand Test
Hashimoto's thyroiditis
hearing threshold
hemagglutination titer
high tension
home treatment
hospital treatment
Hubbard tank
Huhner test
hydrotherapy
hyperopia, total
hypertension (see also HTN)
hyperthyroidism
hypodermic tablet
H.T. Histotechnologist
5-HT serotonin (5-hydroxytryptamine)
ht heart
heat
height (also H)
HTA human thymocyte antigen
3-hydroxytryptamine
HTAR hepatic testosterone 5-alpha-A-ring reductase
HTB hot tub bath
HTC hepatoma tissue culture
homozygous typing cell
HTCVD hypertensive cardiovascular disease
HTh hypothalamus
HTHD hypertensive heart disease
HTI hemisphere thrombotic infarction
human tetanus immunoglobulin
HTIG homologous tetanus immune globulin
HTL hearing threshold level
histotechnologist
human T cell leukemia
human T cell lymphoma
HTLA human T lymphocyte antigen
HTLV human T leukemia virus
human T lymphoma virus
HTN hypertensive (see also HT)
HTO tritiated water
5-HTO 5-hydroxytryptamine
5-HTOL 5-hydroxytryptophol
HTP House, Tree, Person
5-HTP 5-hydroxytryptophan
HTPN home total parenteral nutrition
HTS human thyroid stimulator
hTSAb human thyroid stimulating antibody
HTSCA human tumor stem cell assay
HTSH human thyroid-stimulating hormone
HTT hand thrust test
HTV herpes-type virus
HU hemagglutinin unit
Hounsfield unit
hydroxyurea
hyperemia unit
HUI headache unit index
HURT hospital utilization review team
HUS hemolytic uremic syndrome
HUV human umbilical vein
HV hepatic vein
Herpesvirus
high volume
hospital visit
hyperventilation
H&V hemigastrectomy and vagotomy
HVA Herpesvirus ateles
homovanillic acid
HVD hypertensive vascular disease
hypoxic ventilatory drive
HVE hepatic venous effluence
high-voltage electrophoresis
HVF hepatocycle volume fraction
HVFP hepatic vein free pressure
HVG hematoxylin and van Gieson
HVH Herpesvirus hominis
HVID horizontal visible iris diameter
HVL half-value layer
HVLP high volume, low pressure
HVM high-velocity missile
hypothalamic ventromedial nucleus
HVPG hepatic venous pressure gradient
HVR hypoxic ventilatory response
HVS Herpesvirus saimiri
herpes virus sensitivity
HVSD hydrogen-detected ventricular septal defect
HVT herpes virus of turkeys
HVWP Hospitalized Veterans Writing Project
HW heart weight
hemisphere width
hw housewife
HWE hot water extract
HWRS Habits of Work and Recreation Survey
HWS hot water soluble
HX histocytosis X
Hx history
HXIS hard x-ray imaging spectrometer

HXM hexamethylmelamine

Hy hyperopia

HYD hydralazine

Hyd hydrocortisone
hydrostatics

Hyg hygiene

Hyp hydroxyproline
hypnosis
hypoxanthine

Hypo hypodermic (also H)

Hys hysteria

HZ herpes zoster

Hz Hertz

HZV herpes zoster virus

I

I implantation
incisor, permanent
independent
induction
inosine (also INO)
inspired gas
insulin
intake
intensity of magnetism
Iodamoeba
iodine
Isopora
Ixodes
luminous intensity
sulfafurazole

^{123}I radioactive isotope of iodine

^{124}I radioactive isotope of iodine

^{125}I radioactive isotope of iodine

^{126}I radioactive isotope of iodine

^{129}I radioactive isotope of iodine

^{130}I radioactive isotope of iodine

^{131}I radioactive isotope of iodine

^{132}I radioactive isotope of iodine

^{133}I radioactive isotope of iodine

i incisor, deciduous
optically inactive

IA immune adherence
impedance angle
inactive alcoholic
inhibitory antigen
intra-alveolar
intra-arterial
isonicotonic acid

Ia immune associated

IAA indoleacetic acid
iodoacetic acid

IAAAM International Association for Aquatic Animal Medicine

IAASG International Aplastic Anemia Study Group

IAASM International Academy of Aviation and Space Medicine

IAB Interspecialty Advisory Board

IABC intraaortic balloon counterpulsation (also IABP)

IABP intraaortic balloon counterpulsation (also IABC)
intraaortic balloon pump

IAC internal auditory canal
International Academy of Cytology

IACAPAP
International Association for Child and Adolescent Psychiatry and Allied Professions

IACD intraatrial conduction defect

IACME International Association of Coroners and Medical Examiners

IACP intraaortic counterpulsation

IACR Inter-American College of Radiology
International Association of Cancer Registries

IACRLRD
International Association for Comparative Research on Leukemia and Related Diseases

IACS International Academy of Cosmetic Surgery

IACVF International Association of Cancer Victims and Friends

IADFA International Association of Dento-Facial Abnormalities

IADH inappropriate antidiuretic hormone

IADHS inappropriate antidiuretic hormone syndrome

IADR International Association for Dental Research

IADS International Association of Dental Students

IAEA International Atomic Energy Agency

IAET International Association for Enterostomal Therapy

IAFI infantile amaurotic familial idiocy

IAG International Association of Gerontology

IAGP International Association of Geographic Pathology

IAGUS International Association of Genito-Urinary Surgeons

IAH idiopathic adrenal hyperplasia

IAHA idiopathic autoimmune hemolytic anemia
immune adherence hemagglutination

IAHCSM
International Association of Hospital Central Service Management

IAHD idiopathic acquired hemolytic disease

IAHS International Association for Hospital Security

IALP International Association of Logopedics and Phoniatrics

IAM internal auditory meatus
International Academy of Metabology
International Academy of Myodontics

IAMAT International Association for Medical Assistance to Travelers

IAMFES
International Association of Milk, Food and Environmental Sanitarians

IAMLT International Association of Medical Laboratory Technologists

IAMM International Association of Medical Museums

IAMS International Association of Microbiological Societies

IAN idiopathic aseptic necrosis

IANC International Anatomical Nomenclature Committee

IANS Institute of Applied Natural Science

IAO intermittent aortic occlusion
International Association of Orthodontics

IAOE International Association of Optometric Executives

IAP immunosuppresive acidic protein
innervated antral pouch
inosinic acid pyrophosphorylase
intermittent acute porphyria
International Academy of Pathology (also IAPath)
International Academy of Proctology
islet-activating protein

IAPath
International Academy of Pathology (also IAP)

IAPB International Association for Prevention of Blindness

IAPD International Association of Parents of the Deaf

IAPM International Academy of Preventive Medicine

IAPP International Association of Pacemaker Patients
International Association for Preventive Pediatrics

IAR immediate asthmatic reaction
inhibitory anal reflex
iodine-azide reaction

IARASM
Institute for Advanced Research in Asian Science and Medicine

IARC International Agency for Research on Cancer

IARS International Anesthesia Research Society

IAS interatrial septum
internal anal sphincter
intra-amniotic saline

IASD interatrial septal defect

IASP International Association of Social Psychiatry
International Association for the Study of Pain

IASSMD
International Association for the Scientific Study of Mental Deficiency

IAT immunoaugmentative therapy
International Association of Trichologists
iodine-azide test

IAVM intramedullary arteriovenous malformation

IB immune balance
immune body
immunobeads
inclusion body
index of body build

IBA isobutyric acid

IBB intestinal brush border

IBBBA International Bundle Branch Block Association

IBC iron-binding capacity

IBD inflammatory bowel disease

IBI intermittent bladder irrigation
ischemic brain infarction

ibid in the same place (ibidem)

IBL immunoblastic lymphadenopathy

IBM inclusion body myositis

IBMX isobutyl methylxanthine

Ibo ibotenic acid

IBP iron-binding protein

IBQ Illness Behavior Questionnaire

IBR infectious bovine rhinotracheitis

IBRO International Brain Research Organization

IBS inside bathing solution
International Bronchoesophagological Society
Interpersonal Behavior Survey
irritable bowel syndrome

IBSA iodinated bovine serum albumin

iBSA immunoreactive bovine serum albumin

IBU ibuprofen
international benzoate unit

IBV infectious bronchitis virus

IBW ideal body weight

IC immune complex
immune cytotoxicity
impedence cardiogram
incomplete diagnosis
indirect calorimetry
individual counseling
inferior colliculus
inhibiting concentration
inspiratory capacity
intensive care
intercostal
intermediate care
intermittent claudication
internal capsule
internal carotid
internal cholecystectomy
interstitial cell
intracamerally
intracavitary
intracellular
intracellular concentration
intracerebral
intracisternal
intracranial
intracutaneous
irritable colon
isovolumetric colon
isovolumetric contraction

ICA internal carotid artery
International Chiropractors Association
International College of Anesthetics
intracranial aneurysm
islet cell antibody (also ICAb)

ICAA International Council on Alcoholism and Addiction

ICAAC Interscience Conference on Antimicrobial Agents and Chemotherapy

ICAb islet cell antibody (also ICA)

ICAF internal carotid artery flow

ICAMI International Committee Against Mental Illness

ICAN International College of Applied Nutrition

ICAng International College of Angiology

ICBP intracellular binding protein

ICC immunocompetent cell
Indian childhood cirrhosis
intensive coronary care
interchromosomal crossing-over
intermediate cell column
Interstate Commerce Commission

ICCE intracapsular cataract extraction

ICCU intensive coronary care unit
intermediate coronary care unit

ICD Institute for Crippled and Disabled
intercanthal distance
International Classification of Diseases
International College of Dentists
intrauterine contraceptive device (also IUCD)
ischemic coronary disease

isocitric dehydrogenase (also ICDH)
ICDA International Classification of Diseases, Adapted
ICDCD International Classification of Diseases and Causes of Death
ICDH isocitric dehydrogenase (also ICD)
ICD-O International Classification of Diseases for Oncology
ICDRG International Contact Dermatitis Research Group
ICDS Integrated Child Development Scheme
ICE ice, compression, elevation
Institute of Cancer Epidemiology
ICEA International Childbirth Education Association
ICF intensive care facility
intercellular fluorescence
interciliary fluid
intermediate care facility
International Cardiology Foundation
intracellular fluid (also IF)
intravascular coagulation fibrinolysis
ICG indocyanine green
ICGN immune complex mediated glomerulonephritis
ICH infectious canine hepatitis
intracerebral hemorrhage
intracerebral hypertension
intracranial hemorrhage
intracranial hypertension
ICHD Intersociety Commission for Heart Disease
ICI intracardiac injection
ICIDH International Classification of Impairments, Disabilities and Handicaps
ICIS International Council for Infant Survival
ICLM International Christian Leprosy Mission
ICM inner cell mass
intercostal margin
intracytoplasmic membrane
ipsilateral competing message
ICMMP International Committee of Military Medicine and Pharmacy
ICMPH International Center of Medicine and Psychological Hypnosis
ICN intensive care nursery
International Council of Nurses
ICNC intracerebellar nuclear cell
ICNND Interdepartmental Committee on Nutrition for National Defense
ICNV International Committee on Nomenclature of Viruses
ICOI International Congress of Oral Implantologists
ICP inductively coupled plasma
infectious cell protein
intracranial pressure
ICPDS International Cancer Patient Data Exchange System
ICPEMC
International Commission for Protection Against Environmental Mutagens and Carcinogens
ICPI Intersociety Committee on Pathology Information
ICPM International College of Psychosomatic Medicine
ICPMM incisor, canine, premolar, molar
ICPS Interpersonal Cognitive Problem-Solving
ICR Immunodeficiency Cancer Registry
Institute for Cancer Research
international calibrated ratio
ion cyclotron resonance
ICRC International Committee of the Red Cross
ICRDB International Cancer Research Data Bank
ICRFSDD
Independent Citizens Research Foundation for the Study of Degenerative Diseases
ICRO International Cell Research Organization
ICRP International Commission on Radiological Protection
ICRTT International Cancer Research Technology Transfer
ICRU International Commission on Radiological Units and Measurement
ICS ileo-cecal sphincter
immotile alia syndrome
impulse conducting system
intercostal space
International Cardiovascular Society
International College of Surgeons
International Congress of Surgeons
intracranial self-stimulation (also ICSS)
ICSA International Correspondence Society of Allergists
islet cell surface antibody
ICSC idiopathic central serous chorioretinopathy
ICSH International Committee for Standardization in Hematology
interstitial cell-stimulating hormone
ICSOG International Correspondence Society of Obstetricians and Gynecologists
ICSS intracranial self-stimulation (also ICS)
ICSU International Council of Scientific Unions
ICT icteric
immunoglobulin consumption test
indirect Coombs' test
indirect Coombs' titer
inflammation of connective tissue
insulin coma therapy
intensive conventional therapy
interstitial cell tumor
intraoral cariogenicity test
isovolumic contraction time
iCT immunoreactive calcitonin
ICTA International Commission on Technical Aids, Housing and Transportation
ICTH International Committee on Thrombosis and Haemostasis
ICTS idiopathic carpal tunnel syndrome
ICTV International Committee on the Taxonomy of Viruses
ICU infant care unit
intensive care unit
intermediate care unit
ICV intracellular volume
icv intracerebroventricular
ICVS International Cardiovascular Society
ICW intact canal wall
intensive care ward
intercellular water
intracellular water
ICX immune complex
ID identification
immunodiffusion
inappropriate disability

induction delivery
infant death
infectious disease
infective dose
inhomogeneous deposition
initial dose
inner (or inside) diameter
insufficient data
internal diameter
interstitial disease
intradermal
intraduodenal
isosorbide dinitrate
I&D incision and drainage
ID_{50} median infective dose
Id idiotypic
id the same (idem)
IDA image display and analysis
iminodiacetic acid
insulin degrading activity
iron dificiency anemia
id ac the same as (idem ac)
IDAMIS
Integrated Drug Abuse Management System
IDB Investigational Drug Branch
IDC idiopathic dilated cardiomyopathy
interdigitilating cell
IDD insulin-dependent diabetes
IDDF investigational drug data form
IDDM insulin-dependent diabetes mellitus
IDDS investigational drug data sheet
IDDT immuno-double diffusion test
IDE Investigational Device Exemption
IDEALS
Institute for the Development of Emotional and Life Skills
IDES isodesmosine
IDG intermediate-dose group
IDH-M isocitrate dehydrogenase, mitochondrial
IDH-S isocitrate dehydrogenase, soluble
IDI induction delivery interval
IDK internal derangement of knee
IDL difference limen for intensity
intermediate density lipoprotein
IDM idiopathic disease of the myocardium
immune defense mechanism
infant of diabetic mother
intermediate-dose methotrexate
IDMC interdigestive motility complex
interdigestive motor complex
IDMEC interdigestive myoelectric complex
IDP initial dose period
inosine diphosphate
IDPase
inosine diphosphatase
IDPN beta-iminodipropionitrile
IDR intradermal reaction
IDS immune deficiency state
intraduodenal stimulation
investigational drug service
Investigative Dermatological Society
IDSA Infectious Disease Society of America
IDU idoxuridine (also IDUR, IUDR)
iododeoxyuridine
Ivy dog unit
IDUR idoxuridine (also IDU, IUDR)
IDV intermittent demand ventilation
IDVC indwelling venous catheter
IdX cross-reactive idiotype
IE immunizing unit (immunitats Einheit)
infective endocarditis
intraepithelial
isoeugenol
I/E inspiratory/expiratory
i.e. that is (id est)
IEA International Epidemiological Association
intravascular erythrocyte aggregation
IEC International Electrotechnical Commission
intraepithelial carcinoma
IEEE Institute of Electrical and Electronics Engineers
IEF International Eye Foundation
isoelectric focusing
IEI isoelectric interval
IEL internal elastic lamina
intimal elastic lamina
intraepithelial lymphocyte
IEM immunoelectron microscopy
IEMG integrated electromyogram
IEP immunoelectrophoresis
individual education plan
Individualized Educational Program
IES ingressive-egressive sequence
IESS-I
Intergroup Ewing's Sarcoma Study I
IF idiopathic fibroplasia
immersion foot
immunofluorescence (also IFL)
inferior facet
interferon (also IFN)
Interferon Foundation
intermediate filament
intermediate frequency
internal fixation
internal friction
interstitial fluid
intracellular fluid (also ICF)
intrinsic factor
involved field
IFA immunofluorescent antibody
immunofluorescent assay
indirect fluorescent antibody
International Filariasis Association
IFAT indirect fluorescent antibody test
IFC Infant Formula Council
inspiratory flow cartridge
IFCC International Federation of Clinical Chemistry
IFCL intermittent flow centrifugation leukapheresis
IFCR International Foundation for Cancer Research
IFE interfollicular epidermis
IFGO International Federation of Gynecology and Obstetrics
IFGS interstitial fluids and ground substance
IFHPMSM
International Federation for Hygiene, Preventive Medicine, and Social Medicine
IFL immunofluorescence (also IF)
IFL-rA
recombinant leukocyte A interferon
IFM Institute of Forensic Medicine
IFMSA International Federation of Medical Students Associations
IFN immunoreactive fibronectin
interferon (also IF)
IFN-a human leukocyte interferon
IFN-C partially pure human leukocyte interferon

IFOS International Federation of Ophthalmological Societies
IFP intrapatellar fat pad
IFPRA International Family Planning Research Association
IFR inspiratory flow rate
IFRA indirect fluorescent rabies antibody
IFRP International Fertility Research Program
IFS interstitial fluid space
IFSC International Federation of Surgical Colleges
IFSECN International Federation of Societies for Electroencephalography and Clinical Neurophysiology
IFSM International Federation of Sports Medicine
IFSSH International Federation of Societies for Surgery of the Hand
IFT immunofluorescence technique
immunofluorescent test
international frequency tables
IFV interstitial fluid volume
intracellular fluid volume
IG immature granule
intragastric
I-G insulin-glucagon
Ig immunoglobulin
IgA immunoglobulin A
IGD interglobal distance
IgD immunoglobluin D
IGDM infant of gestational diabetic mother
IGE International Guiding Eyes
IgE immunoglobulin E
IGF insulin-like growth factor
IgG immunoglobulin G
IGIV intravenous immunoglobulin
IgM immunoglobulin M
IGR immediate generalized reaction
integrated gastrin response
IgSC immunoglobulin secreting cell
IGSP Institute for Gravitational Strain Pathology
IGT impaired glucose tolerance
interpersonal group therapy
intragastric titration
IGTT intravenous glucose tolerance test
IGV intrathoracic gas volume
IH incomplete healing
infectious hepatitis
in hospital
inner half
intermittent heperization
IHA idiopathic hyperaldosteronism
indirect hemagglutination
IHBP iodohydroxybenzylpendolol
IHBTD incompatible hemolytic blood transfusion disease
IHC idiopathic hemochromatosis
idiopathic hypercalciuria
inner hair cell
intrahepatic cholestosis
IHCA isocapneic hyperventilation with cold air
IHCP Institute on Hospital and Community Psychiatry
IHD in-center hemodialysis
ischemic heart disease
IHDA incertohypothalamic dopamine
IHEA International Health Evaluation Association
IHF Industrial Health Foundation
International Hospital Federation
IHG ichthyosis hystrix gravior
IHH idiopathic hypogonadotropic hypogonadism
IHHS idiopathic hyperkinetic heart syndrome
IHO idiopathic hypertrophic osteoarthropathy
IHP idiopathic hypoparathyroidism
idiopathic hypopituitarism
inositol hexaphosphate
IHPA intrahepatic portal hypertension
IHPC intrahepatic cholestasis
IHR intrahepatic resistance
intrinsic heart rate
IHRA isocapneic hyperventilation with room air
IHS infrahyoid strap (also IS)
Institute of Hypertension Studies
International Health Society
IHSA iodinated human serum albumin
IHSS idiopathic hypertrophic subaortic stenosis
IHT ipsilateral head turning
IIBA International Institute for Bioenergetic Analysis
IIC integrated ion current
IID insulin-independent diabetes
IIDM insulin-independent diabetes mellitus
IIE idiopathic ineffective erythropoiesis
IIF indirect immunofluorescent
IIIVC infrahepatic interruption of inferior vena cava
IIP idiopathic interstitial pneumonia
idiopathic intestinal pseudoobstruction
indirect immunoperoxidase
IIS intensive immunosuppression
International Institute of Stress
IIT ineffective iron turnover
IJ intrajejunal
IJD inflammatory joint disease
IJP internal jugular pressure
IJV internal jugular vein
IK immobilized knee
immune bodies (immune Koerper)
immunoconglutinin
infusoria killing
IL independent laboratory
insensible loss
inspiratory loading
intensity level
intestinal lymphocyte
intralipid
I-L intensity-latency
IL-2 interleukin-2
Il illinium
ILA insulin-like activity
International Leprosy Association
ILAE International League Against Epilepsy
ILAR Institute of Laboratory Animal Resources
International League Against Rheumatism
ILBBB incomplete left bundle branch block
ILBW infant, low birth weight
ILD interstitial lung disease
ischemic leg disease
ischemic limb disease
isolated lactase deficiency
Ile isoleucine
ILGF insulin-like growth factor
illic lag
stopper the bottle (illico lagena)

illic lag obturat
stopper the bottle immediately (illico lagena obturatur)
ILM internal limiting membrane
ILS increase in life-span
intralobular sequestration
ILSS intraluminal somatostatin
IM indomethacin
infectious mononucleosis
inner membrane
innocent murmur
inspiratory muscle
intermediate megaloblast
internal mammary
internal medicine
intestinal mesenchyme
intramedullary
intramuscular
IMA Industrial Medical Association
inferior mesenteric artery
internal mammary artery
IMAA iodinated macroaggregated albumin
IMAI internal mammary artery implant
IMB intermenstrual bleeding
IMBC indirect maximum breathing capacity
IMC interdigestive migrating complex
interdigestive migrating contraction
interdigestive myoelectric complex
intestinal mucosal mast cell
IMCU intermediate care unit
ImD_{50} immunizing dose to protect 50 percent
IMDC intramedullary metatarsal decompression
IME independent medical examiner
IMET isometric endurance time
IMF idiopathic myelofibrosis
intermaxillary fixation
intermediate filament
IMG internal medicine group
IMH idiopathic myocardial hypertrophy
IMHT indirect microhemagglutination test
IMI imipramine
immunologically measurable insulin
impending myocardial infarction
indirect membrane immunofluorescence
inferior myocardial infarction
intermeal interval
intramuscular injection
IMIBG iodinated metaiodobenzylguanidine
IML internal mammary lymphoscintigraphy
IMLA intramural left anterior descending (also IMLAD)
IMLAD intramural left anterior descending (also IMLA)
ImmU immunizing unit
IMP idiopathic myeloid proliferation
inosine monophosphate
intramembrane particle
imp important
impression
improved
IMPA incisal mandibular plane angle
IMPEX immediate postexercise
IMPS Inpatient Multidimensional Psychiatric Scale
IMR infant mortality rate
infectious mononucleus receptor
IMRC Instructional Materials Reference Center
IMRD introduction, methods, results, discussion
IMRF International Medical and Research Foundation
IMS incurred in military service
IMSS inflight medical support system
IMT indomethacin
IMU international milliunit
IMV inferior mesenteric vein
intermittent mandatory ventilation
IMViC indol, methyl red, Voges-Proskauer, citrate
IMX isobutyl methyl xanthine
IN impetigo neonatorum
incidence
incompatibility number
indacrinone
intermediate nucleus
interstitial nephritis
intranasal
In indium
^{111}In radioactive isotope of indium
^{114}In radioactive isotope of indium
^{116}In radioactive isotope of indium
in inch
INA inferior nasal artery
International Naturopathic Association
International Neurological Association
INAD infantile neuroaxonal dystrophy
INAH isonicotinic acid hydrazide
INB ischemic necrosis of bone
INC interstitial nucleus of Cajal
inc incisional
incomplete
inconclusive
increase
incurred
INCAP Institute of Nutrition of Central America and Panama
IncB inclusion body
incid cut (incide)
IND indapamide
indomethacin
Investigational New Drug
in d daily (in dies)
INDM infant of nondiabetic mother
Ind-Med
industrial medicine
Ind-Surg
industrial surgery
INE infantile necrotizing encephalomyelopathy
Inf infant
infected
inferior
infusion
inf pour in (infunde)
INFORM
International Reference Organization in Forensic Medicine and Sciences
ing inguinal
INH isoniazid (isonicotinic acid hydrazide)
INI intranuclear inclusion
Inj inject
inj enem
let an enema be injected (injiciatur enema)
INMT indolamine N-methyltransferase
INN international nonproprietary name
INO inosine (also I)
internuclear ophthalmoplegia
INOC inoculate
INPC isopropyl-N-phenyl carbamate (also IPC, IPPC)
INPH iproniazide phosphate
INPV intermittent negative pressure-assisted ventilation

INQ inferior nasal quadrant
INR international normalized ratio
INS idiopathic nephrotic syndrome
INSERM
Institut de la Sante et de la Recherche Medicale
insol insoluble
inspir
inspiration
int intermediate
intermittent
intern
internal
int cib
between meals (inter cibos)
IntlMA
International Medical Association
IntlSN
International Society of Nephrology
int noct
during the night (inter noctem)
INV inferior nasal vein
inv inversion
involv
coat (involve)
involvement
IO inferior olive
internal os
intestinal obstruction
intraocular
I&O intake and output
Io ionium
IOA inner optic anlage
International Office for Audiophonology
International Osteopathic Association
International Ostomy Association
IOAT International Organization Against Trachoma
IOC in our culture
intern on call
IOD interorbital distance
IOFB intraocular foreign body
IOH idiopathic orthostatic hypotension
IOL intraocular lens
IOM Institute of Medicine
IOMP International Organization for Medical Physics
IOP intraocular pressure
IOR information outflow rate
IOT intraocular tension
IOU intensive therapy observation unit
IP immunoblastic plasma
immunoperoxidase
implantation test
inactivated pepsin
incisoproximal
incontinentia pigmenti
incubation period
induction period
industrial population
infusion pump
in-patient
instantaneous pressure
International Pharmacopoeia
interpeduncular nucleus
interpharyngeal
interpositus nucleus
intestinal pseudoobstruction
intracellular proteolysis
intraperitoneal
isoelectric point
isoproterenol
IPA incontinentia pigmenti achromians
Independent (or Individual) Practice Association
indole, pyruvic acid
International Phonetic Alphabet
International Psychoanalytic Association
intrapulmonary artery
IPAA International Psycho-Analytical Association
IPAT Institute for Personality and Aptitude Testing
Iowa Pressure Articulation Test
IPC isopropyl chlorophenyl
isopropyl-N-phenyl carbamate (also INPC, IPCC)
IPD immediate pigment darkening
incurable problem drinker
inflammatory pelvic disease
intermittent peritoneal dialysis
interpupillary distance
IPE injury pulmonary edema
interstitial pulmonary emphysema
IPF idiopathic pulmonary fibrosis
infection-potentiating factor
interstitial pulmonary fibrosis
IPG impedence plethysmography
inspiratory phase gas
IPH idiopathic pulmonary hemosiderosis
inflammatory papillary hyperplasia
intraparenchymal hemorrhage
IPI Imagined Process Inventory
interphonemic interval
IPL inner plexiform layer
intrapleural
IPM infant passive mitt
IPMANA
Interstate Postgraduate Medical Association of North America
IPN interpeduncular nucleus
interpenetrating polymer network
IPn interstitial pneumonitis
IPNA N-isopropylnoradrenaline
IPO improved pregnancy outcome
International Parents' Organization
IPOF immediate postoperative fitting
IPOP immediate postoperative prosthesis
IPP independent practice plan
inorganic pyrophosphate
inosine, pyruvate, inorganic phosphate
inositol pentaphosphate
intermittent positive pressure
intrahepatic portal pressure
intrapleural pressure
IPPB intermittent positive-pressure breathing
IPPC isopropyl-N-phenyl carbamate (also INPC, IPC)
IPPD isopropyl paraphenylenediamine
IPPF International Planned Parenthood Federation
IPPI interruption of pregnancy for psychiatric indications
IPPO intermittent positive-pressure inflation with oxygen
IPPR integrated pancreatic polypeptide response
intermittent positive-pressure respiration
IPPUAD
immediate postprandial upper abdominal distress

IPPV intermittent positive-pressure ventilation

IPR insulin production rate
interval patency rate
intraparenchymal resistance
iproniazid

IPRL isolated, perfused rabbit lung

IPRT interpersonal reaction test

IPS infundibular pulmonary stenosis
initial prognostic score
intermittent photic stimulation
Interpersonal Perception Scale
para-iodophenylsulfonyl

ips inches per second

IPSB intrapartum stillbirth

IPSC-E Inventory of Psychic and Somatic Complaints in the Elderly

IPSID immunoproliferative small intestinal disease

IPSP inhibitory postsynaptic potential

IPSS International Pilot Study of Schizophrenia

IPT immunoprecipitation
interpersonal psychotherapy
ipratropium

IPTG isopropyl thiogalactoside

IPTH immunoreactive parathyroid hormone

IPTP Impaired Physician Treatment Program

IPU in-patient unit

IPV inactivated poliovirus
inactivated poliovirus vaccine
incompetent perforator vein
infectious pustular vaginitis
intrapulmonary vein

IPVD index of pulmonary vascular disease

IPW interphalangeal width

IQ intelligence quotient

IR ileal resection
immune response
immunoreactive
index of response
infrared
inside radius
inspiratory resistance
insulin receptor
insulin requirement
insulin response
integer ratio
internal resistance
inversion recovery
irritant reaction
isovolumetric relaxation

Ir iridium

^{192}Ir radioactive isotope of iridium

^{194}Ir radioactive isotope of iridium

IRA immunoradioassay

IRB institutional review board

IRBBB incomplete right bundle branch block

IRBC infected red blood cell

iRBC immature red blood cell

IRC inspiratory reserve capacity
instantaneous resonance curve

IRCA intravascular red cell aggregation

IRCU intensive respiratory care unit

IRD isorhythmic dissociation

IRDS idiopathic respiratory distress syndrome
infant respiratory distress syndrome

IRECA International Rescue and Emergency Care Association

IRET Institute for Rational-Emotive Therapy

IRF idiopathic retroperitoneal fibrosis

IRG immunoreactive gastrin
immunoreactive glucagon

IRGH immunoreactive growth hormone

IRH Institute for Research in Hypnosis
intraretinal hemorrhage

IRhCG immunoreactive human chorionic gonadotropin

IRhCS immunoreactive human chorionic somatomammotropin

IRhPL immunoreactive human placental lactogen

IRI immunoreactive insulin
insulin radioimmunoassay

IRI/G immunoreactive insulin to glucose ratio

IRIS International Research Information Service

IRL Institute for Rational Living

IRM innate (or inherited) release mechanism

IRMA immunoradiometric assay
intraretinal microvascular abnormality

IROS ipsilateral routing of signal

IRP immunoreactive plasma
incus replacement prosthesis
inhibitor of radical processes
insulin-releasing polypeptide
International Reference Preparation

IRPH immunoreactive prolyl hydroxylase

IRR infrared refractometry
intrarenal reflux

Irr irradiation
irritant

IRRD Institute for Research of Rheumatic Diseases

IRS immunoreactive secretin
infrared spectrophotometry
insulin receptor species
Intergroup Rhabdomyosarcoma Study
International Rhinologic Society

IRSA idiopathic refractory sideroblastic anemia
iodinated rat serum albumin

IRSD idiopathic respiratory distress syndrome

IRT immunoreactive trypsin
Institute for Reality Therapy
interresponse time

IRTO immunoreactive trypsin output

IRV inferior radicular vein
inspiratory reserve volume

IS ilial segment
immediate sensitivity
immune serum
incentive spirometer
index of sexuality
infrahyoid strap (also IHS)
initial segment
insertion sequence
in situ
insulin secretion
intercellular space
intercostal space
interictal spike
internal standard
interstitial space
intraspinal
Ionescu-Shiley
Irvine syndrome
ischemic score
isoproterenol
Israels syndrome

is interspace

ISA Instrument Society of America

International Society of Audiology
intrinsic sympathomimetric activity
iodinated serum albumin
irregular spiking activity

ISAC International Society for Autistic Children
ISADH inappropriate secretion of antidiuretic hormone
ISAP International Society of Art and Psychopathology
ISBI International Society for Burn Injuries
ISBT International Society of Blood Transfusion
ISC immunoglobulin-secreting cell
intensive supportive care
International Society of Cardiology
International Statistical Classification
intersystem crossing
irreversibly sickled cell
ISCCO intersternocostoclavicular ossification
ISCF interstitial cell fluid
ISCLP International Society of Clinical Laboratory Pathologists
ISCLT International Society for Clinical Laboratory Technology
ISCM International Society of Cybernetic Medicine
ISCN International System for Human Cytogenetic Nomenclature
ISCP infection surveillance and control program
International Society of Comparative Pathology
ISD immunosuppresive drug
interventricular septal defect
isosorbide dinitrate (also ISDN)
ISDB indirect self destructive behavior
ISDN isosorbide dinitrate (also ISD)
ISE integrated square error
International Society for Electrostimulation
International Society of Endocrinology
ISED Interview Schedule for Events and Difficulties
ISEK International Society of Electrophysiological Kinesiology
ISF interstitial fluid
ISFC International Society and Federation of Cardiology
ISFET ion specific field effect transducer
ISG immune serum globulin
ISGE International Society of Gastro-Enterology
ISH icteric serum hepatitis
International Society of Hematology
International Society of Hypertension
ISHAM International Society for Human and Animal Mycology
ISHM International Society of the History of Medicine
ISHR International Society for Heart Research
ISHSS International Standard for Human Syphilitic Serum
ISI initial slope index
international sensitivity index
ISIH interspike interval histogram
ISIM International Society of Internal Medicine
ISKDC International Study of Kidney Disease in Children
ISM International Society of Microbiologists
intersegmental muscle
ISMED International Society on Metabolic Eye Disease
ISMHC International Society of Medical Hydrology and Climatology
ISMR Independent Snowmobile Medical Research
ISO International Standards Organization
isoproterenol
ISOS International Southern Ocean Studies
ISOST International Society of Orthopaedic Surgery and Traumatology
ISOX isoxsuprine
ISP immunoreactive substance P
Independent Study Program
ISPI Iowa Structured Psychiatric Interview
ISPN International Society for Pediatric Neurosurgery
ISPO International Society of Prosthetics and Orthotics
ISPOUSC
International Society for Prosthetics and Orthotics--U.S. Committee
ISPX Ionescu-Shiley pericardial xenograft
ISR insulin secretion rate
International Society of Radiology
ISRM International Society of Reproductive Medicine
ISRRT International Society of Radiographers and Radiological Technicians
ISRT International Spinal Research Trust
ISS Injury Severity Scale
International Society of Surgery
IST insulin sensitivity test
insulin shock therapy
International Society on Toxicology
interstitiospinal tract
ISTC International Stress and Tension Control Association
ISTD insulin standard
International Society of Tropical Dermatology
ISTH International Society on Thrombosis and Hemostasis
ISTS International Society for Twin Studies
ISU International Society of Urologists
ISW interstitial water
ISWI incisional surgical wound infection
IT immunotherapy
implantation test
information technology
inhalation test
inhalation therapy
insulin treatment
intensive therapy
internal thoracic
interstitial tissue
intolerance and toxicity
intracellular tachyzoite
intradermal test
intrathecal
intrathoracic
intratracheal
intratracheal tube
intratumor
isomeric transition
I.T. Inhalation Therapist
ITA inferior temporal artery
International Transpersonal Association
International Tuberculosis Association
itaconic acid

ITAA International Transactional Analysis Association
ITC imidazolyl thioguanine chemotherapy
ITD insulin-treated diabetic
ITE intrapulmonary interstitial emphysema
ITET isotonic endurance test
ITH intrathecal
ITHI International Travelers Health Institute
ITIR International Tumor Immunochemotherapy Registry
ITLC instant thin layer chromatography
ITLC-SG instant thin layer chromatography-silica gel
ITM intrathecal methotrexate
ITP idiopathic thrombocytopenic purpura
immune thrombocytopenic purpura
inosine triphosphate
ITPA Illinois Test of Psycholinguistic Ability
ITPase inosine triphosphatase
ITQ inferior temporal quadrant
ITSHD isolated thyroid stimulating hormone deficiency
ITT identical twins raised together
inhalation therapy technician
insulin tolerance test
ITU intensive therapy unit
International Telecommunications Union
ITV inferior temporal vein
ITX intertriginous xanthoma
ITyr monoiodotyrosine
IU immunizing unit
international unit
intrauterine
IUAC International Union Against Cancer (also UICC)
IUB International Union of Biochemistry
IUCD intrauterine contraceptive device (also ICD)
IUD intrauterine death
intrauterine device
IUDR idoxuridine (also IDU, IDUR)
IUFB intrauterine foreign body
IUFD intrauterine fetal demise
IUFGR intrauterine fetal growth retardation
IUG intrauterine growth
IUGR intrauterine growth retardation
IUHPS International Union of the History and Philosophy of Science
IUIS International Union of Immunological Societies
IUM internal urethral meatus
intrauterine malnourishment
intrauterine membrane
IUNS International Union of Nutritional Sciences
IUP International Union of Phlebology
intrauterine pregnancy
intrauterine pressure
IUPAC International Union of Pure and Applied Chemistry
IUSSP International Union for Scientific Study of Population
IUT intrauterine transfusion
IUVDT International Union Against Venereal Diseases and Treponematoses
IV ichthyosis vulgaris
interventricular
intervetebral
intravascular
intravenous
intraventricular
invasive
in vitro
in vivo
iodine value
IVACG International Vitamin A Consultative Group
IVAP in vivo adhesive platelet
IVAR insulin variable
IVB intraventricular block
intravitreal blood
IVC inferior vena cava
inspiratory vital capacity
integrated vector control
intravascular coagulation
intravenous cholangiography
IVCC intravascular consumption coagulopathy
IVCD intraventricular conduction defect
intraventricular conduction delay
IVCP inferior vena cava pressure
IVCT isovolumic contraction time
IVD intervetebral disk
IVF intravascular fluid
in vitro fertilization
in vivo fertilization
IVGTT intravenous glucose tolerance test
IVH intravenous hyperalimentation
intraventricular hemorrhage
IVJC intervertebral joint complex
IVM Immediate Visual Memory
intravascular mass
IVMP intravenous methyl prednisolone
IVN intravenous nutrition
IVP intravenous pyelogram
intraventricular pressure
intravesical pressure
IVPB intravenous piggyback
IVS intact ventricular septum
interventricular septum
intervillous space
IVSD interventricular septal defect
IVSE interventricular septal excursion
IVT index of vertical transmission
intravenous transfusion
intraventricular
isovolumic time
IVTTT intravenous tolbutamide tolerence test
IVU intravenous urogram
IVV influenza virus vaccine
IW inner wall
IWHC International Women's Health Coalition
IWI interwave interval
IWL insensible water loss
IWMI inferior wall myocardial infarction
IWS Index of Work Satisfaction
IYDP International Year for Disabled Persons
IZ infarction zone
IZS insulin zinc suspension

J

J flux
Jewish
joint (also jt)
Joule's equivalent

j juice
JA juvenile atrophy
JAI juvenile amaurotic idiocy
JBE Japanese B encephalitis
JBIA Jewish Braille Institute of America
JC joint contracture
JCA juvenile chronic arthritis
JCAH Joint Commission on Accreditation of Hospitals
JCAHPO Joint Commission on Allied Health Personnel in Ophthalmology
JCML juvenile chronic myelocytic leukemia
JCP juvenile chronic polyarthritis
JCPD Joint Commission on Prescription Drugs
jct junction
JCV JC virus
JD Janet's disease
jejunal diverticulitis
JDC Joslin Diabetes Center
JDF Juvenile Diabetes Foundation
JDM juvenile diabetes mellitus
JE Japanese encephalitis
junctional escape
jej jejunum
jentac breakfast (jentaculum)
JEV Japanese encephalitis virus
JF jugular foramen
junctional fold
JFS jugular foramen syndrome
JG juxtaglomerular
JGA juxtaglomerular apparatus
JGB Jewish Guild for the Blind
JGC juxtaglomerular cell
JGCT juxtaglomerular cell tumor
JGI jejunogastric intussusception
juxtaglomerular index
JH juvenile hormone
JHMV JHM virus
JHR Jarisch-Herxheimer reaction
JIB jejunoileal bypass
JIF Janus Information Facility
JIH joint interval histogram
JJ jaw jerk
JKD Junius-Kuhnt disease
JLP juvenile laryngeal papilloma
JM josamycin
JMR Jones-Mote reactivity
JNA Jena Nomina Anatomica
JND just noticeable difference
JOD juvenile-onset diabetes
JODM juvenile-onset diabetes mellitus
JP juvenile periodontitis
JPD juvenile plantar dermatosis
JPMA Juvenile Product Manufacturers Association
JPS joint position sense
JPSA Jewish Pharmaceutical Society of America
Joint Project for the Study of Abortion
JR Jolly's reaction
JRA juvenile rheumatoid arthritis
JRCRTE Joint Review Committee for Respiratory Therapy Education
JrNAD Junior National Association for the Deaf
JS jejunal segment
Job syndrome
junctional slowing
JSU Junkman-Schoeller unit
jt joint (also J)
JV jugular vein
JVD jugular vein distension
JVP jugular venous pressure
jugular venous pulse

K

K absolute zero
cathode (kathode)(also CA, KA, Ka)
electrostatic capacity
kanamycin (also KM)
Kell
Kelvin
kerma
ketotifen
kidney
Klebsiella
knee (also Kn)
phylloquinone
potassium (kalium)
^{42}K radioactive isotope of potassium
^{43}K radioactive isotope of potassium
k constant
kilo
thousand
KA cathode (kathode) (also CA, K, Ka)
kainic acid
ketoacidosis
King-Armstrong
kynurenic acid
K/A ketogenic to antiketogenic ratio
Ka cathode (also CA, K, KA)
K_a dissociation constant of an acid
KAAD kerosene, alcohol, acetic acid, dioxane
KAB knowledge, attitude, behavior
KABC Kaufman Assessment Battery for Children
KAFO knee-ankle-foot orthosis
KAP knowledge, attitude, practice
KAST Kindergarten Auditory Screening Test
KAU King-Armstrong unit
KB ketone body
KB5 potassium pentaborate
K_b dissociation constant of a base
KBM Kondylen Betrung Munster
KBS Kluver-Bucy syndrome
KC cathodal (kathodal) closing
keratoma climacterium
knees to chest
knuckle cracking
Kupffer cell
kc kilocycle
Kcal kilocalorie
KCC cathodal (kathodal) closing contraction
KCG kinetocardiogram
KCi kilocurie
kcps kilocycles per second
KCS keratoconjunctivitis sicca
KCT cathodal (kathodal) closing tetanus
kaolin cephalin time
KD cathodal (kathodal) duration
KDA known drug allergy
KDO keto-deoxyoctonic acid
2-keto-3-deoxyoctulosonic acid
KDP potassium dihydrogen phosphate
KDT cathodal (kathodal) duration tetanus

KE kinetic energy
KEC Klebsiella, Enterobacter, Citrobacter
KED Kendrick extrication device
KEL constant elimination rate
KeV kiloelectron volts
Kf flocculation speed
KFAB kidney-fixing antibody
KFD kinetic family drawing
KFS Klippel-Feil syndrome
kG kilogauss
kg kilogram
KGDHC ketoglutarate dehydrogenase complex
kg-m kilogram-meter
KGS ketogenic steroid
KHb potassium hemoglobinate
KHC Karen Horney Clinic
kinetic hemolysis curve
KHD kinky hair disease
KHF Korean hemorrhagic fever
KHN Knoop hardness number
KHz kilohertz
KI Kronig's isthmus
KIA Kligler iron agar
KIC keto-isocaproic acid
KICB killed intracellular bacteria
KIDS Kent Infant Development Scale
KIMSA Kirsten murine sarcoma virus
KISS key integrative social system
KIT Kahn Intelligence Tests
KIU kallikrein inhibitor unit
KIV keto-isovalerate
KJ kilojoule
kj knee jerk
kk knee kick
KL Klebs-Loffler
kl kiloliter
7-KLCA
7-ketolithocholic acid
KLH keyhole limpet hemocyanin
KLS kidney, liver, spleen
KLST Kindergarten Language Screening Test
KM kanamycin (also K)
Kato-Muira
K_m Michaelis constant
km kilometer
kMc kilomegacycle
kMcps kilomegacycles per second
KMEF keratin, myosin, epidermin, fibrin
kmps kilometers per second
KMV killed measles virus vaccine
Kn knee (also K)
KO keep open
KOC cathodal (kathodal) opening contraction
KP keratitic precipitate
keratitis punctata
kidney protein
KPB ketophenylbutazone
potassium phosphate buffer
KPM kilopondmeter
KPR Kuder Preference Record
KPV killed parenteral vaccine
KR knowledge of results
Kr krypton
^{79}Kr radioactive isotope of krypton
^{83}Kr radioactive isotope of krypton
^{85}Kr radioactive isotope of krypton
KRBB Krebs-Ringer bicarbonate buffer
KRBG Krebs-Ringer bicarbonate buffer with glucose
KRBS Krebs-Ringer bicarbonate solution
KRP Kolmer-Reiter protein
Krebs-Ringer phosphate

KS Kaposi's sarcoma
Kartagener syndrome
Kawasaki syndrome
keratan sulfate
ketosteroid
Klinefelter's syndrome
Kveim-Siltzbach
17-KS 17-ketosteroid
KSA knowledge, skills, and abilities
KSP kidney-specific protein
7-KT 7-ketocholesterol
KTSA Kahn Test for Symbol Arrangement
KTVS Keystone Telebinocular Visual Survey
KU Karmen unit
Kimbrel unit
KUB kidney, upper bladder
kidney, ureter, bladder
KV kanomycin-vancomycin
killed vaccine
kv kilovolt
KVA kilovolt-ampere
KVCP kilovolt constant potential
KVE Kaposi's varivelliform eruption
KVLB kanamycin-vancomycin laked blood
KVO keep vein open
KVp kilovolt peak
KW Keith-Wagener
kw kilowatt
KWB Keith, Wagener, Barker
KW-hr kilowatt-hour
KWIC key word in context
KWOC key word out of context
KYB Know Your Body

L

L coefficient of induction
Lactobacillus
Lambert
Latin
left (also lt)
left eye (also LE)
Legionella
Leishmania
length
Leptospira
Leptotrichia
lethal
Leuconostoc
levorotatory
lewisite
licensed
lidocaine
ligament (also lig)
light (also, lev, lt)
limes (or limit)
lincomycin (also LM)
Listeria
liter (also l)
liver
Loa
low
lumbar
lumen (also lm)
lung (also Lu)
lymph (also LYM)
lymphocyte (also LY)

lymphogranuloma
lysosome
L_0 limes null
L1...L5
lumbar nerves 1 through 5
L1...L5
lumbar vertebrae 1 through 5
L_+ limes death
l liter (also L)
LA lactic acid
language age
latex agglutination
left angle
left arm
left atrium
left auricle
leucine aminopeptidase
leukemia antigen
levator ani
lichen amyloidosis
linguoaxial
local anesthesia
long-acting
low anxiety
Ludwig angina
L&A light and accommodation
La lanthanum
^{140}La radioactive isotope of lanthanum
la according to the art (lege artis)
LAA left auricular appendage
leukemia-associated antigen
leukocyte ascorbic acid
LAAAD L-aromatic amino acid decarboxylase
LAAM L-alpha-acetylmethadol
LAAO L-amino acid oxidase
Lab laboratory
LABAD Laboratory Bases Automated Diagnosis
LABS Laboratory Admission Baseline Study
LABVT left atrial ball-valve thrombus
LAC low amplitude contraction
lac laceration
lactation
LACAT Legislative Alliance of Creative Arts Therapies
LACT lecithin, cholesterol, acyltransferase
LAD lactic acid dehydrogenase
language acquisition device
left anterior descending
left axis deviation
LADA laboratory animal dander allergy
LAE left atrial enlargement
LAF laminar air flow (also LAM)
leukocyte activating factor
lymphocyte activating factor
LAFB left anterior fascicular block
LAFR laminar air flow room
LAG labiogingival
lymphangiography
lag flask (lagena)
LAH lactalbumin hydrolysate
left anterior hemiblock
left atrial hypertrophy
L.A.H.
Licentiate of Apothecaries Hall
LAHV leukocyte-associated herpes virus
LAI labioincisal
leukocyte adherence inhibition
LAIF leukocyte adherence inhibition factor
LAIT latex agglutination-inhibition test
LAL Limulus amebocyte lysate
low air loss
LAM laminar air flow (also LAF)
laminectomy
left anterior measurement
left atrial myxoma
LA-MAX
maximal left atrial dimension
LAMO Local Area Management Organization
LAN long-acting neuroleptic
LAO left anterior oblique
left atrial overloading
L.A.O.
Licentiate in Obstetric Science
LAP left atrial pressure
leucine aminopeptidase
leukocyte alkaline phosphatase
lyophilized anterior pituitary
lap laparotomy
LAPA leukocyte alkaline phosphatase activity
$LAPF_4$ low affinity platelet factor 4
LAPOCA
L-asparaginase, prednisone, vincristine (Oncovin), cytosine arabinoside, doxorubicin (Adriamycin)
LAPW left atrial posterior wall
LAR late asthmatic response
left arm recumbent
lar laryngology
LARC leukocyte automatic recognition computer
LAS laxative abuse syndrome
left anterior superior
linear alkylate sulfonate
linear alkylbenzenesulfonate
lower abdominal surgery
lysine acetylsalicylate
LASA Laboratory Animal Science Association
LASER light amplification by stimulated emission of radiation
LASFB left anterior-superior fascicular block
LASH left anterior superior hemiblock
LASS labile aggregation stimulating substance
Linguistic Analysis of Speech Samples
LAT latex agglutination test
lat lateral
LAT-A latrunculin A
lat admov
let it be applied to the side (lateri admoveatum)
LAT-B latrunculin B
LATP left atrial transmural pressure
LATS long-acting transmural stimulator
LATS-P
long-acting thyroid stimulator-protector
LAW left atrial wall
LB lamellar body
large bowel
left bundle
lipid body
live birth
liver biopsy
Living Bank
loose body
low back
low breakage
lung biopsy
lb pound (also lib)
LBA left basal artery
LBB left bundle branch
LBBB left bundle branch block
LBC lidocaine blood concentration
LBCD left border of cardiac dullness

LBCF Laboratory Branch Complement Fixation
LBD large bile duct
left border dullness
LBF Lactobacillus bulgaricus factor
limb blood flow
LBH length, breath, height
LBI low serum-bound iodine
LBM lean body mass
LBN Lewis-Brown-Norway
LBNP lower body negative pressure
LBP low back pain
low blood pressure
LBRF louse-borne relapsing fever
LBT low back trouble
lupus band test
LBTI lima bean trypsin inhibitor
LBW lean body weight
low birth weight
LBWI low birth weight infant
LBWR lung-body weight ratio
LC lamina cortex
Langerhans cell
left circumflex
lethal concentration
light chain
light coagulation
lining cell
lipid cytosome
liquid chromotography
live clinic
liver cirrhosis
living children
locus ceruleus
long chain
longus capitus
longus colli
lung cancer
lung cell
lymph capillary
lymphocyte count
lymphocytotoxin
lymphoma culture
LCA left circumflex artery
left coronary artery
lithocholic acid
lymphocyte chemoattractant activity
lymphocytotoxic antibody
LCAT lecithin-cholesterol acyltransferase
LCBF local cerebral blood flow
LCC left common carotid
left coronary cusp
LCCA late cortical cerebellar atrophy
left common carotid artery
LCCP limited channel-capacity processes
LCD liquid crystal display
liquor carbonis detergens
LCDD light chain deposition disease
LCEC liquid chromatography with electro-chemical detection
LCF least common factor
linear correction factor
low-frequency current field
LCFA long-chain fatty acid
LCFAO long-chain fatty acid oxidation
LCFU leukocyte colony-forming units
LCG Langerhans cell granule
LCGU local cerebral glucose utilization
L.Ch. Licentiate in Surgery
LCI length complexity index
LCIS lobular carcinoma in situ
LCL Levinthal-Coles-Lillie
lower confidence limit
lymphoblastoid cell line
lymphocytic lymphosarcoma
lymphoid cell line
LCM left costal margin
leukocyte-conditioned medium
lowest common multiple
lymphatic choriomeningitis
lymphocytic choriomeningitis
LCME Liaison Committee on Medical Education
LCMV lymphocytic choriomeningitis virus
LCN lateral cervical nucleus
LCPD Legg-Calve-Perthes disease
LCQG left caudal quarter ganglion
LCR leurocristine (also VCR--vincristine)
LCT liver cell tumor
long-chain triglyceride
lymphocytotoxicity test
LCU life change unit
LCX left circumflex
LD labyrinthine defect
lactic dehydrogenase (also LDH)
L-dopa
learning disability
learning disorder
left deltoid
Legionnaire's disease
Leishman-Donovan
lethal dose
light-dark
light difference
limited disease
linguodistal
lithium discontinuation
liver disease
living donor
loading dose
Lombard-Dowell
low density
low dose
lung destruction
lymphocyte defined
LD_{50} median lethal dose
LD_{100} completely lethal dose
LDA laser Doppler anemometry
left dorsoanterior
linear displacement analysis
lymphocyte-dependent antibody
LDB Leader Dogs for the Blind
Legionnaire's disease bacillus
LDD light-dark discrimination
LDE lauric diethamide
LDG long-distance group
low-dose group
LDH lactate dehydrogenase (also LD)
LDH_6 lactate dehydrogenase isoenzyme
LDIH left direct inguinal hernia
LDL loudness discomfort level
low-density lipoprotein
low-density lymphocyte
LDLC low-density lipoprotein cholesterol
LDP left dorsoposterior
LDS ligating, dividing stapler
L.D.S. Licentiate in Dental Surgery
LDU long double upright
LDUB long double upright brace
LDV lactate dehydrogenase-elevating virus
laser doppler velocimetry
LE left ear (also AS)
left eye (also L)
leukocyte elastase
leukoerythrogenetic

live embryo
Long-Evans
lower extremity
lupus erythematosus

Le Leonard
Lewis

LEA language experience approach
lower extremity amputation

LEB lupus erythematosus body

LECP low-energy charged particle

LED light-emitting diode
lowest effective dose
lupus erythematosus disseminatus

LEED low-energy electron diffraction

LEEP left end-expiratory pressure

LEER lower extremity equipment related

LEF Life Extension Foundation
leukokinesis enhancing factor
lupus erythematosus factor

Leg Com
legally committed

LEJ ligation of the esophagogastric junction

LEM lateral eye movement
leukocyte endogenous mediator
light electron microscope

LEMS Lambert-Eaton myasthenic syndrome

lenit gently (leniter)

LEP low egg passage

LE prep
lupus erythematosus preparation

LES Life Experience Survey
local excitatory state
lower esophageal segment
lower esophageal sphincter
lower esophageal stricture

LESA liposomally entrapped second antibody

LESG Late Effects Study Group

LESP lower esophageal sphincter pressure

LET language enrichment therapy
linear energy transfer
low energy transfer

LETD lowest effective toxic dose

LETS large external transformation sensitive

Leu leucine

lev light (levis) (also L, lt)

levit lightly (leviter)

LEX lactate extraction

LF labile factor
laryngofissure
lavage fluid
leaflet
leucine flux
limit of flocculation
low fat
low frequency

Lf limes flocculation

LFA left femoral artery
left frontoanterior
leukotactic factor activity

LFB lingual-facial-buccal

LFC left frontal craniotomy
low fat and cholesterol

LFD lactose-free diet
large for date
least fatal dose
low fat diet
low fiber diet
low forceps delivery

LFECT loose fibroelastic connective tissue

LFI Lebanese Fear Inventory

LFL left frontolateral

LFN lactoferrin

LFP left frontoposterior

L.F.P.S.
Licentiate of the Faculty of Physicians and Surgeons

LFS limbic forebrain structure

LFT latex flocculation test
left frontotransverse
liver function test

LFTSW left foot switch

LFV Lassa fever virus
low frequency ventilation

LG lactoglobulin
lamellar granule
laryngectomy
left gluteal
leucylglycine
linguogingival
little gastrin
liver graft
low glucose

Lg large
leg

LGA large for gestational age
left gastric artery

LGB Landry-Guillain-Barre
lateral geniculate body

LGBS Landry-Guillain-Barre-Strohl

LGH lactogenic hormone

LGL large granular lymphocyte
Lown-Ganong-Levine

LGN lateral geniculate nucleus

LGV large granular vesicle
lymphogranuloma venereum

LH late healed
lateral hypothalamus
left hand
liver homogenate
lues hereditaria
lung homogenate
luteinizing hormone

LHA lateral hypothalamic area
left hepatic artery

LHb lateral habenular

LHBV left heart blood volume

LHCG luteinizing hormone-chorionic gonadotropin hormone

LHF left heart failure
ligament of the head of the femur

LHFA lung Hageman factor activator

LHHS Lutheran Hospitals and Homes Society of America

LHL left hepatic lobe

LHM lisuride hydrogen maleate

LHN lateral hypothalamic nucleus

LHNCBC
Lister Hill National Center for Biomedical Communications

LHPZ lower esophageal high-pressure zone

LHR liquid holding recovery

LH-RF luteinizing hormone-releasing factor (also LRF)

LH-RH luteinizing hormone-releasing hormone (also LRH)

LHS left hand side
left heart strain
lymphatic and hematopoietic system

LHTP L-5-hydroxytryptophan

LHV lady health visitor

LI labeling index
lactose intolerance
lamellar ichthyosis

large intestine
learning impaired
life island
linguoincisal
lithogenic index
low impulsiveness

Li lithium
LIA leukemia inhibitory associated
lysine iron agar
LIAC light-induced absorbance change
LIAF lymphocyte-induced angiogenesis factor
LIAFI late infantile amaurotic familial idiocy
lib pound (libra) (also lb)
LIBC latent iorn-binding capacity
LIC left internal carotid
limiting isorrheic concentration
LICA left internal carotid artery
LICC lectin-induced cellular cytotoxicity
LICD lower intestinal Crohn's disease
LICM left intercostal margin
Lic.Med.
Licentiate in Medicine
LID late-onset immunoglobulin deficiency
lymphocytic infiltrative disease
LIDC low intensity direct current
LIF left iliac fossa
leukocyte infiltration factor
leukocyte inhibitory factor
LIFE Longitudinal Interval Follow-up Evaluation
LIFT lymphocyte immunofluorescence test
lig ligament (also L)
LIH left inguinal hernia
LIHA low impulsiveness, high anxiety
LILA low impulsiveness, low anxiety
LIMA left internal mammary artery
lin liniment
LINAC linear accelerator
LIO left inferior oblique
LIP lymphocytic interstitial pneumonia
LIPO Laboratory Improvement Program Office
LIPS Leiter International Performance Scale
liq liquid
liquor
LIRBM liver, iron, red bone marrow
LIS lithium diiodosalicylate
lobular in situ
LISS low ionic strength solution
LIV left innominate vein
LIVC left inferior vena cava
LIVIM lethal intestinal virus of infant mice
LK left kidney
lichenoid keratosis
LK$^+$ low potassium ion
LKM liver-kidney microsomal
LKPD Lillehei-Kaster pivoting disk
L.K.Q.C.P.I.
Licientate of the King and Queen's College of Physicians of Ireland
LKS liver, kidney, spleen
LL large local
large lymphocyte
Lean Line
left lateral
left leg
left lower
left lung
lingual lipase
loudness level
lower lid
lower lobe
lung length
lymphocytic lymphoma
lysolecithin
LLA Limulus lysate assay
LLAT lysolecithin acyl transferase
LLB left lower border
long leg brace
lower lobe bronchus
LLBCD left lower border of cardiac dullness
LLBP long leg brace with pelvic band
LLC Lewis lung carcinoma
long leg cast
LLD Lactobacillus lactis Dorner
left lateral decubitus
long-lasting depolarization
LLDF Lactobacillus lactis Dorner factor
LLE left lower extremity
LLF Laki-Lorand factor
LLL left liver lobe
left lower lid
left lower lobe
LLLE lower lid left eye (also LLOS)
LLLM low liquid level monitor
LLLNR left lower lobe, no rales
LLM localized leukocyte mobilization
LLO Legionella-like organization
LLOD lower lid, right eye (oculus dexter) (also LLRE)
LLOS lower lid, left eye (oculus sinister) (also LLLE)
LLP late luteal phase
LLQ left lower quadrant
LLR large local reaction
left lateral rectus
LLRE lower lid right eye (also LLOD)
LLS lateral loop suspensor
LLSB left lower sternal border
LLT left lateral thigh
Limulus lysate test
LLV lymphoid leukosis virus
LLW low-level waste
LM lactose malabsorption
left main
left median
legal medicine
light microscopy
light minimum
lincomycin (also L)
linguomesial
lipid mobilizer
longitudinal muscle
L.M. Licentiate in Midwifery
lm lumen (also L)
LMA left mentoanterior
limbic midbrain area
liver membrane antibody
liver membrane autoantibody
LMB Laurence-Moon-Biedl
LMC lymphocyte-mediated cytolysis
lymphocyte-mediated cytotoxicity
lymphocyte microcytotoxicity
LMCA left main coronary artery
left middle cerebral artery
LMD left main disease
local medical doctor
low molecular weight dextran (also LMWD)
LMDF lupus miliaris disseminatus faciei
LME left mediolateral episiotomy
leukocyte migration enhancement
LMF leukocyte mitogenic factor
lymphocyte mitogenic factor

LMG lethal midline granuloma
low mobility group
LMH lipid-mobilizing hormone
LMI leukocyte migration inhibition
LMIF leukocyte migration inhibitory factor
LMIR leukocyte migration inhibition reaction
LMIT leukocyte migration inhibition test
LML left mediolateral
LMM light meromyosin
LMN lower motor neuron
LMNL lower motor neuron lesion
LMP last menstrual period
left mentoposterior
lymphoproliferative malignancy
LMR left medial rectus
log magnitude ratio
L.M.R.C.P.
Licentiate in Midwifery of the Royal College of Physicians
L.M.S.
Licentiate in Medicine and Surgery
L.M.S.S.A.
Licentiate in Medicine and Surgery of the Society of Apothecaries
LMSV left maximal spatial voltage
LMT left mentotransverse
LMTA Language Modalities Test for Aphasia
LMW low molecular weight
LMWD low molecular weight dextran (also LMD)
LN lamina neuropile
Lesch-Nyhan
lipoid nephrosis
lupus nephritis
lymph node
ln natural logarithm
LNA leucyl-napthylamine
LNC lymph node cell
LND Lesch-Nyhan disease
LNG liquified natural gas
LNI log neutralization index
LNL lower normal limit
LNMP last normal menstrual period
LNNB Luria-Nebraska Neuropsychological Battery
LNP large neuronal polypeptide
LNPF lymph node permeability factor
LO leucine oxidation
linguo-occlusal
lysyl oxidase
LOA leave of absence
left occipitoanterior
LOB Loyal Order of the Boar
LOC laxative of choice
level of consciousness
Locus of Control
loss of consciousness
LOC-C Locus of Control-Chance
loc dol
to the painful spot (loco dolenti)
LOC-E Locus of Control-External
LOC-I Locus of Control-Internal
LOC-PO
Locus of Control-Powerful Others
log logarithm
LOI level of incompetence
Leyton Obsessive Inventory
LOIH left oblique inguinal hernia
LOL left occipitolateral
LOM limitation of motion
loss of motion
LOMPT Lincoln-Oseretsky Motor Performance Test
LOMSA left otitis media suppurative, acute
LOMSC left otitis media suppurative, chronic
LOP leave on pass
left occipitoposterior
POQ lower outer quadrant
LOR lorazepam
lorcainide
LOS length of stay
low output syndrome
LOT lateral olfactory tract
left occipitotransverse
lengthened off time
lot lotion
LOV large opaque vesicle
LP laboratory procedure
lamina propria
latency period
lateral plantar
latex particle
leading pole
Legionella pneumophila
leukocyte poor
levator palati
lichen planus
ligamentum patella
lightly padded
light perception
linguopulpal
lipoprotein
low potency
low power
low pressure
low protein
lumbar puncture
lumboperitoneal
lung parenchyma
lymphocyte predominant
lymphoid plasma
L/P lactate to pyruvate ratio
lymph to plasma ratio
LPA larval photoreceptor axon
latex particle agglutination
left pulmonary artery
L-PAM melphalan (L-phenylalanine mustard)
LPB lipoprotein B
low profile bioprosthesis (also LPBP)
LPBP low profile bioprosthesis (also LPB)
LPC late positive component
lysophosphatidyl choline
LPE lipoprotein electrophoresis
LPF leukocytosis-promoting factor
lipopolysaccharide factor
localized plaque formation
low power field
lymphocytosis-promoting factor
LPFB left posterior fascicular block
LPFN low pass filtered noise
LPFS low pass filtered signal
LPG liquified petroleum gas
LPH left posterior hemiblock
lipotrophin
LPI left posterior inferior
long process of incus
LPIFB left posterior inferior fascicular block
LPIH left posterior inferior hemiblock
LPK liver pyruvate kinase
LPL lamina propria lymphocyte
lichen planuslike lesion
lipoprotein lipase
LPLA lipoprotein lipase activity
LPM lateral pterygoid muscle

liver plasma membrane
localized pretibial myxedema
lpm liters per minute
LPN Licensed Practical Nurse
LPO left posterior oblique
light perception only
LPOA lateral preoptic area
LPP lateral pterygoid plate
LPPH late postpartum hemorrhage
LPR late phase response
LPS levator palpebrae superioris
linear profile scan
lipopolysaccharide
London Psychogeriatric Scale
lps liters per second
L.P.T.
Licensed Physical Therapist
LPV left portal view
left pulmonary vein
lymphopathia venereum
lpw lumens per watt
LQ lower quadrant
LR laboratory reference
large reticulocyte
latency reaction
lateral recess
ligand receptor
light reaction
lymphocyte recruitment
L/R left to right
Lr lawrencium (also Lw)
limes reacting
LRA low right atrium
LRC Lipid Research Clinics
locomotor-respiratory coupling
L.R.C.P.
Licentiate of the Royal College of Physicians
L.R.C.P.E.
Licentiate of the Royal College of Physicians, Edinburgh
L.R.C.P.I.
Licentiate of the Royal College of Physicians, Ireland
L.R.C.P.S.I.
Licentiate of the Royal College of Physicians and Surgeons, Ireland
L.R.C.S.
Licentiate of the Royal College of Surgeons
L.R.C.S.E.
Licentiate of the Royal College of Surgeons, Edinburgh
LRD living related donor
LRE lymphosarcoma reticuloendothelial
LREH low renin essential hypertension
LRF latex and resorcinol formaldehyde
liver residue factor
luteinizing hormone-releasing factor (also LHRF)
L.R.F.P.S.
Licentiate of the Royal Faculty of Physicians and Surgeons
LRH luteinizing hormone-releasing hormone (also LHRH)
LRI lower respiratory illness
lower respiratory infection
lymphocyte reactivity index
LRN lateral reticular nucleus
LRNA low renin, normal aldosterone
LRM left radical mastectomy
LRP lichen ruber planus
LRQ lower right quadrant
LRQG left rostal quarter ganglion
LRR labyrinthine righting reflex
lymphatic return rate
LRS lactated Ringer's solution
LRSF lactating rat serum factor
liver regenerating serum factor
LRSP long-range systems planning
LRT lower respiratory tract
LRTI lower respiratory tract illness
LS lateral septal
lateral suspensor
left septum
left side
legally separated
lesser sac
Libman-Sacks
light sleep
liminal sensitivity
linear scleroderma
lipid synthesis
liver and spleen
lower segment
lumbosacral
lung strip
lymphosarcoma
L-S lipid-saccharide
L/S lecithin to sphingomyelin ratio
LSA left sacroanterior
left subclavian artery
Leukemia Society of America
leukocyte-specific activity
lichen sclerosus et atrophicus
L.S.A.
Licentiate of Society of Apothecaries
LSB left sternal border
LSC late systolic click
LSCA left scapuloanterior
lower segment caesarean section
LSCL lymphosarcoma cell leukemia (also LSL)
LSCP left scapuloposterior
LSCS lower segment cesarean section
LSD least significance difference
low salt diet
lysergic acid diethylamide
LSEP left somatosensory evoked potential
LSG Lymphoma Study Group
LSH lutein-stimulating hormone
LSIZ Life Satisfaction Index Z
LSK liver, spleen, kidney
LSKM liver, spleen, kidney megalia
LSL left sacrolateral
lymphosarcoma cell leukemia (also LSCL)
LSM late systolic murmur
lysergic acid morpholide
LSN left sympathetic nerve
LSP left sacroposterior
liver-specific protein
LSp life-span
LSQ least square
LSRA low septal right atrium
LSS Life Span Study
Life Study Sample
life support station
LSSA lipid soluable secondary antioxidant
LST lateral spinothalamic tract
left sacrotransverse
local sojourn time
LSTC laparoscopic tubal cautery
LSTL laparoscopic tubal ligation
LSU lactose, saccharose, urea
LSV lateral sacral vein

left subclavian vein
LSWA large-amplitude slow-wave activity
LT labile toxin
laminar tomography
left thigh
lethal time
leukotriene
levothyroxine
long-term
lymphocyte transformation
lymphocyte transitional
lymphotoxin
lt left (also L)
light (also L, lev)
low tension
LTA leukotriene A
lipoteichoic acid
lymphocyte transforming activity
LTAS lead trtra-acetate Schiff
LTB laryngotracheobronchitis
leukotriene B
LTC leukotriene C
lidocaine tissue concentration
long-term care
lysed tumor cell
LTCF long-term care facility
LTD leukotriene D
long-term disability
LTE laryngotracheoesophageal
leukotriene E
LTF lipotropic factor
lymphocyte transformation factor
LTH lactogenic hormone
low-temperature holding
luteotropic hormone
LTI low temperature isotropic
lupus-type inclusion
LTM long-term memory
LTP leukocyte thromboplastin
long-term potentiation
LTPP lipothiamide pyrophosphate
LTR long terminal repeat
lymphocyte transfer reaction
LTS long-term storage
long-term surviving
LTT lactose tolerance test
lymphoblastic transformation test
lymphocyte transformation test
LTV Lucke tumor virus
lung thermal volume
LU left upper
leucomycin
L&U lower and upper
Lu lung (also L)
lutetium
^{177}Lu radioactive isotope of lutetium
LUA left upper arm
luc prim
at daybreak (luce primo)
LUE left upper extremity
LUL left upper lobe
LUMO lowest unoccupied molecular orbital
LUOQ left upper outer quadrant
LUQ left upper quadrant
LUSB left upper sternal border
lut yellow (luteum)
LUTT lower urinary tract tumor
LV lacto-ovo-vegetarian
laryngeal vestibule
lateral ventricle
left ventricle
leucovorin
leukemia virus
levulinate
live virus
lividomycin
low volume
lumbar vertebra
lung volume
LVA left vertebral artery
LVAD left ventricle assist device
LVAS left ventricular assist system
LVBP left ventricle bypass pump
LVD left ventricular dysfunction
LVDP left ventricular diastolic pressure
LVDT linear variable differential transformer
LVE left ventricular enlargement
LVEDD left ventricular end-diastolic dimension
LVEDP left ventricular end-diastolic pressure
LVEDV left ventricular end-diastolic volume
LVEF left ventricular ejection fraction
LVESD left ventricular end-systolic dimension
LVESV left ventricular end-systolic volume
LVET left ventricular ejection time
LVF left ventricular failure
left ventricular function
low voltage fast
low voltage focus
LVH left ventricular hypertrophy
LVI left ventricular insufficiency
left ventricular ischemia
LVID left ventricular internal diastolic
left ventricular internal dimension
LVIDP left ventricular initial diastolic pressure
LVIV left ventricular infarct volume
LVM lateral ventromedial nucleus
left ventricular mass
LVMF left ventricular minute flow
L.V.N.
Licensed Vocational Nurse
LVOT left ventricular outflow tract
LVP large volume parenteral
left ventricular pressure
levator veli palatini
lysine-vasopressin
LVPEP left ventricular preejection period
LVPSP left ventricular peak systolic pressure
LVPW left ventricle posterior wall
LVR limb vascular resistance
LVS left ventricular strain
LVSI left ventricular systolic index
LVSO left ventricular systolic output
LVSP left ventricular systolic pressure
LVSV left ventricular stroke volume
LVSW left ventricular stroke work
LVSWI left ventricular stroke work index
LVV live varicella vaccine
LVW lateral ventricular width
left ventricular wall
left ventricular work
LVWI left ventricular work index
LVWMA left ventricular wall motion abnormality
LVWMI left ventricular wall motion index
LW lacerating wound
lateral wall
Lee-White
lung weight
lung width
L&W living and well
Lw lawrencium (also Lr)

LWCT Lee-White clotting time
LWD living with disease
LWMEL Leonard Wood Memorial for the Eradication of Leprosy
LWP lateral wall pressure
LX local irradiation
Lx latex
lux
LY lactoalbumin-yeastolate
lymphocyte (also L)
lyophilization
ly Langley
lying
LYEL lost years of expected life
LYG lymphomatoid granulomatosis
LYM lymph (also L)
LYP lower yield point
Lys lysine
Lzm lysozyme

M

M Macaca
macerate (also mac)
male
malignant
Mansonia
manual
married
mass
massage
matt
mature
mean
meatus
media
median (also Med)
medical (also Med)
memory
metal
metastasis
meter (also m)
mexiletine
Microbacterium
Micrococcus
Microsporum
mitochondria
molar concentration (also molc)
molar, permanent
mole (also mol)
molecular weight (also MW)
molsidomine
Monday
monocyte (also Mono)
month (also mo)
Moraxella
morgan
Morganella
morphine
mother
movement response to human figure
mucoid
Mucor
multiceps
multipara
murmur
Musca
muscle
Mycobacterium
Mycoplasma
myopia
myosin
thousand (mil)
M_1 mitral first sound, slight dullness
M_2 mitral second sound, marked dullness
M_3 mitral third sound, absolute dullness
m handful (manipulus) (also Man)
melts at
meter (also M)
minim (also Min)
minute (also min)
mix
mixture (also mist)
molar, deciduous
m^2 square meter
m^3 cubic meter
MA cefamandole
mafenide acetate
mandelic acid
massater
maternal aunt
medical assistance
medical audit
megaloblastic anemia
megestrol acetate
Melia Azedarach
membrane antigen
menstrual age
mental age
Mexican American
microaneurysm
microcytotoxicity assay
Miller-Abbott
mitochondrial antibody
mitogen activation
moderately advanced
monoamine
monoclonal antibody
multiple action
myelinated axon
M.A. Master of Arts
M/A mood and affect
Ma masurium
ma meter-angle
milliampere
MAA macroaggregated albumin
Medical Assistance for the Aged
microaggregated albumin
MAAC Medical Assistants Advisory Council
MAACL Multiple Affect Adjective Checklist
MAB Metropolitan Asylums Board
Modified Ascending Bekesy
N-methyl-4-aminoazobenzene
MABI Mother's Assessment of the Behavior of Her Infant
MABP mean arterial blood pressure
MAC malignancy associated change
maximum acid concentration
maximum allowable concentration
maximum allowable cost
methotrexate, actinomycin D, cyclophosphamide
midarm circumference
minimal antibiotic concentration
minimum alveolar concentration
mitral anular calcium
multidimensional acturarial classification
Multipurpose Arthritis Center

mac macerate (also M)
MACB 2-methylamino-5-chlorobenzophenone
MACC methotrexate, doxorubicin (Adriamycin), lomustine (CCNU), cyclophosphamide
Mobility, Affect, Cooperation, and Communication
MACE methylchloroform chloroacetophenone
M.A.C.P.
Master of the American College of Physicians
MACR mean axillary count rate
MAD maximum allowable dose
methandriol
myoadenylate deaminase
MADD Mothers Against Drunk Driving
MADDS monoacetyldapsone
MADRS Montgomery and Asberg Depression Rating Scale
MADU 2'-deoxy-5-(methylamino)uridine
MAE Multilingual Aphasia Examination
MAF macrophage activation factor
minimum audible field
MAFA midarm fat area
MAFH macroaggregated ferrous hydroxide
MAFI Medic Alert Foundation International
MAG myelin-associated glycoprotein
mag large (magnus)
magnification
MAGE mean amplitude of glycerine excursion
MAgF macrophage aggregation factor
MAHA microangiopathic hemolytic anemia
microangiopathic hemolytic aneurysm
MAI Morbid Anxiety Inventory
MAIN Midwest Alliance in Nursing
MAIS Mycobacterium avium intercellulare scrofulaceum
MAKA major karyotypic abnormality
MAL midaxillary line
MALG Minnesota antilymphoblast globulin
MALT mucosa-associated lymphoid tissue
MAM methylazoxymethanol
M+Am myopic astigmatism
mam milliampere minute
MAMA midarm muscle area
MAMC mean arm muscle circumference
midarm muscle circumference
MAMCS Michigan Ambulatory Medical Care Survey
MAmg medial amygdaloid nucleus
mAMSA 4'-(9-acridinylamino) methanesulfon-m-anisidide
Man handful (manipulus) (also m)
manipulation (also Manip)
mannose
man morning (mane)
Manip manipulation (also Man)
MANOVA
multivariate analysis of variance
man pr
early in the morning (mane primo)
MAO maximal acid output
monoamine oxidase
M.A.O.
Master of Arts in Obstetrics, Dublin
MAODP Medic Alert Organ Donor Program
MAOI monamine oxidase inhibitor
MAP maximal aerobic power
mean aortic pressure
mean arterial pressure
megaloblastic anemia of pregnancy
mercapturic acid pathway
microtubule-associated protein
monophasic action potential
muscle action potential
MAPC migrating action potential complex
MAPS Make a Picture Story
measurement of air pollution from satellites
MAR marasmus
marrow
maximal aggregation ratio
medication administration record
minimal angle resolution
mixed antiglobulin reaction
MARC Medical Air Rescue Corps
marg margin
MARS Mathematics Anxiety Rating Scale
MARS-A
Mathematics Anxiety Rating Scale--Adolescents
MARTI mobile advanced real-time image
MAS Manifest Anxiety Scale
Maternal Attitude Scale
meconium aspiration syndrome
minor axis shortening
mobile arm support
motion analysis system
mas milliampere second
masc mass concentration
MASER microwave amplification by stimulated emission of radiation
MASF Melcher's acid soluble fraction
MASH Mobile Army Surgical Hospital
multiple automated sample harvester
mas pil
pill mass (massa pilularum)
MAST Medical Antishock Trousers
Michigan Alcoholism Screening Test
Military Antishock Trousers
Military Assistance to Safety and Traffic
MAT manual arts therapist
mean absorption time
medication administration team
methionine adenosyltransferase
Metropolitan Achievement Test
microagglutination test
Motivation Analysis Test
multifocal atrial tachycardia
MATRIS
Medical Manpower and Training Information System
MATSA Marek's associated tumor-specific antigen
matut in the morning (matutinus)
MAV mechanical auxiliary ventricle
minimum apparent viscosity
movement arm vector
MAVA multiple abstract variance analysis
MAVR mitral and aortic valve replacement
max maxillary
maximum
MB Mallory body
mamillary body
mercury bougie
mesiobuccal
methyl bromide
methylene blue
myocardial band
M.B. Bachelor of Medicine
2-MB 2-methylbutyrate
Mb mandible body
myoglobin
mb millibar
mix well (misce bene)

MBA nitrogen mustard (also HN_2)
M-BACOD
methotrexate, bleomycin, doxorubicin (Adriamycin), cyclophosphamide, vincristine (Oncovin), dexamethasone
MBB modified barbital buffer
MBC maximum bladder capacity
maximum breathing capacity
minimum bactericidal concentration
MBCU metallic bead-chain urethrocystograph
MBD Mental Deterioration Battery
methotrexate, bleomycin, cisplatin (DDP)
methylene blue dye
minimal brain damage
minimal brain dysfunction
Morquio-Brailsford disease
MBF medullary blood flow
muscle blood flow
myocardial blood flow
MBFLB monaural bifrequency loudness balance
MBG mean blood glucose
MBGS Morphine-Benzedrine Group Scale
MBH medial basal hypothalamus
MBI Marine Biomedical Institute
MBK methyl-n-butyl ketone
MBL minimal bactericidal level
MBM mineral base medium
MBO mesiobucco-occlusal
MbO_2 oxymyoglobin
MBP major basic protein
mean blood pressure
melitensis bovine, porcine
mesiobuccopulpal
myelin basic protein
MBq megabecquerel
MBRT methylene blue reaction time
MBS monobromosalicylanilide
MBSA methylated bovine serum albumin
MBSD maple bark stripper disease
MBT mercaptobenzothiazole
MBTI Myers-Briggs Type Indicator
MBTS mercaptobenzthiazyl ether
MC mass casualty
mast cell
maximum concentration
medium chain
medulla cortex
medullary cavity
megacurie (also MCi)
megacycle (also Mc)
melanoma cell
meningeal carcinomatosis
Merkel cell
mesenteric collateral
mesocaval shunt
metacarpal
metacyclin
methyl cellulose
methylcholanthrene (also MCA)
microcilary clearance
microcirculation
midcapillary
midcarpal
mitomycin C (also MMC)
mitotic cycle
mitral commissurotomy
mixed cellularity
monkey cell
mononuclear cell
mouth care
myocarditis
M.C. Master of Surgery (Magister Chirurgiae) (also M.Ch.)
Medical Corps
M&C morphine and cocaine
3-MC 3-methylcholanthrene
Mc mandible coronoid
megacycle (also MC)
mC millicoulomb
millicurie (also mCi)
MCA Manufacturing Chemists Association
Maternity Center Association
medical care administration
Medical Correctional Association
methylcholanthrene (also MC)
middle cerebral artery
monocarboxylic acid
monoclonal antibody
Multiple Classification Analysis
multiple congenital abnormality
multiple congenital anomaly
MCAR mixed cell agglutination reaction
MCAT Medical College Admissions Test
Medical College Aptitude Test
MCB membraneous cytoplasmic body
monochlorobenzidine
MCBMT muscle capillary basement membrane thickening
MCBR minimum concentration of bilirubin
MCC marked co-contraction
mean corpuscular concentration
medial cell column
metastatic cord compression
microcrystalline collagen
mucocutaneous candidiasis
MCCD minimum cumulative cardiotoxic dose
MCCU mobile coronary care unit
MCD mean cell diameter
mean corpuscular diameter
medullary cystic disease
minimal change disease
muscle carnitine deficiency
MCDP mast cell degranulating peptide
MCDT multiple choice discrimination test
MCE medical care evaluation
MCES multiple cholesterol emboli syndrome
MCF macrophage chemotactic factor
macrophage cytotoxicity factor
Medical Care Foundation
medium corpuscular fragility
monocyte leukotactic factor
mononuclear cell factor
most comfortable frequency
myocardial contractile force
MCFA medium-chain fatty acid
miniature centrifugal fast analyzer
MCFP mean circulating filling pressure
MCG magnetocardiogram
membrane-coating granule
mcg microgram
MCGF mast cell growth factor
MCGN mesangiocapillary glomerulonephritis
MCH maternal and child health
mean cell hemoglobin (also MCHg)
mean corpuscular hemoglobin (also MCHg)
methacholine
M.Ch. Master of Surgery (Magister Chirurgiae) (also M.C.)
mch millicurie hour (also mchr)
MCHC maternal and child health care
mean cell hemoglobin concentration
mean corpuscular hemoglobin concentration

M.Ch.D.
Master of Dental Surgery
MCHg mean cell hemoglobin (also MCH)
mean corpuscular hemoglobin (also MCH)
mchr millicurie-hour (also mch)
MCI mean cardiac index
methicillin
MCi megacurie (also MC)
mCi millicurie (also mC)
mCid millicuries destroyed
MCK2 macrocreatine kinase-2
MCL maximum comfort level
maximum containment laboratory
medial collateral ligament
midclavian line
midcostal line
minimal change lesion
mixed leukocyte culture
most comfortable listening
most comfortable loudness
MCLD Mycobacterium chelonei-like organism
MCLL most comfortable listening level
most comfortable loudness level
MCLS mucocutaneous lymph node syndrome
MCMHA Metropolitan College Mental Health Association
MCMI Millon Clinical Multiaxial Inventory
MCMN 1-methyl-5-nitroimidazole-2-methanol carbamate
MCMV mouse cytomegalovirus
murine cytomegalovirus
MCN minimal change nephropathy
MCNS minimal change nephrotic syndrome
MCO medical care organization
mcoul millicoulomb
MCP maximal closure pressure
melanosis circumscripta precancerosa
metacarpophalangeal (also MP)
methyl-accepting chemotaxis protein
2-methyl-4-chlorophenoxyacetic acid (also MCPA)
metoclopramine
mitotic control protein
MCPA 2-methyl-4-chlorophenoxyacetic acid (also MCP)
mcps megacycles per second
MCQ multiple choice question
MCR message to competition ratio
metabolic clearance rate
MCRS Medicare Cognitive Reimbursement System
MCS malignant carcinoid syndrome
Marlow-Crowne Social Desirability Scale
mesocaval shunt
MCSP Member of the Chartered Society of Physiotherapists
MCT mean circulation time
mean corpuscular thickness
medium-chain triglyceride
medullary carcinoma of the thyroid
monocrotaline
MCTC metrizamide computed tomography cisternography
MCTD mixed connective tissue disease
MCV mean cell volume
mean clinical value
mean corpuscular volume
motor conduction velocity
MCZ miconazole
MD macula densa
maintenance dose
malate dehydrogenase (also MDH)
malrotation of the duodenum
manic depressive
Mantoux diameter
Marek's disease
maternal deprivation
mean deviation
mean diastolic
measurable disease
Meckel's diverticulum
medialis dorsalis
mediastinal disease
mediodorsal
medium dosage
mentally deficient
mentally depressed
Minamata disease
mitral disease
moderate disability
movement disorder
muscular dystrophy
myeloproliferative disease
myocardial damage
myocardial disease
M.D. Doctor of Medicine (Medicinae Doctor)
Md mendelevium
md as directed (more dicto)
MDA malondialdehyde
manual dilation of the anus
mentodextra anterior
methylenedioxyamphetamine
Mission Doctors Association
motor discriminative acuity
Muscular Dystrophy Association
MDAA Medical Devices Associations of America
Muscular Dystrophy Association of America
MDAP Medical Devices Applications Program
MDB Molecular Disease Branch
MDBDF March of Dimes Birth Defects Foundation
MDBSS Mischell-Dutton balanced salt solution
MDC minimum detectable concentration
monodansyl cadaverine
MDCEF Medical-Dental Committee on Evaluation of Fluroidation
MDCK Madin-Darby canine kidney
MDD major depressive disorder
mean daily dose
mean day of death
Microseal drug delivery
M.D.D.
Doctor of Dental Medicine
MDDA Minnesota Differential Diagnosis of Aphasia
MDE major depressive episode
MDEBP mean daily erect blood pressure
MDF mean dominant frequency
myocardial depressant factor
MDGF macrophage-derived growth factor
MDH malate dehydrogenase (also MD)
medullary dorsal horn
MDHM malate dehydrogenase, mitochondrial
MDHS malate dehydrogenase, soluble
MDHV Marek's disease herpesvirus
MDI diphenylmethane diisocyanate
metered dose inhaler
Multiscore Depression Inventory
MDIBL Mount Desert Island Biological Laboratory
MDIT mean disintegration time
MDM methyloldimethylhydantoin
mid-diastolic murmur
minor determinant mixture
MDMH monomethyloldimethylhydantoin

MDMP 2-(4-methyl-2,6-dinitroanilino)-N-methyl proprionamide
MDN methadinitrobene
MDNB mean daily nitrogen balance
MDP manic-depressive psychosis
maximum deliverable pressure
mentodextra posterior
methylene diphosphate
muramyl dipeptide
MDPI maximum daily permissible intake
MDQ memory deviation quotient
MDR median duration of response
minimum daily requirement
MDRH multidisciplinary rehabilitation hospital
MDS medical data screen
medical data system
multidimensional scaling
M.D.S.
Master of Dental Surgery
MDSBP mean daily supine blood pressure
MDT mast cell degeneration test
mean dissolution time
median detection threshold
mentodextra transversa
multidisciplinary team
MDTR mean diameter thichness ratio
MDUO myocardial disease of unknown origin
MDV Marek's disease virus
multiple dose vial
ME Mache Einkeit (also MU--Mache unit)
macular edema
magnitude estimation
male equivalent
malic enzyme
manic episode
median eminence
medical education
medical examination
Medical Examiner
meningoencephalitis
mercaptoethanol
metamyelocyte
methyleugenol
meticillin
microembolization
middle ear
muscle examination
M/E myeloid to erythroid ratio
ME_{50} 50 percent maximal effect
Me methyl
MEA mercaptoethylamine
multiple endocrine adenomatosis
MEA I multiple endocrine adenopathy, type I
MeB methylene blue
MEC mecillinam
median effective concentration
minimal effective concentration
myoepithelial cell
5-MeC 5-methylcytosine
MECCNU
semustine (methyl-1-(2-chloroethyl-3-4-methylcyclohexyl)-1-nitrosourea
MECT maximum extrapolated clotting time
MECTA mobile electroconvulsive therapy apparatus
MECY methyltrexate, cyclophosphamide
MED median erythrocyte diameter
minimal effective dose
minimal erythema dose
Med median (also M)
medical (also M)
medication
medicine
MEDICS
Medical Education Information and Career Service
Michael E. DeBakey International Cardiovascular Society
MEDLARS
Medical Literature Analysis and Retrieval System
MEDLINE
MEDLARS on-line
MEE methylethyl ether
middle ear effusion
MEF maximal expiratory flow
migration enhancement factor
mouse embryo fibroblast
MEF_{50} mean maximum expiratory flow
MEFR maximum expiratory flow rate
MEFV maximum expiratory flow volume
MEFVC maximum expiratory flow volume curve
mechanical expiratory flow volume curve
MEG magnetoencephalogram
megakaryocyte
mercaptoethylguanidine
Meg megacycle
MEGX monoethylglycine xylidide
3-MEH 3-methylhistidine
MEK methylethylketone
MEL murine erythroleukemia
MELI met-enkephalin-like immunoreactivity
MEM macrophage electrophoretic mobility
methyl-2-acetoxyethyl-2'-chloroethylamine
minimum essential medium
MEm mitochondrial malic enzyme
MEMA methyl methacrylate
MEMPP 4-methyl-2-(2-morpholinoethyl)-6-phenyl-3(2H)-pyridazinone
MEN methylethylnitrosamine
multiple endocrine neoplasia
MEND Medical Education for National Defense
MEO 3'-deamino-3-(4-methoxy-1-piperdinyl)-daunorubicin
malignant external otitis
MEOS microsomal ethanol oxidizing system
MEP maximal expiratory pressure
mean effective pressure
motor end-plate
Mep meperidine
MEPC miniature end-plate current
MEPP miniature end-plate potential
MePr methylprednisolone
mEq milliequivalent
MER mean ejection rate
mersalyl acid
methanol extraction residue
molar esterification rate
multimodality evoked response
MERB met-enkephalin receptor binding
MES maintenance electrolyte solution
maximal electroshock
maximal electroshock seizure
Medical Electronics Society
Metrazol-electroshock seizure
morpholino-ethane-sulfonic acid
muscle in elongated state
myoelectric signal
Mes mesencephalon
MESGN mesangial glomerulonephritis
MeSH Medical Subject Headings
MET metoprolol

midexpiratory time
oxygen consumption of 3.5 ml per kg per minute (metabolic equivalent)
Met metaramicol
methionine
MetHb methemoglobin
m et n
morning and night (mane et nocte)
m et sig
mix and label (misce et signa)
METT maximum exercise tolerance test
m et v
morning and evening (mane et vespere)
MEV maximal exercise ventilation
MeV million electron volts
MEX mexiletine
MF mass fragmentography
meat free
medium frequency
megafarad
melamine formaldehyde
methanol formaldehyde
methoxyflurane
microfibrile
microfilament
microfilia
microscopic factor
mitogenic factor
mossy fiber
multifactorial
multiplying factor
mycosis fungoides
myelin figure
myelofibrosis
myocardial fibrosis
M/F male to female ratio
M&F mother and father
mf microfilaria
millifarad
MFA multifunctional acrylic
MFAT multifocal atrial tachycardia
MFB medial forebrain bundle
metallic foreign body
MFC mean frequency of compensation
minimal fungicidal concentration
MFD Memory for Designs
midforceps delivery
milk-free diet
minimal fatal dose
mfd microfarad
MFG modified heat-degraded gelatin
MFH malignant fibrous histiocytoma
MF-IFGR
Michael Fund-International Foundation for Genetic Research
m flac
membranae tympani (membrana flaccida)
MFM millipore filter method
N-methyl-formimino-methylester
MFO mixed function oxidase
MFP melphalan, 5-fluorouracil, medroxyprogesterone acetate
monofluorophosphate
MFR mean flow rate
mucus flow rate
MFRL maximum force at rest length
MFS medical fee schedule
Merthiolate-formaldehyde solution
Minnesota Follow-up Study
MFT multifocal atrial tachycardia
muscle function test
m ft make a mixture (mistura fiat)
MFU medical follow-up
MFW multiple fragment wound
MG membraneous glomerulonephritis
mesiogingival
methyl glucoside
methylguanidine
minigastrin
monoclonal gammopathy
monoglyceride
mucigen granule
mucous granule
muscle group
myasthenia gravis (also MyG)
myoglobin
Mg magnesium
^{28}Mg radioactive isotope of magnesium
mg milligram
MGA medical gas analyzer
MGB medial geniculate body
mg-el milligram element
MGF macrophage growth factor
maternal grandfather
mother's grandfather
Myasthenia Gravis Foundation
MGG May-Gruenwald-Giemsa
mouse gamma globulin
MGGH methylglyoxal guanylhydrazone
mgh milligram hour
MGI macrophage and granulocyte inducer
MGM maternal grandmother
mother's grandmother
mgm See mg
MGN membranous glomerulonephritis
MGP marginated granulocyte pool
mucin glycoprotein
mucous glycoprotein
MGR modified gain ratio
multiple gas rebreathing
MGSA melanoma growth-stimulating activity
MGUS monoclonal gammopathy of undetermined significance
MH maleic hydrazide
malignant histiocytosis
malignant hyperthermia (or hyperpyrexia)
mammotropic hormone
mannoheptulose
marital history
medial hypothalamus
medical history
melanophore hormone
Mended Hearts
menstrual history
mental health
mercuri-hematoporphyrin
mutant hybrid
mylohyoid
Mh mandible head
mh millihenry
MHA Mental Health Association
methemalbumin
microangiopathic hemolytic anemia
microhemagglutination
middle hepatic artery
mixed hemadsorption assay
Mueller-Hinton agar
MHA-TP
microhemagglutination-Treponema pallidum
MHB maximum hospital benefit
m-hydroxybenzoate
MHb medial habenular

methemoglobin
myohemoglobin

MHC major histocompatibility complex
mental health clinic
multiphasic health check-up

MHD maintenance hemodialysis
mean hemolytic dose
minimum hemolytic dose

MHDPS Mental Health Demographic Profile System

MHEC multiphasic health examination clinic

MHFB Mental Health Film Board

m Hg millimeters of mercury

MHI malignant histiocytosis of the intestine

MHIFM Milton Helpern Institute of Forensic Medicine

MHIP methoxyphenoxy-hydroxy-isopropylaminopropane

MHMC Mental Health Materials Center

MHN massive hepatic necrosis

MHNTG multiheteronodular toxic goiter

MHO microsomal heme oxygenase

MHP maternal health program
mecurihydroxypropane

MHPA mild hyperphenylalaninemia
Minnesota-Hartford Personality Assay

MHPG 3-methoxy-4-hydroxyphenylethyleneglycol

MHR major histocompatibility region
maximal heart rate
methemoglobin reductase

MHSA microaggregated human serum albumin

MHT multiphasic health testing

MHTI minor hypertensive infant

MHV minimal height velocity
mouse hepetitis virus

MHV_3 mouse hepetitis virus 3

MHz megahertz

MI maturation index
mental illness
mercaptoimidazole
metaproterenol inhaler
methyl indole
migration index
mikamycin
mild irritant
mitotic index
mitral incompetance
mitral insufficiency
mononucleosis infectiosa
morphologic index
motility index
myocardial infarction
myocardial ischemia
myoinositol

Mi mitomycin

MIA medically indigent adult

MIAA microaggregated albumin

MIAP modified innervated antral pouch

MIBG meta-iodobenzylguanidine

MIBK methyl isobutyl ketone

MIBT methylisatin-beta-thiosemicarbasone

MIC maternal and infant care
methacholine inhalation challenge
minimal isorrheic concentration
minimum inhibitory concentration

mic pan
bread crumb (mica panis)

MICR methacholine inhalation challenge response

MICU medical intensive care unit
mobile intensive care unit

MID maximum inhibiting dilution
mesioincisodistal
midazolam
minimal infecting dose
minimum inhibitory dilution
minimum irradiation dose
multiinfarct dementia
multiple ion detection

MIE methylisoeugenol

MIF macrophage inhibiting factor
melanocyte inhibiting factor
methylene-iodine-formalin
micro-immunofluorescence
migration inhibiting factor
mixed immunofluorescence
mullerian inhibiting factor

MIFR maximal inspiratory flow rate

MIFT Merthiolate iodine formaldehyde technique

MIG measles immune globulin

MIGW maximum increment in growth and weight

MIH methylhydrazine methyl isopropylbenzamide
minimal intermittent dosage of heparin
monoiodohistidine

mil milliliter (also ml)

MILP mitogen-induced lymphocyte proliferation

MIME mean indices of meal excursions

Min minim (also m)
minimal

min minute (also m)

MIO minimum identifiable odor

MIP maximun inspiratory pressure

MIPI Medicine in the Public Interest

MIRD medical internal radiation dose

MIRF macrophage immunogenic antigen recruiting factor
Myopia International Research Foundation

MIRU myocardial infarction research unit

MIS mullerian inhibiting substance

MISG modified immune serum globulin

MISIP Minority Institutions Science Improvement Program

MISS Modified Injury Severity Scale

MISSGP
mercury in Silastic strain gauge plethysmography

mist mixture (mistura) (also m)

MIT Male Impotence Test
marrow iron turnover
melodic intonation therapy
metabolism inhibition test
miracidial immobilization test
monoiodotyrosine

mit send (mitte)

mitt sang
bleed (mitte sanguinem)

mitt tal
send such (mitte tales)

MIU milli-international unit

MIX 3-isobutyl-1-methylxanthine

MJ marijuana
megajoule

MJA mechanical joint apparatus

MJT Meade Johnson tube
Mowlem-Jackson technique

MK main kitchen
menaquinone (also MQ)
monkey kidney

MK-6 vitamin K_2

MK-7 vitamin K_2(35)
mkg meter-kilogram
mks meter-kilogram-second
MKSAP Medical Knowledge Self-Assessment Program
MKTC monkey kidney tissue culture
MKV killed measles vaccine
ML marked latency
maximal left
meningeal leukemia
mesiolingual
middle lobe
midline
molecular layer
motor latency
muscular layer
M.L. Licentiate in Medicine
M/L monocyte to lymphocyte ratio
mother-in-law
mL millilambert
ml milliliter (also mil)
MLA Medical Library Association
medium long-acting
mentolaeva anterior
mesiolabial
monocytic leukemia, acute
multilanguage aphasia
MLAI mesiolabialincisal
MLAP mean left atrial pressure
MLB monaural loudness balance
MLb macrolymphoblast
MLBP mechanical low back pain
MLC Marginal Line Calculus
minimum lethal concentration
mixed leukocyte concentration
mixed leukocyte culture
mixed lymphocyte concentration
mixed lymphocyte culture
multilamellar cytosome
myelomonocytic leukemia, chronic
MLCW mixed lymphocyte culture, weak
MLD masking level difference
median lethal dose
metachromatic leukodystrophy
minimum lethal dose
MLD_{50} median lethal dose
MLF medial longitudinal fasciculus
MLI mesiolinguoincisal
motilin-like immunoreactivity
MLL malignant lymphoma, lymphoblastic type
MLN mesenteric lymph node
MLNS mucocutaneous lymph node syndrome
MLO mesiolinguo-occlusal
MLP Mayo Lung Project
mentolaeva posterior
mesiolinguopulpal
MLR mean length of response
middle latency response
mixed leukocyte reaction
mixed leukocyte response
mixed lymphocyte reaction
mixed lymphocyte response
MLS macrolide-lincosamide-streptogramin B
mean life-span
median life-span
median longitudinal section
myelomonocytic leukemia, subacute
Mls minor histocompatibility locus
MLT median lethal time
medical laboratory technician
mentolaeva transversa
MLTC mixed leukocyte-trophoblast culture
MLTI mixed lymphocyte target interaction
MLU mean length of utterance
MLV Moloney's leukomogenic virus
monitored live voice
mouse leukemia virus
murine leukemia virus
MM macromolecule
malignant melanoma
manubrium of the malleus
Marshall-Marchetti
medial malleolus
megamitochondria
meningococcic meningitis
methadone maintenance
methenamine mandelate
methyacryl methylate
middle molecule
milk, molasses
missmatch
morbidity, mortality
mucous membrane
Muller maneuver
multiple myeloma
muscularis mucosa
myeloid metaplasia
Mm mandible mentum
mM millimole
mm millimeter
muscles
mm^2 square millimeter
mm^3 cubic millimeter (also cmm, cu mm)
MMA methylmalonic acid
methylmercuric acetate
methyl methacrylate
MMAD mass median aerodynamic diameter
MMC migrating motor complex
migrating myoelectric complex
minimum medullary concentration
mitomycin C (also MC)
MMD methyl mercury dicyanimide
minimum morbidostatic dose
myotonic muscular dystrophy
MMDA methyoxymethylene dioxyamphetamine
MME mouse mammary epithelium
MMECT multiple monitored electroconvulsive treatment
M.Med Master of Medicine
MMEF maximum midexpiratory flow
MMEFR See MMFR
MMF magnetomotive force
mean maximum flow
MMFG mouse milk fat globule
MMFR maximum midexpiratory flow rate
MMFV maximum midexpiratory flow volume
MMH monomethylhydrazine
MMI macrophage migration index
methylmercaptoimidazole
MMIS Medicaid Management Information System
MMK Marshall-Marchetti-Krantz
MML myelomonocytic leukemia
MMM myelofibrosis with myeloid metaplasia
myelosclerosis with myeloid metaplasia
mmm micromillimeter
millimicron
MMMF man-made mineral fiber
MMOA maxillary and mandibular odontectomy and alveolectomy
mmol millimole
MMPG 3-methoxy-4-hydroxyphenylglycol
MMPI Minnesota Multiphasic Personality Inventory
mmpp millimeters partial pressure

MMPR 6-methylthio-9-B-d-ribofuranosyl-9H-purine
MMPT monomethylphenyltriazene
MMR mass miniature radiography
measles-mumps-rubella
mobile mass x-ray
monomethylolrutin
myocardial metabolic rate
MMS methyl methane sulfonate
M.M.S.
Master of Medical Science
MMSA Medical Mycological Society of the Americas
M.M.S.A.
Master of Midwifery of the Society of Apothecaries
MMSE mini-mental state examination
MMSEL mini-mental state examination, language
MMT alpha-methyl-m-tyrosine
methoxymethyltrioxsalen
manual muscle test
mouse mammary tumor
MMTP Methadone Maintenance Treatment Program
MMTV mouse mammary tumor virus
MMU mercaptomethyl uracil
mmu millimass unit
MMWR Morbidity and Mortality Weekly Report
MN malignant nephrosclerosis
medulla neuropil
membranous nephropathy
mesenteric node
modiolus nucleus
mononuclear
motor neuron
mucosal neurolysis
multinodular
myoneural
M.N. Master in Nursing
M/N midnight
M&N morning and night
Mn manganese
^{52}Mn radioactive isotope of manganese
^{53}Mn radioactive isotope of manganese
^{54}Mn radioactive isotope of manganese
^{56}Mn radioactive isotope of manganese
mN millinormal
MNA maximum noise area
MNAP mixed nerve action potential
MNC mononuclear cell
MNCV motor nerve conduction velocity
MND minimum necrosing dose
motor neuron disease
MNL maximum number of lamellae
mononuclear leukocyte
MNMK maximum number of microbes killed
MNNG N-methyl-N^{1}-nitro-N-nitrosoguanidine
MNO minocycline
MNP mononuclear phagocyte
MNPA methoxy-naphthyl proprionic acid
MNSER mean normalized systolic ejection rate
MNU methylnitrosourea
MNWLT Modified New World Learning Test
MNZ metronidazole
MO manual of operation
medical office
mesio-occlusal
mineral oil
minute output
monooxygenase
morbidly obese
sulfamethoxine
MO_2 myocardial oxygen consumption
Mo mode
molybdenum
^{99}Mo radioactive isotope of molybdenum
mO See mOsm
mo month (also M)
MOA mechanism of action
MOCA 4,4'-methylene-bis-(2-chloroaniline)
MoCM molybdenum-conditioned medium
MOD maturity-onset diabetes (see also MODM)
mesio-occlusodistal
mod moderate
MODM maturity-onset diabetes mellitus (see also MOD)
mod praesc
as prescribed (modo praescripto)
MODS Medically Oriented Data System
MODY maturity onset diabetes of the young
MOF marine oxidation/fermentation
methoxyflurane
MOH Medical Officer of Health
MOI maximun oxygen intake
MOL molecular layer
mol mole (also M)
molecule
molc molar concentration (also M)
moll soft (mollis)
mol wt
molecular weight (also MW)
MOM milk of magnesia
mucoid otitis media
MOMA methoxyhydroxymandelic acid
Mono monocyte (also M)
mononucleosis
MOP major organ profile
methotrexate, vincristine (Oncovin), prednisone
8-MOP 8-methoxypsoralen (also 8-MP)
MOPEG 3-methoxy-4-hydroxyphenylethylene glycol
MOPP mechlorethamine, vincristine (Oncovin), procarbazine, prednisone (also MVPP)
MOPV monovalent oral poliovirus vaccine
MORA mandibular orthopedic repositioning appliance
MORC Medical Officers Reserve Corps
mor dict
as directed (moro dicto)
mor sol
in the usual way (moro solito)
MOS myelofibrosis osteosclerosis
mOsm milliosmole
MOT mini-object test
MOVC membraneous obstruction of vena cava
MOVE medically oriented vocational education
MOX moxalactam
MP macrophage
mean pressure
medial plantar
melting point
membrane potential
menstrual period
mentum posterior
mesiopulpal
metacarpophalangeal (also MCP)
metatarsophalangeal
3-methyl-pentane
methylprednisolone
modulator protein
monophosphate
mouthpiece
mouth pressure

mucopolysaccharide
multiparous
muscle potential
myenteric plexus
6-MP 6-mercaptopurine
8-MP 8-methoxypsoralen (also 8-MOP)
mp early in the morning (mane primo)
MPA main pulmonary artery
medial preoptic area
medroxyprogesterone acetate
methylprednisolone acetate
minor physical anomaly
mycophenolic acid
MPa megapascal
MPAP mean pulmonary arterial pressure
MPB male pattern baldness
MPC marine protein concentrate
maximum permissible concentration
meperidine, promethazine, chlorpromazine
minimum mycoplasmacidal concentration
minimum protozoacidal concentration
myeloblast-promyelocyte compartment
MPCC 2-(2-methyl-4-chlorophenoxy) propionic acid
MPCD minimum perceptible color difference
MPCN microscopically positive, culturally negative
MPCUR maximum permissible concentration of unidentified radionuclides
MPD main pancreatic duct
maximum permissible dose
minimal papular dose
minimal phototoxic dose
minimum perceptible difference
minimum port diameter
Minnesota Percepto-Diagnostic
multiplanar display
myeloproliferative disorder
MPDS myofascial pain dysfunction syndrome
MPDT Minnesota Percepto-Diagnostic test
MPDW mean percent desirable weight
MPE maximal possible effect
methidiumpropyl ethylenediaminetetra-acetic acid
MPEC monopolar electrocoagulation
MPED minimal phototoxic erythema dose
MPEH methylphenylethylhydantoin
MPF maturation promoting factor
Medical Passport Foundation
MPFM mini-Wright peak flow meter
MPG magnetopneumography
MPGN membranoproliferative glomerulonephritis
MPH male pseudohermaphrodite
M.P.H.
Master of Public Health
mph miles per hour
M.Pharm.
Master in Pharmacy
MPhysA
Member of the Physiotherapist Association
MPI mannose phosphate isomerase
Maudsley Personality Inventory
maximum point of impulse
Multiphasic Personality Inventory
Multivariate Personality Inventory
MPIDP Medical Practice Information Demonstration Project
MPJ metacarpophalangeal joint
metatarsophalangeal joint
MPL maximum permissible level
mesiopulpolabial
mesiopulpolingual
MPM medial pterygoid muscle
multiple primary malignancy
MPMP methylpiperidyl methylphenothiazine
MPMT Murphy-Punch Manoeuver Test
MPMV Mason-Pfizer monkey virus
MPN most probable number
MPO maximum power output
myeloperoxidase
MPOA medial preoptic area
MPOS myeloperoxidase system
MPP massive periretinal proliferation
maximum perfusion pressure
medial pterygoid plate
mercaptopyrazidopyrimidine
MPPG microphotoelectric plethysmography
MPPP 1-methyl-4-phenyl-4-propinonoxy piperidine
MPPT methylprednisolone pulse therapy
MPQ McGill Pain Questionnaire
MPR massive preretinal retraction
maximum pulse rate
MPRC Metropolitan Peer Review Council
MPRE minimum pure radium equivalent
MPS Member of the Pharmaceutical Society of Great Britain
methylprednisolone
mononuclear phagocyte system
movement-produced stimulus
mucopolysaccharide
mucopolysaccharidosis
multiphasic screening
MPS I...VI
mucopolysaccharidosis I through VI
MPSI Mental Process Short Inventory
MPSRT matched pairs signed rank test
MPT alpha-methyl-p-tyrosine
maximum predicted phonation time
MPTAH Mallory's phosphotungstic acid hematoxylin
MPTP 1-methyl-4-phenyl-1,2,5,6-tetrahydropyridine
MPU Medical Practitioner's Union
MPV mean platelet volume
MQ memory quotient
menaquinone (also MK)
MQC microbiologic quality control
MR mandibular reflex
mannose-resistant
maximal right
may repeat
medial rectus
median raphe
medical rehabilitation
medication responder
medium range
menstrual regulation
mentally retarded
mental retardation
mesencephalic raphe
metabolic rate
methemoglobin reductase
methyl red
milk ring
mitral reflux
mitral regurgitation
mortality rate
mortality ratio
multicentric reticulohistiocytosis
multiplication rate

multiplicity reactivation
myotatic reflex
Mr mandible ramus
M_r molecular weight ratio
mr milliroentgen
MRA main renal artery
Medical Record Administrator
multivariate regression analysis
MRACP Member of the Royal Australasian College of Physicians
M.Rad.
Master of Radiology
mrad millirad
MRAP maximal resting anal pressure
mean right atrial pressure
MRAS mean renal artery stenosis
Member of the Royal Academy of Sciences
MRBC monkey red blood cell
MRC Medical Research Council
Medical Reserve Corps
methylrosaniline chloride
MRCGP Member of the Royal College of General Practitioners
MRCOG Member of the Royal College of Obstetricians and Gynecologists
MRCP Member of the Royal College of Physicians
MRCPE Member of the Royal College of Physicians of Edinburgh
MRCPI Member of the Royal College of Physicians of Ireland
MRCS Member of the Royal College of Surgeons
MRCSE Member of the Royal College of Surgeons of Edinburgh
MRCSI Member of the Royal College of Surgeons of Ireland
MRCVS Member of the Royal College of Veterinary Surgeons
MRD 3'-deamino-3'(4-morhobinyl) daunorubicin
method of rapid determination
minimal reacting dose
minimal renal disease
mrd millirutherford
MRE maximun risk estimate
mrem millirem
MRF medical record form
melanocyte releasing factor
mesencephalic reticular formation
midbrain reticular formation
mitral regurgitation flow
moderate renal failure
monoclonal rheumatoid factor
mullerian regression factor
mRF monoclonal rheumatoid factor
MRFC mouse rosette-forming cells
MRFIT Multiple Risk Factor Intervention Trial
MRHA mannose-resistant hemagglutination
MRHT modified rhyme hearing test (see also MRT)
MRI Mental Research Institute
MRIH melanocyte hormone-release inhibiting factor
MRL Medical Record Librarian
MRM modified radical mastectomy
MRN malignant renal neoplasm
mRNA messenger ribonucleic acid
MRO muscle receptor organ
MRP maximum reimbursement point
mean resting potential
MRPAH mixed reverse passive antiglobulin hemagglutination
MRR maximal relaxation rate
MRS mania rating scale
median range score
MRSA methicillin-resistant Staphylococcus aureus
MRSH Member of the Royal Society for the Promotion of Health
MRT major role therapy
mean residence time
median recognition threshold
median relapse time
medical records technology
milk ring test
modified rhyme test (see also MRHT)
MRU measure of resource use
minimal reproductive unit
MRUS maximun rate of urea synthesis
MRVP mean right ventricular pressure
methyl red, Voges-Proskauer
MRW Metropolitan Relative Weight
MS main scale
mannose-sensitive
mass spectrometry
mean score
menopause syndrome
mental status
metaproterenol sulfate
methyl sternol
Mikulicz syndrome
mitral stenosis
modal sensitivity
molar solution
morphine sulfate
multilaminated structure
multiple sclerosis
muscle shortening
muscle strength
musculoskeletal
M.S. Master of Science (also M.Sc.)
Master of Surgery
Ms masrium
ms millisecond (also msec)
MSA major serologic antigen
mannitol salt agar
Medical Services Administration
membrane-stabilizing activity
mine safety appliance
mouse serum albumin
multichannel signed averager
Multidimensional Scalogram Analysis
multiplication stimulating activity
MSAP mean systemic arterial pressure
MSAT Medical School Aptitude Test
MSB Martius scarlet blue
mid-small bowel
MSC multiple sib case
M.Sc. Master of Science (also M.S.)
MSCLC mouse stem cell-like cell
MSCP mean spherical candle power
MSCU medical special care unit
MSD mild sickle cell disease
M.S.D.
Master of Science in Dentistry
MSE mental status examination
msec millisecond (also ms)
MSER mean systolic ejection rate
Mental Status Examination Record
MSF macrophage slowing factor
Mediterranean spotted fever
migration stimulating factor
modified sham feeding
MSG monosodium glutamate

MSH medical self-help
melanocyte-stimulating hormone
melanophore-stimulating hormone
MSHA mannose-sensitive hemagglutination
MSHIF melanocyte-stimulating hormone-inhibiting factor
MSHRF melanocyte-stimulating hormone-releasing factor
MSK medullary sponge kidney
MSKP Medical School Knowledge Profile
MSL midsternal line
multiple symmetric lipomatosis
MSLA mouse-specific lymphocyte antigen
MSLES Medical School Learning Environment Survey
MSLR mixed skin cell leukocyte reaction
MSN medial septal nucleus
mildly subnormal
M.S.N.
Master of Science in Nursing
MSO methionine sulfoximine
M.S.P.H.
Master of Science in Public Health
MSQ Mental Status Questionnaire
MSR mitral steno-regurgitation
monosynaptic reflex
MSRPP multidimensional scale for rating psychiatric patients
MSRT Minnesota Spatial Relations Test
MSS medical social service
Medical Superintendents' Society
Mental Status Schedule
Metabolic Support Service
minor surgery suite
mucous-stimulating substance
multiple sclerosis susceptibility
MSSST Meeting Street School Screening Test
MST mean (or median) survival time
$MsTh_1$ mesothorium-1
$MsTh_2$ mesothorium-2
MSU midstream urine
monosodium urate
myocardial substrate uptake
MSUD maple syrup urine disease
MSUM monosodium urate monohydrate
MSUSM Medical Society of the United States and Mexico
MSV mean scale value
Moloney sarcoma virus
murine sarcoma virus
MSVC maximal sustained ventilatory capacity
MSVL maximal spatial vector to the left
MSW medical social worker
multiple stab wounds
M.S.W.
Master of Social Work
MSX L-methionine-D,L-sulfoximine
MT malignant teratoma
mammary tumor
mastoid tip
maximal therapy
medial thalamus
medial thickness
medical technologist
medical treatment
melatonin
membrane thickness
membrana tympani
mesangial thickening
metallothionein
metatarsal
methyltyrosine
microtuble
midtrachea
muscle test
music therapy
sulfamethomidine
M/T myringotomy with tubes inserted
5-MT 5-methoxytryptamine
MTA mammary tumor agent
myoclonic twitch activity
MTAC mass transfer-area coefficient
MTAL medullary thick ascending limb
MTB Mycobacterium tuberculosis
MTBE methyl-tert butyl ether
MTC Make Today Count
mass transfer coefficient
medullary thyroid carcinoma
metoclopramide
MTCA 2-methylthiozolidine-r-carboxylic acid
MTD maximum tolerated dose
membrane tympani dextra
metastatic trophoblastic disease
multiple tic disorder
Munroe tidal drainage
mtd send such doses (mitte tales doses)
MTDDA Minnesota Test for the Differential Diagnosis of Aphasia
mtDNA mitochondrial deoxyribonucleic acid
MTDT modified tone decay test
MTE medical toxic environment
MTET modified treadmill exercise testing
MTF maximum terminal flow
modulation transfer factor
modulation transfer function
MTg mouse thyroglobulin
MTHF methyltetrahydrofolic acid
2-MTHF
2-methyltetrahydrofuran
MTI malignant teratoma intermediate
minimum time interval
MTLP metabolic toxemia of late pregnancy
MTM modified Thayer-Martin
MTO 3-O-methyldopa (also OMD)
MTP maximum tolerated pressure
medial tibial plateau
metatarsophalangeal
MTPJ metatarsophalangeal joint
MTQ methaqualone
MTR Meinicke turbidity reaction
metronidazole
monosyllabic, trocher, spondee
Registered Music Therapist
MTS membrana tympani sinestra
monosyllabic, trochee, spondee
MTT 3-(4-5-dimethyl-2 thiazolyl)-2,5-diphenyl-2H-tetrazolium bromide
malignant teratoma trophoblastic
maximal treadmill testing
mean transit time
monotetrazolium
MTU malignant teratoma undifferentiated
methylthiouracil
MTV mammary tumor virus
MTX methotrexate
MU Mache unit
maternal uncle
Montevideo unit
mouse unit
4-MU 4-methylumbelliferone
mU milliunit
mu micron
MUA middle uterine artery
multiple unit activity

MUAP motor unit action potential
MUC maximum urinary concentration
muc mucilage
MUD minimal urticarial dose
MUGA multiple gated image acquisition analysis
MUGB 4-methylumbelliferyl-guanidinobenzoate
MuLV murine leukemia virus
MuMTV murine mammary tumor virus
MUO myocardiopathy of unknown origin
MUP maximal urethral pressure
motor unit potential
MURD 5-mercapto, 2-deoxyuridine
MUST medical unit self-contained and transportable
MUU mouse uterine unit
MUW mouse uterine weight
MV measles virus
mechanical ventilation
megavolt
microvillus
minute ventilation
minute volume
mitral valve
mixed venous
multivesicular
M.V. veterinary physician (Medicus Veterinarius)
2-MV 2-methylvalerate
Mv mendelevium
mv millivolt
MVA mechanical ventricular assistance
mitral valve area
modified vaccinia virus, Ankara
motor vehicle accident
moving vehicle accident
MVB multivescicular body
MVC maximum voluntary contraction
MVD Marburg virus disease
mitral valve disease
mouse vas deferens
multivessel disease
MVE mitral valve leaflet excursion
Murray Valley encephalitis
MVH massive variceal hemorrhage
MVI multivalvular involvement
multivitamin infusion
MVII Minnesota Vocational Interest Inventory
MVM microvillus membrane
MVN medial ventromedial nucleus
MVO maximum venous outflow
MVO_2 maximum oxygen consumption
myocardial oxygen consumption
mVO_2 minute oxygen consumption
MVOS mixed venous oxygen saturation
MVP microvascular pressure
mitral valve prolapse
MVPP mustine, vincristine, procarbazine, prednisone (also MOPP)
MVPS mitral valve prolapse syndrome
MVR massive vitreous retraction
mitral valve replacement
multiple valve replacement
MVV maximum voluntary ventilation
MW mean weight
microwave
molecular weight (also M)
Munich Wistar
mw milliwatt
MWCB manufacturer's working cell bank
MWIA Medical Women's International Association
MWLT Modified Word Learning Test
MWMT Monotic Word Memory Test
MWPC multiwire proportional chamber
Mx Medex
My myopia
myxedematous
my mayer
Myco See M (Mycobacterium)
MYD myotonic dystrophy
myel myelin
MyG myasthenia gravis (also MG)
Myg myriagram
Myl myrialiter
Mym myriameter
MZ mezlocillin
monozygotic
MZA monozygotic twins reared apart
MZT monozygotic twins reared together

N

N index of refraction
nasal
Necator
negative (also neg)
Negro
Neisseria
neomycin
nerve
neurology
Neurospora
newton
Nitrobacter
nitrogen
Nocardia
node
noon
normal (also Nl)
nucleoside
nucleus (also Nu)
number
NI...NXII
cranial nerves 1 through 12
^{15}N radioactive isotope of nitrogen
n born (natus)
haploid
nano
night
unit of neutron dosage
2n diploid
3n triploid
4n tetraploid
NA nalidixic acid
Narcotics Anonymous
native American
neuraminidase
neurologic age
neutralizing antibody
nicotinamide
nitric acid
Nomina Anatomica
nonadherent
nonalcoholic
nonanionic
nonmyelinated axon
noradrenaline
not admitted

not antagonized
not applicable
not attempted
not available
nuclear antibody
nucleic acid
nucleus accumbens
numeric aperture
nurse's aide
nursing action

Na sodium (natrium)

^{22}Na radioactive isotope of sodium

^{24}Na radioactive isotope of sodium

NAA N-acetyl-L-aspartate
naphthaleneacetic acid
neutron activation analysis
nicotinic acid amide
no apparent abnormalities

NAACLS National Association of American Clinical Laboratory Services

NAACOG Nurses Association of the American College of Obstetricians and Gynecologists

NAALBWV National Association for the Advancement of Leboyer's Birth Without Violence

NAAMM North American Academy of Manipulative Medicine

NAANAD National Association of Anorexia Nervosa and Associated Disorders

NAAP N-acetyl-4-aminophenazone
National Association for Accreditation in Psychoanalysis

NAAPABAC National Association for the Advancement of Psychoanalysis and the American Boards for Accreditation and Certification

NAB novarsenobenzol

NABP National Association of Boards of Pharmacy

NABS National Alliance of Blind Students

NAC N-acetylcysteine
National Accreditation Council
National Asthma Center
National Audiovisual Center
nitrogen mustard, doxorubicin (Adriamycin), lomustine (CCNU)
nonadherent cell

NACC Narcotic Addicition Control Commission
National Advisory Cancer Council

NACDG North American Contact Dermatitis Group

NACDS North American Clinical Dermatological Society

NACEHC National Accreditation Council for Environmental Health Curricula

NACHC National Association of Community Health Centers

NACHM National Advisory Commission of Health Manpower

NACHO National Association of County Health Officials

NACHRI National Association of Children's Hospitals and Related Institutions

NACMC National Association of Christian Marriage Counselors

NACOR National Advisory Committee on Radiation

NAD National Association of the Deaf
nicotinamide-adenine dinucleotide
nicotinic acid dehydrogenase
no acute distress
no appreciable disease
normal axis deviation
nothing abnormal detected

NAD+ oxidized nicotinamide-adenine dinucleotide

NADA National Association of Dental Assistants

NADC National Animal Disease Center

NADE National Association of Disability Examiners

NADG nicotinamide-adenine dinucleotide glycohydrolase

NADH reduced nicotinamide-adenine dinucleotide

NADH-TR nicotinamide-adenine dinucleotide-tetrazolium reductase

NADL National Association of Dental Laboratories

NADP nicotinamide-adenine dinucleotide phosphate (also TPN)

NADP+ oxidized nicotinamide-adenine dinucleotide phosphate

NADPH reduced nicotinamide-adenine dinucleotide phosphate

NAE net acid excretion

NaE exchangeable sodium

NAEC National Advisory Eye Council

NAEHCA National Association of Employers on Health Care Alternatives

NAEL National Association of Earmold Laboratories

NAEMT National Association of Emergency Medical Technicians

NAF nafcillin
National Abortion Federation
National Association for the Feeble-Minded
National Ataxia Foundation
normal auditory reflex

NAFPD National Association of Family Planning Doctors

NAFV National Association of Federal Veterinarians

NAG N-acetylglucosamine (also GlcNAc)
N-acetylglutamate (also AGA)
nonagglutinating

NAGS N-acetylglutamate synthetase (also AGAS)

NAHC National Advisory Heart Council

NAHCS National Association of Health Career Schools

NAHD National Association for Hospital Development

NAHHA National Association of Home Health Agencies

NAHN National Association of Hispanic Nurses

NAHPMM National Association of Hospital Purchasing Materials Management

NAHSA National Association for Hearing and Speech Action

NAHSE National Association of Health Services Executives

NAI net acid input

neuraminidase inhibition
NAIRS National Athletic Injury/Illness Reporting System
NALP neuroadenolysis of the pituitary
NALSF National Amyotrophic Lateral Sclerosis Foundation
NALSI National Association of Life Science Industries
NAMCS National Ambulatory Medical Care Survey
NAME National Association of Medical Examiners
NAMH National Association for Mental Health
NAMI National Alliance for the Mentally Ill
NAMN nicotinic acid mononucleotide
NAMT National Association for Music Therapy
NAN N-acetylneuraminic acid (also NANA)
NANA N-acetylneuraminic acid (also NAN)
NANB non-A, non-B
NANHC National Association of Neighborhood Health Centers
NANM N-allylnormorphine
NANP National Association of Naturopathic Physicians
NANR National Association of Nurse Recruiters
NAO National Academy of Opticianry
NAOO National Association of Optometrists and Opticians
NAP nasion, point A, pogonion
nerve action potential
neutrophil alkaline phosphatase
Nomina Anatomica Parisiensia
nucleic acid phosphorus
NAPA N-acetyl-p-aminophenol
N-acetylprocainamide
NAPAP N-acetyl-p-aminophenol
NAPCC National Association for Poison Control Centers
NAPG sodium pregnanediolglucuronide
NAPHT National Association of Patients on Hemodialysis and Transplantation
NAPN National Association of Physicians' Nurses
NAPNAP
National Association of Pediatric Nurse Associates and Practitioners
NAPNES
National Association for Practical Nurse Education and Services
NAPPH National Association of Private Psychiatric Hospitals
NAPT National Association of Physical Therapists
National Association for the Prevention of Tuberculosis
NAQAP National Association of Quality Assurance Professionals
NAR nasal airway resistance
National Amniocentesis Registry
NARC Narcotics Addiction Rehabilitation Center
National Association for Retarded Citizens
NARD National Association of Retail Druggists
NARF National Association of Rehabilitation Facilities
NARI National Association of Residents and Interns
NARIC National Rehabilitation Information Center
NARS National Acupuncture Research Society
NART National Association of Recreational Therapists
NAS N-acetylserotonin
National Academy of Sciences
neonatal airleak syndrome
neuroallergic syndrome
no added salt (also NSA)
normalized alignment score
NASA National Aeronautics and Space Administration
North American Student Association
NASADAD
National Association of State Alcohol and Drug Abuse Directors
NASAHP
National Association of Schools of Allied Health Professions
NASAR National Association for Search and Rescue
NASCD National Association for Sickle Cell Disease
NASE National Association for the Study of Epilepsy
NASMHPD
National Association of State Mental Health Program Directors
NASMV National Association on Standard Medical Vocabulary
NAS-NRC
National Academy of Sciences, National Research Council
NASPE North American Society of Pacing and Electrophysiology
NASPG North American Society for Pediatric Gastroenterology
NASTPHV
National Association of State and Territorial Public Health Veterinarians
NASW National Association of Social Workers
NAT N-acetyltransferase
nonaccidental trauma
NATM sodium aurothiomalate
NAVA National Association for Veterinary Acupuncture
NAVPC National Association of Vision Program Consultants
NB nail bed
Negri bodies
nervi buccalis
newborn
nitrous oxide-barbiturate
note well (nota bene)
novobiocin
nutrient broth
N/B neopterin to biopterin ratio
Nb niobium
^{95}Nb radioactive isotope of niobium
NBA National Braille Association
NBAD N-beta-alanyldopamine
NBBP National Blood Bank Program
NBCCGA
National Bladder Cancer Collaborative Group A
NBCDL National Board for Certification of Dental Laboratories
NBCDT National Board for Certification in Dental Technology
NBCP National Bladder Cancer Project
NBD neurologic bladder dysfunction
no brain damage
NBE northern bean extract

NBEO National Board of Examiners in Optometry
NBEOPS
National Board of Examiners for Osteopathic Physicians and Surgeons
NBF not breast fed
NBI neutrophil bactericidal index
no bone injury
NBIE National Burn Information Exchange
NBM nothing by mouth (also NPO)
nucleus basalis of Meynert
NBME National Board of Medical Examiners
normal bone marrow extract
NBN narrow band noise
NBNA National Black Nurses Association
NBO nonbed occupancy
NBP National Braille Press
NBRA National Biomedical Research Association
NBRF National Biomedical Research Foundation
NBRP National Blood Resource Program
NBRT National Board for Respiratory Therapy
NBS National Bureau of Standards
N-bromosuccinimide
Neri-Barre syndrome
normal bowel sounds
normal brainstem
normal burro serum
NBT nitroblue tetrazolium
NBTE nonbacterial thrombotic endocarditis
NBTG nitrobenzylthioguanosine
NBTS National Blood Transfusion Service
NBW normal birth weight
NC nabothian cyst
nasal clearance
natural cytotoxicity
neonatal cholestasis
neurologic check
neurologic control
nevus comedonicus
nitrocellulose
nitrosocarbazole
no casualty
no change
noise criterion
noncirrhotic
noncontributory
normal control
normocephalic
noseclip
not classified
not cultured
Nurse Corps
N/C no complaints
nC nanocurie (also nCi)
NCA National Certification Agency for Medical Lab Personnel
National Clearinghouse on Alcoholism
National Council on Aging
National Council on Alcoholism
neurocirculatory asthenia
neutrophil chemotactic activity
nodulocystic acne
nonspecific cross-reacting antigen
NCALI National Clearinghouse for Alcohol Information
N-CAM nerve cell adhesion molecule
NcAMP nephrogenous cyclic adenosine monophosphate
NCAR National Center for Atmospheric Research
NCB Narcotic Control Board
NCC noncoronary cusp
nucleus caudalis centralis
NCCC National Cancer Cytology Center
NCCD National Council on Communicative Disorders
NCCDS National Cooperative Crohn's Disease Study
NCCEA Neurosensory Center Comprehensive Examination for Aphasia
NCCLS National Committee for Clinical Laboratory Standards
NCCLVP
National Coordinating Committee on Large Volume Parenterals
NCCMHC
National Council of Community Mental Health Centers
NCCMHS
National Consortium for Child Mental Health Services
NCCPA National Commission on Certification of Physician's Assistants
NCCSC National Cancer Chemotherapy Screening Center
NCD National Council on Drugs
nitrogen clearance delay
normal childhood disease
not considered disabling
NCDAI National Clearinghouse for Drug Abuse Information
NCDS National Cooperative Dialysis Study
NCDV Nebraska calf diarrhea virus
NCE new chemical entity
NCF National Cancer Foundation
neutrophil chemotactic factor
no cold fluids
NCFRF National Cystic Fibrosis Research Foundation
NCFS National College of Foot Surgeons
NCGL nucleus corporis geniculati lateralis
NCGS National Cooperative Gallstone Study
NCH National Center for Homoeopathy
NCHC National Council of Health Centers
NCHCT National Center for Health Care Technology
NCHLS National Council on Health Laboratory Services
NCHS National Center for Health Statistics
NCHSR National Center for Health Services Research
NCI National Cancer Institute
nucleus colliculi inferioris
nCi nanocurie (also nC)
NCL neuronal ceroid lypofuscinosis
NCMC natural cell-mediated cytotoxicity
NCMF National Capitol Medical Foundation
NCMH National Committee for Mental Hygiene
NCMI National Committee Against Mental Illness
NCN National Council of Nurses
NCNCA normochromic normocytic anemia
NCP National Caries Program
NCPCC National Clearinghouse for Poison Control Centers
NCPE noncardiogenic pulmonary edema
NCPG National Catholic Pharmacists Guild of the United States
NCPIE National Council on Patient Information and Education
NCQHC National Committee for Quality Health Care
NCR National Cancer Registry

National Committee for Research in Neurological and Communicative Disorders
neutrophil chemotactic response

NCRP National Council on Radiation Protection and Measurements

NCRSR National Congenital Rubella Syndrome Registry

NCS National Council of Stutterers
newborn calf serum
noncured sarcoidosis
noncurrent serum

NCSAB National Council of State Agencies for the Blind

NCT number connection test

NCTC National Collection of Type Cultures

NCTIP National Committee on the Treatment of Intractable Pain

NCTR National Center for Toxicological Research

NCV nerve conduction velocity
noncholera vibrios

NCWAS National Coal Workers' Autopsy Study

NCWTM National Council on Wholistic Therapeutics and Medicine

NCYC National Collection of Yeast Cultures

ND nasal deformity
nasolacrimal duct
neonatal death
neoplastic disease
neurotic depression
neutral density
Newcastle disease
nifedipine
no data
no disease
nondiabetic
nondisabling
normal delivery
normal deposition
not detectable
not detected
not determined
not done
nothing done
nucleus of Darkschewitsch
nurse's diagnosis

N_D refractive index

Nd neodymium
number of dissimilar

^{147}Nd radioactive isotope of neodymium

^{149}Nd radioactive isotope of neodymium

NDA National Dental Association
New Drug Application
no data available
no demonstrable antibodies

NDAB National Diabetes Advisory Board

NDBA N-nitrosodibutylamine

NDC National Drug Code
nuclear dehydrogenating Clostridia

NDCOP N-demethyl-chlordiazepoxide

NDDG National Diabetes Data Group

NDDR National Digestive Disease Foundation

NDE near death experience
nondiabetic extremity

NDEA N-nitrosodiethylamine

NDF neutral detergent fiber
neutrophil diffraction factor
new dosage form

NDGA nordihydroguaiaretic acid

NDI naphthalenediisocyanate
nephrogenic diabetes insipidus

NDMA N-nitrosodimethylamine
p-nitrosodimethyl aniline

NDP net dietary protein

NDPA N-nitrosodipropylamine

NDR neonatal death rate
normal detrusor reflex
nucleus dorsalis raphe

NDT noise detection threshold

NDTA National Dental Technicians Association

NDV Newcastle disease virus

NE necrotic enteritis
neomycin (also NM)
nerve ending
nerve excitability
neuroendocrine
neuroepithelium
neurologic examination
neutrophil elastase
never exposed
no effect
nonelastic
nonendogenous
norepinephrine
not enlarged
not evaluated
not examined
nutcracker esophagus

Ne neon

NEB neuroendocrine body

neb a spray (nebula)

NEC necrotizing enterocolitis
neuroendocrine cell
not elsewhere classified
not enough cells

NECA 5'-N-ethylcarboxamide

NED no evidence of disease

NEEP negative end-expiratory pressure

NEF Nurses' Educational Fund

NEFA nonesterified fatty acid

NEG neglect

neg negative

NEHA National Environmental Health Association

NEI National Eye Institute

NEISS National Electronic Injury Surveillance Systems

NEJ neuroeffector junction

NEM N-ethylmaleimide (also NEME)
no evidence of malignancy
nutritional milk unit (Nahrungs Einheit Milch)

NEMA National Eclectic Medical Association
National Electrical Manufacturers' Association

NEMD nonspecific esophageal motility disorder

NEME N-ethylmaleimide (also NEM)

NEP noise-equivalent power

NEPCC North East Pacific Culture Collection

NEPHGE nonequilibrium pH gradient gel electrophoresis

NERF National Eye Research Foundation

NERO noninvasive evaluation of radiation output

NESS national excess sodium syndrome

NET nasoendotracheal tube
netilmicin
norethisterone

NETEN norethisterone enanthate

n et m night and morning (nocte et mane)

ne tr s num
do not deliver unless paid (ne tradas sine nummo)

NEU N-ethylurea

neu neurilemma (also nu)

NEYA neomycin egg yolk agar

NF nafcillin
nasopharyngeal fibroma
National Formulary
National Foundation
nephritic factor
neurofibromatosis
neurofilament
neutral fraction
nitrofurantoin
nonfluent
nonfront
nonfunction
normal flow
not found
Nutrition Foundation
nylon fiber

N/F Negro female

NFA National Foundation for Asthma

NFB National Federation of the Blind
nonfermenting bacteria
Nonfunctional Behavior

NFCPG National Federation of Catholic Physicians Guilds

NFCR National Foundation for Cancer Research

NFD neurofibrillary degeneration

NFE nonferrous extract

NFIC National Foundation for Ileitis and Colitis

NFID National Foundation for Infectious Diseases

NFIP National Foundation for Infantile Paralysis

NFJGD National Foundation for Jewish Genetic Diseases

NFLPN National Federation of Licensed Practical Nurses

NFM northern fowl mite

NFME National Fund for Medical Education

NFMLP N-formyl-methionine-leucine-phenylalanine

NFP National Federation of Parents
natural family planning
19-nortestosterone furylpropionate

NFMP N-formyl-methionyl-phenylalanine

NFPOD National Foundation for the Prevention of Oral Disease

NFPRHA
National Family Planning and Reproductive Health Association

NFRM National Foundation for Research in Medicine

NFS nonfire setter

NFT neurofibrillary tangles

NFTA N-(4-(5-nitro-2-furyl)-2-thiozolyl)-acetamide

NFTD normal full-term delivery

NFZ 5-nitro-2-furaldehyde semicarbazone

NG nasogastric
nodose ganglion
no good
no growth
nongenetic
nongroupable

ng nonogram

NGA nutrient gelatin agar

NGC nucleus gigantocellularis

NGCND National Group for Classification of Nursing Diagnosis

NGCP National Guild of Catholic Psychiatrists

NGF National Genetics Foundation
nerve growth factor

NGI nuclear globulin inclusion

NGR narrow gauze roll

NGS National Geriatrics Society

NGT normal glucose tolerance

NGU nongonococcal urethritis

NH nodular histiocytic
nonhuman
nursing home

NH_2 nitrogen mustard (also NM)

$^{13}NH_3$ radioactive ammonia

NHA National Hearing Association
nonspecific hepatocellular abnormality

NHANES
National Health and Nutrition Examination Survey

NHAS National Hearing Aid Society

NHBPCC
National High Blood Pressure Coordinating Committee

NHBPEP
National High Blood Pressure Education Program

NHC National Health Council
neighborhood health center
neonatal hypocalcemia
nursing home care

NHDA National Huntington's Disease Association

NHF National Health Federation
National Hemophilia Foundation

NHHI Nursing Home Hearing Handicap Index

NHI National Health Insurance
National Heart Institute

NHIP National Health Insurance Plan

NHK normal human kidney

NHL nodular histiocytic lymphoma
non-Hodgkin's lymphoma

NHLBI National Heart, Lung, and Blood Institute

NHLI National Heart and Lung Institute

NHMRC National Health and Medical Research Council

NHO National Hospice Organization

NHP nonhemoglobin protein
normal human plasma
nursing home placement

NHPRO N-nitrosohydroxyproline

NHR net histocompatibility ratio

NHS National Health Service
normal horse serum
normal human serum

NHSC National Health Service Corps

NHSI New Haven Schizophrenia Index

NHTSA National Highway Traffic Safety Administration

NI neuraminidase inhibition
nitroxoline
no information
not identified
not isolated
nucleus intercalatus

Ni nickel

^{63}Ni radioactive isotope of nickel

^{65}Ni radioactive isotope of nickel

NIA National Institute of Allergy
National Institute on Aging

neutrophil-inducing activity
niacin
no information available
Nutrition Institute of America
NIAAA National Institute on Alcohol Abuse and Alcoholism
NIADDK National Institute of Arthritis, Diabetes and Digestive and Kidney Diseases
NIAID National Institute of Allergy and Infectious Diseases
NIAMD National Institute of Arthritis and Metabolic Disease
NIAMDD National Institute of Arthritis, Metabolism and Digestive Diseases
NIB National Industries for the Blind
noninvolved bone
NIBM National Institute of Burn Medicine
NIBS nearly ideal binary solvent
NIBSC National Institute for Biological Standards and Control
NIC Nomarsky interference contact
nurse interim care
NICEDD National Institute for Continuing Education in Developmental Disabilities
NICHD National Institute of Child Health and Human Development
NICHHD See NICHD
NICSH National Interagency Council on Smoking and Health
NICU neonatal intensive care unit
neurosurgical intensive care unit
nonimmunologic contact urticaria
NIDA National Institute on Drug Abuse
NIDD noninsulin-dependent diabetes
NIDDM noninsulin-dependent diabetes mellitus
NIDR National Institute of Dental Research
NIDS nonionic detergent soluble
NIEHS National Institute of Environmental Health Sciences
NIF neutrophil immobilizing factor
nifedipine
nifuroquine
nonintestinal fibroblast
NIGMS National Institute of General Medical Sciences
NIH National Institutes of Health
NIHL noise-induced hearing loss
NIHR National Institute of Handicapped Research
NIL noise interference level
nothing in light
NIMH National Institute of Mental Health
NINCDS National Institute of Neurological and Communicative Disorders and Stroke
NINDB National Institute of Neurological Diseases and Blindness
NINDS National Institute of Neurological Diseases and Stroke
NIOSH National Institute for Occupational Safety and Health
NIP nitroiodophenyl
NIPDWR National Primary Drinking Water Regulations
NIPP Nutrition Intervention Pilot Project
NIPS noninvolved psoriatic skin
NIPTS noise-induced permanent threshold shift
NISM bed nucleus of the stria medullaris
NIST bed nucleus of the stria terminalis
NIT 5'-nucleotidase
NITD noninsulin-treated disease
NITTS noise-induced temporary threshold shift
NJ nasojejunal
NJPC National Joint Practice Commission
NK natural killer
Nomenklatur Kommission
not known
N/K name not known
NKA no known allergies
NKC nonketotic coma
NKDA no known drug allergies
NKF National Kidney Foundation
NKH nonketotic hyperosmotic
NKHD nonketotic hyperglycemia
NKTS natural killer target structure
NL neural lobe
neutral lipids
nodular lymphoma
norlorcainide
normolipemic
Nl normal (also N)
nl nanoliter
NLA National Leukemia Association
neuroleptanalgesia
neuroleptanesthesia
normal lactase activity
NLAA naphthoxylactic acid
NLB needle liver biopsy
NLD necrobiosis lipoidica diabeticorum
NLDL normal low density lipoprotein
NLEF National Lupus Erythematosus Foundation
NLM National Library of Medicine
NLMC nocturnal leg muscle cramp
NLN National League for Nursing
NLP nodular liquefying panniculitis
no light perception
NLPD nodular lymphocytic, poorly differentiated
NLPNEF National Licensed Practical Nurses Educational Foundation
NLSD normal lifespan for dogs
NLT Names Learning Test
normal lymphocyte transfer
nucleus lateralis tuberis
NLX naloxone (also NX)
NM neomycin (also NE)
neuromuscular
nitrogen mustard (also NH_2)
nodular mixed
nonmalignant
nonmotile
normetanephrine (also NMN)
not measurable
not measured
not mentioned
nuclear medicine
N/M Negro male
nM nanomolar
nm nanometer
nutmeg (nux moschata)
NMA National Malarial Association
National Medical Association
National Midwives Association
neurogenic muscular atrophy
N-methyl aspartate
NMAC National Medical Audiovisual Center
NMBA nitrosomethylbenzylamine

NMC National Mastitis Council
National Medical Care
neuromuscular control
NMD N-methyl-D-aspartate (also NMDA)
NMDA National Medical and Dental Association
N-methyl-D-aspartate (also NMD)
NMEA N-nitrosomethylethylamine
nmEq millimicron equivalent
NMF National Medical Fellowships
National Migraine Foundation
NMHA National Mental Health Association
NMI no mental illness
no middle initial
NMJ neuromuscular junction
NML nodular mixed lymphoma
NMLN N-methyl levonantradol
NMN nicotinamide mononucleotide
N-methylnicotinamide
no middle name
normetanephrine (also NM)
NMNA National Male Nurse's Association
NMO nitrogen mustard N-oxide
nmol nanomole
NMOR N-nitrosomorpholine (also NOM)
NMP neutral metallopeptidase
normal menstrual period
NMR Neill-Mooser reaction
neonatal mortality rate
nuclear magnetic resonance
NMRI Naval Medical Research Institute
nuclear magnetic resonance imaging
NMS neuroleptic malignant syndrome
neuromuscular spindle
N-methyl scopolamine
normal mouse serum
NMSIDS
near miss sudden infant death syndrome
NMSS National Multiple Sclerosis Society
NMT neuromuscular transmission
N-methyltransferase
nuclear medicine technician
NMTD nonmetastatic trophoblastic disease
NMTS neuromuscular tension state
NMU neuromuscular unit
N-nitroso-N-methyluria
NMUT nitrosomethylurethane (see also NNNMU)
NMVA N-nitrosomethylvinylamine
NN normally nourished
nn nerves
NNC National Nutrition Consortium
National Nutrition Council
NND neonatal death
New and Nonofficial Drugs
NNDA N-nitrosodiethylamine
NNE neonatal necrotizing enterocolitis
NNFF National Neurofibromatosis Foundation
NNI noise and number index
NNICC National Narcotics Intelligence Consumers Committee
NNIS National Nosocomial Infection Study
NNM neonatal mortality
NNNMU N-nitroso-N-methylurethane (see also NMUT)
NNN Nicolle-Novy-MacNeal
nitrosonornicotine
n nov new name (nomen novum) (also nov n)
NNP neonatal nurse practitioner
NNPHW National New Professional Health Workers
NNR New and Nonofficial Remedies
NNT neonatally tolerant
nuclei nervi trigemini

NO none obtained
nonobese
No nobelium
number
NOA National Optometric Association
NOBT nonoperative biopsy technique
Noc nocturia
noc night (nocte)
noct maneq
at night and in the morning (nocte maneque)
NOD nonobese diabetic
NOF National Osteopathic Foundation
2-nitrosofluorene
NOGA National Osteopathic Guild Association
NOHA N-hydroxyamphetamine
NOK next of kin
NOM N-nitrosomorpholine (also NMOR)
NOMI nonocclusive mesenteric infarction
non rep
do not repeat (non repetatur) (also NR)
non repetat
See non rep
NOPHN National Organization for Public Health Nursing
NOPRI National Orthotic and Prosthetic Research Institute
NOR nucleolar organizing region
NORC National Opinion Research Center
NORGD National Organization for the Rights of Guide Dogs
NORML National Organization for the Reform of Marijuana Laws
NOS not otherwise specified
NOSAC nonsteroidal anti-inflammatory compound
NOSIE Nurses Observation Scale for Inpatient Evaluation
NOT nocturnal oxygen therapy
nucleus of the optic tract
NOTB National Ophthalmic Treatment Board
NOTT nocturnal oxygen therapy trial
Nov novobiocin
nov n new name (novum nomen) (also n nov)
nov sp
new species (novum species)
NOW negotiable order of withdrawal
NP nasopharyngeal
nasopharynx
near point
neuritic plaque
neuropathology
neurophysin
neuropsychiatry
neurotigenic protein
new patient
nifurprazine
nitrophenide
nitroprusside
nonpathologic
nonpaying
nonphagocytic
no phone
no progression
normal plasma
not performed
nucleoplasmic index
nucleoprotein
nucleoside phosphorylase
nurse practitioner
nursing practice
nursing procedure
2-NP 2-nitropropane

Np neper
neptunium
^{237}Np radioactive isotope of neptunium
NPA National Perinatal Association
National Pituitary Agency
N-n-propyl-norapomorphine
N-propylajmaline
nucleus of the pretectal area
NPa nail patella
NPAB N-propylajmaline bitartrate
NPAP National Psychological Association for Psychoanalysis
Np-AVP
vasopressin-associated neurophysin
NPB nodal premature beat
nonprotein bound
NPBF nonplacental blood flow
NPC nasopharyngeal cancer
nasopharyngeal carcinoma
near point of convergence
nucleus of the posterior commissure
NPCN National Poison Center Network
NPCNU neopentyl chloroethyl nitosourea
NPCP National Prostatic Cancer Project
NPD Niemann-Pick disease
nitrogen phosphorus detector
no pathologic diagnosis
NPDES National Pollutant Discharge Elimination System
NPDL nodular poorly differentiated lymphocytic lymphoma
NPE neurogenic pulmonary edema
neuropsychologic examination
NPF nasopharyngeal fiberscope
National Parkinson Foundation
National Pharmaceutical Foundation
National Psoriasis Foundation
no predisposing factor
NPG nonpregnant
NPGS neopentyl glycol succinate
NPH neutral protamine Hagedorn
normal pressure hydrocephalus
NPhA National Pharmaceutical Association
NPHI neutral protamine Hagedorn insulin
NPI National Psychiatric Institutes
Neonatal Perception Inventory
neuropsychiatric institute
NPIP N-nitrosopiperidine
NPL National Physicis Laboratory
NPN nonprotein nitrogen
N-phenyl-1-naphthylamine
NPO nothing by mouth (nulla per os) (also NBM)
NPO/HS
nothing by mouth at bedtime (nulla per os hora somni)
Np-OT oxytocin-associated neurophysin
NPP neuropsychologic performance
2-nitro-1-phenylpropane
NPPNG nonpenicillinase-producing Neisseria gonorrhoeae
NPR nucleoside phosphoribosyl
NPRO N-nitrosoproline
Nps nitrophenylsulfenyl
NPSA normal pilosebaceous apparatus
NPSH nonprotein sulfhydryl
NPT neoprecipitin test
nocturnal penile tumescence
normal pressure and temperature
NPU net protein utilization
NPV negative pressure ventilation
nuclear polyhedrosis virus
NPYR N-nitrosopyrrolidine
NQA nursing quality assurance
4NQO 4-nitroquinoline-1-oxide
NR do not repeat (non repetatur) (also non rep)
neutral red
noise reduction
nonreactive
nonrebreathing
nonreimbursable
no radiation
no reaction
no rehearsal
no response
normal range
not readable
not recorded
not reported
not resolved
nutritive ratio
NRA National Rehabilitation Association
nucleus raphe alatus
NRASF National Registry of Ambulatory Surgical Facilities
NRBC National Rare Blood Club
normal red blood cell
nucleated red blood cell
NRC National Regulatory Commission
noise reduction coefficient
normal retinal correspondence
Nuclear Regulatory Commission
NRCC National Registry in Clinical Chemistry
NRCCS National Research Council Committee on Salmonella
NRCL nonrenal clearance
NRD nonrenal death
NRDC National Resources Defense Council
NREH normal renin essential hypertension
NREM nonrapid eye movement
NREMS nonrapid eye movement sleep
NREMT National Registry of Emergency Medical Technicians
NRF normal renal function
NRFC nonrosette-forming cell
NRFF National Research Foundation for Fertility
NRH nodular regenerative hyperplasia
NRI National Rehabilitation Institute
neutral regular insulin
NRK normal rat kidney
NRM natural remanent magnetization
nucleus raphe magnus
NRMC Naval Regional Medical Center
NRMP National Resident Matching Program
NRMS National Registry of Medical Secretaries
nRNA nuclear ribonucleic acid
nRNP nuclear ribonucloprotein
NRPAT net patient revenue
NRPCA National Rural Primary Care Association
NRPF National Retinitis Pigmentosa Foundation
NRR net reproduction rate
Noise Reduction Rating
NRS nonimmunized rabbit serum
normal rabbit serum
normal reference serum
numerical rating scale
NRSF National Reye's Syndrome Foundation
NRTOT net total revenue
NS needle shower
nephrotic syndrome

nervous system
neurologic survey
neurosurgery
nonsmoker
nonsnorer
nonspecific
nonstutterer
nonsymptomatic
Noonan syndrome
normal saline (also N/S)
normal serum
normal smoking
normal study
Norwegian scabies
no sample
no sequelae
no specimen
not significant
not specified
not stated
not sufficient
nuclear sclerosis
nylon suture

N/S normal saline (also NS)
ns nanosecond (also nsec)
NSA Neurosurgical Society of America
normal serum albumin
no salt added (also NAS)
no serious abnormality
no significant abnormality
NSABP National Surgical Adjuvant Breast Project
NSAC National Society for Autistic Children
NSAE nonsupported arm exercise
NSAIA nonsteroidal anti-inflammatory agent
NSAID nonsteroidal anti-inflammatory drug
NSAR N-nitrososarcosine
NSC nonservice connected
nonspecific suppressor cell
no significant change
NSCC National Society for Crippled Children
NSCD nonservice-connected disability
NSCIF National Spinal Cord Injury Foundation
NSCJ new squamocolumnar junction
NSCLC nonsmall cell lung cancer
NSCPT National Society for Cardiopulmonary Technology
NSD neonatal staphyloccal disease
nominal single dose
nominal standard dose
normal spontaneous delivery
normal standard dose
no significant defect
no significant deviation
no significant difference
no significant disease
NSE neuron-specific enolase
nonspecific esterase
nsec nanosecond (also ns)
NSED nonsurgeon, emergency department
NSEH National Survey of Environment and Health
NSEP National Smallpox Eradication Program
NSF National Sanitation Foundation
National Science Foundation
NSFG National Survey of Family Growth
NSFTD normal spontaneous full-term delivery
NSG nursing
NSGCT nonseminomatous germ cell tumor
NSGCTT
nonseminomatous germ cell testicular tumor
NSG HX
nursing history
NSIDSF
National Sudden Infant Death Syndrome Foundation
NSILA nonsuppressible insulin-like activity
NSILP nonsuppressible insulin-like protein
NSL nonsalt losers
NSLF normal sheep lung fibroblast
NSLP National School Lunch Program
NSM neurosecretory material
neurosecretory motorneurones
nonsmoker
NSMR National Society for Medical Research
NSN nephrotoxic serum nephritis
nicotine-stimulated neurophysin
number of similar negatives
NSNA National Student Nurse's Association
NSND nonsymptomatic, nondisabling
NSol nerve to soleus
NSP number of similar positives
NSPB National Society to Prevent Blindness
NSPS National Society of Professional Sanitarians
NSQ not suffieient quantity
NSR nonsystemic reaction
normal sinus rhythm
nSRBC normal sheep red blood cell
NSS normal saline solution
not statistically significant
nutrition support service
NSSLHA
National Student Speech Language Hearing Association
NST neospinothalamic tract
nonshivering thermogenesis
nonstress test
nutritional status type
NSU neurosurgical unit
nonspecific urethritis
NSV nonspecific vaginitis
NSVD normal spontaneous vaginal delivery
NSVT nonsustained ventricular tachycardia
NT nasotracheal
neotetrazolium
neurotensin
neutralization technique
neutralization test
neutralizing
nicotine tartrate
nontypable
normal tissue
normotensive
nortriptyline
no test
not tested
5'-nucleotidase
N&T nose and throat
Nt niton
NTA National Tuberculosis Association
natural thymocytotoxic autoantibody
nitrilotriacetic acid
NTAB nephrotoxic antibody
NTBR not to be resuscitated
NTC neuroepithelioma teratoides ciliare
NTD neural tube defect
nitroblue tetrazolium dye
noise tone difference
NTE neurotoxic esterase
nontest ear
nuclear track emulsion
NTG nitroglycerine

	N-methyl-N'-nitro-N-nitrosoguanidine
	nontoxic goiter
NTGO	nitroglycerine ointment
NTHH	nontumorous hypergastrinemic hyperchlorhydria
NTI	nonthyroid illness
NTIS	National Technical Information Service
NTLI	neurotensin-like immunoreactivity
NTM	Neuman-Tytell medium
	nontuberculous mycobacteria
NTMI	nontransmural myocardial infarction
NTN	nephrotoxic nephritis
NTP	National Toxicology Program
	nitroprusside
	normal temperature and pressure
NTR	negative therapeutic reaction
	normotensive rat
ntr	nutrition
NTRS	National Therapeutic Recreation Society
NTS	nephrotoxic serum
	nonturning against the self
	nucleus tractus solitarius
	Nutrition Today Society
NTSA	National Tuberous Sclerosis Association
NTSAD	National Tay-Sachs and Allied Diseases Association
NTV	nerve tissue vaccine
NTX	naltrexone
Nu	nucleolus
	nucleus (also N)
nu	nanounit
	neurilemma (also neu)
Nuc	nucleoside
NUG	necrotizing ulcerative gingivitis
NUV	near ultraviolet
NV	naked vision (also Nv)
	negative variation
	new vessel
	nonvaccinated
	nonvegetarian
	nonveteran
	normal volunteers
	norverapamil
N&V	nausea and vomiting
Nv	naked vision (also NV)
nv	nonvolatile
NVA	near visual acuity
NVB	neurovascular bundle
NVC	nonvalved conduit
NVD	nausea, vomiting, and diarrhea
	neck vein distension
	Newcastle virus disease
	new vessels on disk
NVE	neovascularization elsewhere
	new vessels elsewhere
NVG	nonventilated group
NVS	nonvaccine serotype
NW	nasal wash
	nonwithdrawn
NWB	nonweight-bearing
NWDA	National Wholesale Druggists Association
NWDS	Noah Worcester Dermatological Society
NWF	new working formulation
NWHN	National Women's Health Network
NWm	multiple breath nitrogen washout
NWs	single breath nitrogen washout
NWSM	Nocardia water-soluable nitrogen
NWTS	National Wilm's Tumor Study
Nx	naloxone (also NLX)
NY	nystatin
NYD	not yet diagnosed
NYHA	New York Heart Association
NYLS	New York Longitudinal Study
NZ	normal zone
NZB	New Zealand black
NZW	New Zealand white

O

O	eye (oculus)
	none
	nonmotile
	obese (also OB)
	objective
	obstetrics
	occiput
	Ochromonas
	Onchocerca
	Oncomelania
	opening
	operon
	Opisthorchis
	opium
	oral
	orderly
	Ornithonyssus
	orotidine (also Ord)
	osteocyte
	oxidative
	oxygen
	pint (octarius)
	respirations
	suture size
^{15}O	radioactive isotope of oxygen
O_2^-	superoxide
O_2	both eyes
O_3	ozone
OA	object assembly
	obstructive apnea
	occipital artery
	occiput anterior
	old age
	oleic acid
	opiate analgesia
	opsonic activity
	oral alimentation
	orthopedic assistant
	orthophoric acid
	osteoarthritis
	ovalbumin
	overall assessment
	Overeaters Anonymous
	oxalic acid
	oxolinic acid
O_2a	oxygen availability
OAA	old age assistance
	oxaloacetic acid
OAAD	ovarian ascorbic acid depletion
OAAT	o-aminoazotoluene
OABP	organic anion binding protein
OAc	acetate
OAD	obstructive airway disease
	occlusive arterial disease
OADC	oleic aicd, albumin, dextrose, catalase
OAF	open air factor
	Opticians Association of America
	osteoclast activating factor
OAH	ovarian androgenic hyperfunction

OAJ open apophyseal joint
OALF organic acid-labile fluoride
OALL ossification of the anterior longitudinal ligament
o alt hor
every other hour (omnibus alternis horis)
OAM oxyacetate malonate
OAP ophthalmic arterial pressure
osteoarthropathy
vincristine (Oncovin), Ara-C, prednisone
OAR orientation/alertness remediation
other administrative reasons
OARSA oxacillin, aminoglycoside-resistant Staphylococcus aureus
OASDHI
Old Age, Survivors, Disability and Health Insurance Program
OASP organic acid soluble phosphorus
OAV oculoauriculovertebral
OB obese (also O)
objective benefit
obstetrics (also Obs, Obst)
occult blood
olfactory bulb (also OLB)
O&B opium and belladonna
OBB own bed bath
OBD organic brain disease
OBE Order of the British Empire
out-of-body experience
OBF organ blood flow
OBG obstetrics and gynecology (also OB-GYN, OG, O&G)
OB-GYN
obstetrics and gynecology (also OBG, OG, O&G)
Obl oblique
OBS obstetrical service
organic brain syndrome
Obs obstetrics (also OB, Obst)
obs observation
Obst obstetrics (also OB, Obs)
OC occlusocervical
office call
on call
oncology counselor
optic chiasm
oral contraceptive
organ culture
original claim
outer canthus
ovarian cancer
oxygen consumed
O&C onset and course
OCA operant conditioning audiometry
oral contraceptive agent
OCAD occlusive carotid artery disease
OCAW Oil, Chemical, and Atomic Workers
OCC Office of Cancer Communications
Occ occasional
OCD ovarian cholesterol depletion
OCDD o-chlorodibenzo-p-dioxin
OCG oral cholecystography
OCH oral contraceptive hormone
OCI See OX (oxacillin)
OCM oral contraceptive medication
OCOO Osteopathic College of Ophthalmology and Otorhinolaryngology
OCP oral contraceptive pill
OCR ocular counterrolling
ocular countertorsion reflex
oculocerebrorenal
OCS open canalicular system
oral contraceptive steroid
OCT Object Classification Test
octanoate
ornithine carbamyl transferase (also OTC)
oxytocin challenge test
oct a pint (octarius)
OCTD ornithine carbamyl transferase deficiency
OCU observation care unit
OCV ordinary conversational voice
OCVM oculocerebrovasculometer
OD occupational dermatitis
occupational disease
open duct
optical density
optimal dose
organizational development
outside (or outer) diameter
overdose
right eye (oculus dexter)
O.D. Doctor of Optometry
od every day (omni die)
ODA occipitodextra anterior
oxydiacetate
ODAP beta-N-oxalyl-L-alpha,beta-diaminopropionate
ODAT one day at a time
ODB o-dichlorobenzine (also ODCB)
ODC ornithine decarboxylase
oxyhemoglobin dissociation curve
ODCB o-dichlorobenzene (also ODB)
ODD oculodentodigital
ODEPA N-(3-oxapentamethylene)-N',N''-diethylene phosphoramide
ODM ophthalmodynamometry
oxydimalonate
ODP occipitodextra posterior
offspring of diabetic parents
ODT occipitodextra transversa
oculodynamic test
OE on examination
O/E observed to expected
O&E observation and examination
OEE outer enamel epithelium
OEF oil emersion field
OEM opposite ear masked
OEPF Optometric Extension Program Foundation
OER oxygen enhancement ratio
oer See H (oersted)
OF occiptofrontal
osteitis fibrosa
Ovenstone factor
O/F oxidation/fermentation
OFA oncofecal antigen
Orthopedic Foundation for Animals
OFBM oxidation-fermentation basal medium
OFC occipitofrontal circumference
orbitofacial cleft
osteitis fibrosa cystica
OFD orofaciodigital
OG obstetrics and gynecology (also OBG, OB-GYN, O&G)
oligodendrocyte
orange-green
orogastric
O&G obstetrics and gynecology (also OBG, OB-GYN, OG)
OGA orogastric gonoccocal aspirate
OGD oesophagogastroduodenoscopy (also EGD)

OGS oxogenic steroid
OGT oral glucose tolerance
OGTT oral glucose tolerance test
OH obstructive hypopnea
occupational history
out of hospital
11-OH 11-beta-hydroxylase
17-OH 17-alpha-hydroxylase
18-OH 18-hydroxylase
21-OH 21-hydroxylase
oh every hour (omni hora) (also omn hor)
OHA oral hypoglycemic agent
4-OHA 4-hydroxyanisole
17-OHA
17-beta-hydroxyandrogen
19-OH-AE
19-hydroxyandrostenedione
OHB_{12} hydroxocobalamin
18-OH-B
18-hydroxycorticosterone
O_2Hb oxyhemoglobin
3-OHBP
3-hydroxybenzo(a)pyrene
OHC outer hair cell
25-OHC
25-hydroxycalciferol
2-OH-CPA
2-hydroxychlorpropamide
OHCS hydroxycorticosteroid
11-OHCS
11-hydroxycorticosteroid
17-OHCS
17-hydroxycorticosteroid
OHD organic heart disease
25-OHD
25-hydroxyvitamin D
$1,25-(OH)_2D$
1,25-dihydroxyvitamin D
$1,25-(OH)_2D_3$
1,25-dihydroxyvitamin D_3
$24,25-(OH)_2D_3$
24,25-dihydroxyvitamin D_3
$1,alpha-OHD_3$
1-alpha-hydroxyvitamin D_3
OHDA 6-hydroxydopamine
18-OH-DOC
18-hydroxydesoxycorticosterone
OHF Omsk hemorrhagic fever
OHI Occupational Health Institute
ocular hypertension indicator
Oral Hygiene Index
OHIS Simplified Oral Hygiene Index
2-OH-19-OXO-T
2-hydroxy-19-oxotestosterone
OHP hydroxyproline
oxygen under high pressure
17OH Pe
17-alpha-hydroxypregnenolone
17OH Po
17-alpha-hydroxyprogesterone
OHS obesity hypoventilation syndrome
open heart surgery
Optometric Historical Society
Overcontrolled Hostility Scale
17-OHS
17-hydroxycorticosteroid
OHSM office of Health Systems Management
OHT occupational health technician
19-OH-T
19-hydroxytestosterone
OHU hydroxyurea
OI objective improvement
obturator internus
opportunistic infection
opsonic index
osteogenesis imperfecta
ouabain-insensitive
O-I outer-to-inner
OIH orthoiodohippurate
ovulation-inducing hormone
OISB orthoioso sodium benzoate
OIT organic integrity test
OJ orange juice
OKAN optokinetic after nystagmus
OKN optokinetic nystagmus
OKT ornithine-ketoacid transaminase
OL left eye (oculus laevus)
oleandomycin
other location
ol oil (oleum)
OLA occipitolaeva anterior
OLB olfactory bulb (also OB)
open-liver biopsy
OLD obstructive lung disease
OLH ovine lactogenic hormone
OLIB osmiophilic lamellar inclusion body
ol lini s i
cold-drawn linseed oil (oleum lini sine igne)
ol oliv
olive oil (oleum olivae)
OLP occipitolaeva posterior
OLR otology, laryngology, rhinology
ol res
oleoresin
OLSIST
Oral Language Sentence Imitation Screening Test
OLT occiptolaeva transversa
OM occipitomental
occupational medicine
osteomalacia
otitis media
outer membrane
Om every morning (omni mane)
OMAA Occupational Medical Administrators' Association
OMAR Office of Medical Applications of Research
OMB Office of Management and Budget
OMC open mitral commissurotomy
OMCA otitis media catarrhalis, acute
OMCC otitis media catarrhalis, chronic
OMD ocular muscle dystrophy
organic mental disorder
3-OMD 3-O-methyldopa (also MTO)
OME otitis media with effusion
OMI old myocardial infarction
OMM outer mitochondrial membrane
OMN oculomotor nucleus
omn bid
every two days (omni biduo)
omn bih
every two hours (omni bihora)
omn hor
every hour (omni hora)
omn man
every morning (omni mane)
omn noct
every night (omni nocte) (also on)
omn quar hor
every quarter of an hour (omni quadrante hora)
OMP olfactory marker protein

oligo-N-methylmorpholinium propylene oxide
ophthalmic medical practitioner
orotidylic acid (orotidene 5'phosphate)
outer membrane protein

OMPA octamethyl pyrophosphoramide
otitis media purulent, acute

OMPC otitis media purulent, chronic

OMS offshore medical school
Organisation Mondiale de la Sante
otomandibular syndrome

OMSC otitis media suppurating, chronic

ON optic nerve
orthopedic nurse
osteonecrosis

on every night (omni nocte) (also omn noct)

ONC Orthopedic Nursing Certificate

OND orbitonasal dislocation
other neurologic diseases

O.N.D.
Ophthalmic Nursing Diploma

ONP operating nursing procedure

ONPG o-nitrophenyl-beta-galactopyranoside

ONS Oncology Nursing Society

O-O outer-to-outer

OOA outer optic anlage

OOB out of bed

OOC out of control

OOLR ophthalmology, otology, laryngology, rhinology

OOR out of room

OOSS Outpatient Ophthalmic Surgery Society

OP occiput posterior
opening pressure
operation
operative procedure
opponens pollicus
organophosphate
oropharynx
orthostatic proteinuria
osmotic pressure
osteoporosis
outpatient (also OPT)

O&P ova and parasites

op other than psychotic

OPA o-phthaldialdehyde

OPAL vincristine (Oncovin), prednisone, L-asparaginase

OPB outpatient basis

OPC outpatient clinic

OPCA olivopontocerebellar atrophy

OPD obstetric prediabetes
o-phenylenediamine
optical path difference
otopalatodigital
outpatient department
outpatient dispensary

OPDG ocular plethysmodynamography

OPE Office of Planning and Evaluation

OPG oculoplethysmography
oculopneumoplethysmography
oxypolygelatin

OPH obliterative pulmonary hypertension

Oph ophthalmology (also Ophth)

Ophth ophthalmology (also Oph)

OPI oculoparalytic illusion

OPK optokinetic

OPL outer plexiform layer

OPLL ossification of the posterior longitudinal ligament

OPP ovine pancreatic polypeptide
vincristine (Oncovin), procarbazine, prednisone

OPPES oil-associated pneumoparalytic eosinophilic syndrome

OPS outpatient service

OPSA ovarian papillary serous cystadenocarcinoma

OPSI overwhelming postsplenectomy infection

OPT o-phthalaldehyde
outpatient (also OP)
outpatient treatment

OPV oral poliovaccine
oral poliovirus
oral poliovirus vaccine

OPWL opiate withdrawal

Opx orthopyroxene

OR oil retention
operating room
Operations Research
optic radiation
oral rehydration
Organ Recovery
orienting response
oxidized/reduced

O-R oxidation-reduction

O_R rate of outflow
right operator

ORA opiate receptor agonist

ORBC ox red blood cell (see also ORC)

ORC ox red cell (see also ORBC)

ORD optical rotatory dispersion

Ord orotidine (also O)

ORDS Office of Research, Demonstrations, and Statistics

OREF Orthopedic Research and Education Foundation

ORI Optometric Research Institute

ORIF open reduction with internal fixation

ORL otorhinolaryngology

ORM Orientation Remediation Module

ORN L-ornithine

ORNL Oak Ridge National Laboratory

ORO Oropouche

Oro orotic acid

ORPM orthorhythmic pacemaker

OrRS Orthopedic Research Society (also ORS)

ORS oral rehydration salt
oral rehydration solution
oral surgeon
Orthopedic Research Society (also OrRS)
orthopedic surgery

ORT oestrogen replacement technique (also ERT)
operating room technician
oral rehydration therapy

Orth orthopedics (also Ortho)

ORTHO American Orthopsychiatric Association

Ortho orthopedics

OS left eye (oculus sinister)
Obese strain
opening snap
oral surgery
Orton Society
osteoid surface
osteosclerosis
ouabain-sensitive
overall survival
oxygen saturation

Os osmium

^{185}Os radioactive isotope of osmium

^{191}Os radioactive isotope of osmium

^{193}Os radioactive isotope of osmium

OSA obstructive sleep apnea
Optical Society of America
OSAS obstructive sleep apnea syndrome
OSB o-succinylbenzoic acid
OSCE objective structural clinical examination
OSCJ original squamocolumnar junction
OSF outer spinal fiber
overgrowth stimulating factor
OSG Otosclerosis Study Group
OSHA Occupational Safety and Health Administration
OSL Osgood-Schlatter lesion
OSM osmolarity
ovine submaxillary mucin
oxygen saturation meter
osm osmole
OSRVD ophthalmologists subspecializing in retinal vascular disease
OSS osseous
over-shoulder strap
OST object sorting test
OSUK Ophthalmological Society of the United Kingdom
OT objective test
occlusion time
occupational therapy
old term
old terminology
old tuberculin
olfactory tubercle
Orientation Test
orotracheal
otolaryngology
otology (also Oto, Otolar)
oxotremorine
oxytetracycline
oxytocin
O.T. Occupational Therapist
OTA Office of Technology Assessment
orthotoluidine arsenite
OTC ornithine transcarbamylase (also OCT)
over the counter
oxytetracycline
OTD Occupational Therapy Diploma
organ tolerance dose
OTH other
Oto otolaryngology
otology (also OT, Otolar)
Otolar
otology (also OT, Oto)
OTR Ovarian Tumor Registry
O.T.R.
Registered Occupational Therapist
OTS Office of Toxic Substances
OTU olfactory tubercle
OU both eyes (oculi unitas)
each eye (oculus uterque)
observation unit
OURD outer upper right quadrant
OV oculovestibular
oestradiol valerate (also EV)
office visit
osteoid volume
O_v outflow volume
ov egg (ovum)
OVA ovalbumin
OVD occlusal vertical dimension
O_2V_E ventilatory equivalent for oxygen
OVLT organum vasculosum lamina terminalis
OVX ovariectomized
OW once weekly
outer wall
out of wedlock
oval window
O/W oil in water
oil to water ratio
OWR ovarian wedge resection
OX oxacillin
oxalate
Ox oxymel
OXAZ oxazepam
OXEA ox erythrocyte antibody
19-OXO-AE
19-oxoandrostanedione
19-OXO-T
19-oxotestosterone
OXP oxypressin
OXT oxytocin
OYE old yellow enzyme
oz ounce
oz ap apothecary's ounce
oz av avoirdupois ounce

P

P benzylpenicillin
handful (pugillus)
near (proximum)
para
Paragonimus
partial pressure
Pasteurella
Pediculus
pelvis
Penicillium
Peptococcus
percentile
percussion (also percus)
Pfeifferella
pharmacopoeia
phenacetin
phosophorus
Phthirus
Physopsis
Pityrosporon
plan
Planorbis
plasma
Plasmodium
Plebotomus
Pneumocystis
poise
pons
poor
popular response
porcelain
position
positive (also Pos)
posterior (also Post)
postpartum (also PP)
Pott's
premolar
presbyopia (also PR)
pressure
primipara
propranolol (also prop)
Proprionibacterium
protein (also Pr, Prot)

Proteus
Providencia
Pseudomonas
psychiatry (also Psy, Psych)
Pulex
pulse
pupil
pyroplasty
radiant flux
weight (pondus)

^{32}P radioactive isotope of phosphorus

^{33}P radioactive isotope of phosphorus

P_1 first parental generation
pulmonic first sound

P_2 pulmonic second sound
second parental generation

P_4 progesterone

P_{50} oxygen pressure at 50 percent hemoglobin saturation

P_{700} chloroplast pigment bleached by 700 nm

P_{870} bacterial chromatophore pigment bleached by 870 nm

p after (post)
frequency of the more common allele
optic papilla
page
papilla
probability (also Prob)
proton
short arm of a chromosome

PA paralysis agitans
paternal aunt
pathology
pentenoic acid
per annum
periarteritis
periodontal abscess
pernicious anemia
peroxidatic activity
phenylalanine
phosphatidic acid
phosphoarginine
phthalic anhydride
physical assistance
physician assistant
Picture Arrangement
pituitary-adrenal
plasma aldosterone
plasminogen activator
platelet aggregation
polyacrylamide
posteroanterior
prealbumin
pressinamide
primary amenorrhea
primary anemia
proactivator
procainamide
proinsulin antibody
prolonged action
prophylactic antibiotic
propionic acid
prostate antigen
prothrombin activity
Pseudomonas aeruginosa
Pseudosel agar
psychoanalyst
pulmonary artery
pulmonary atresia
pulpoaxial
pyrophosphate arthropathy

P&A percussion and auscultation

Pa pascal
protactinium
unit of blood pressure

^{231}Pa radioactive isotope of protactinium

^{233}Pa radioactive isotope of protactinium

^{234}Pa radioactive isotope of protactinium

PAA partial agonist activity
phosphonoacetic acid
physical abilities analysis
plasma angiotensinase activity
polyacrylic acid

3PAA 3 pyridine acetic acid

paa let it be applied to the affected area (parti affectae applicetur)

$P(A-aDO_2)$
alveolar-arterial oxygen gradient

PAAO Pan-American Association of Ophthalmology

PAB para-aminobenzoic acid (also PABA)
polyacrylamide bead
Positive Attention Behavior
premature atrial beat
purple agar base

PABA para-aminobenzoic acid (also PAB)

PAC cisplatin, doxorubicin (Adriamycin), cyclophosphamide
para-amino-clonidine
phenacetin, aspirin, caffeine
plasma aldosterone concentration
preadmission certification
premature atrial contraction
premature auricular contraction
Progress Assessment Chart of Social and Personal Development
pseudoatrophoderma colli

PACC protein A collodion charcoal

PACE Personal Assessment for Continuing Education
promoting aphasics' communicative effectiveness
pulmonary angiotensin I converting enzyme

$PACO_2$ alveolar carbon dioxide pressure (or tension)

$PaCO_2$ arterial carbon dioxide pressure (or tension)

PAD percutaneous abscess drainage
phenacetin, aspirin, desoxyephedrine
phonological-acquisition devise
primary affective disorder
psychoaffective disorder
pulsatile assist device

PADDS photon-activated drug delivery system

PADP pulmonary artery diastolic pressure

PAE progressive assistive exercise

p ae in equal parts (partes aequales) (also part aeq)

PAEDP pulmonary artery end-diastolic pressure

PAF platelet-activating factor
platelet-aggregation factor
pollen adherence factor
Premenstrual Assessment Form
pulmonary arteriovenous fistula

PA&F percussion, auscultation, and fremitus

PAFD pulmonary artery filling defect

PAFG picric acid formaldehyde-glutaraldehyde

PAFI platelet aggregation factor inhibitor

PAFIB paroxysmal atrial fibrillation

PAG periaqueductal gray
phenylacetylglutamine
pregnancy-associated alpha-glycoprotein
Pro-Leu-Gly-NH_2

PAGE polyacrylamide gel electrophoresis
PAgF platelet aggregating factor
PAGG pentaacetylglucopyranosyl guanine
PAGIF polyacrylamide gel isoelectric focusing
PAGMK primary African green monkey kidney
PAH para-aminohippuric acid (also PAHA)
polycyclic aromatic hydrocarbon
pulmonary arterial hypertension
PAHA para-aminohippuric acid (also PAH)
PAHO Pan American Health Organization
PAHVC pulmonary alveolar hypoxic vasoconstriction
PAIgG platelet-associated immunoglobulin G
PAIR Personal Assessment of Intimacy in Relationships
PAIS Psychosocial Adjustment to Illness Scale
PAL phenylalanine ammonia lyase
posterior axillary line
Profile of Adaptation to Life
pyogenic abscess of the liver
PALST Picture Articulation and Language Screening Test
PAM pancreatic acinor mass
penicillin aluminum monostearate
phenylalanine mustard
pregnancy-associated alpha-macroglobulin
primary amebic meningoencephalitis
pulmonary alveolar macrophage
pulmonary alveolar microlithiasis
pyridine aldoxime methiodide
2-PAM pralidoxime
PAMA Pan American Medical Association
PAMP pulmonary artery mean pressure
PAMWA Pan American Medical Women's Alliance
PAN periarteritis nodosa (also PN)
periodic alternating nystagmus
peroxyacetyl nitrate
polyacrilonitryl
polyarteritis nodosa
puromycin aminonucleoside
PANESS
Physical and Neurological Examination for Soft Signs
PANS puromycin aminonucleoside
PAO peak acid output
psychiatric admitting office
PAO_2 alveolar oxygen pressure (or tension)
PaO_2 arterial oxygen pressure (or tension)
Pao ascending aortic pressure
P_{ao} airway opening pressure
PAOD peripheral arterial occlusive disease
peripheral arteriosclerotic occlusive disease
PAOI peak acid output insulin-induced
PAOx phenylacetone oxime
PAP Papanicolaou
papaverine
para-aminophenol
Patient Assessment Program
peak airway pressure
peroxidase antiperoxidase
placental acid phosphatase
placental alkaline phosphatase
primary atypical pneumonia
private ambulatory patient
prostatic acid phosphatase
pulmonary alveolar proteinosis
pulmonary artery pressure
purified alternate pathway
Pap papillary
PAPF platelet adhesiveness plasma factor
PAPP para-aminopropiophenone
PAPPC pregnancy-associated plasma protein C
PAPS phosphoadenosyl-phosphosulfate
PAPVC partial anomalous pulmonary venous connection
PAPVR partial anomalous pulmonary venous return
PAPW posterior aspect of the pharyngeal wall
PAQ Personal Attributes Questionnaire
PAR Physicians for Abortion Rights
positive attention received
postanesthetic recovery
postanesthetic room
proximal alveolar region
pulmonary arteriolar resistance
Para paraplegic
par aff
the part affected (pars affecta)
PARD platelet-aggregation as a risk of diabetes
PARH plasminogen activator-releasing hormone
PARIS Persantine-Aspirin Reinfarction Study
PARS Personal and Roll Skills
PaRS pararectal space
part aeq
in equal parts (partes aequales) (also p ae)
part dolent
painful parts (partes dolentes)
part vic
in divided doses (partitis vicibus)
PARU postanesthetic recovery unit
PAS para-aminosalicylic acid
Parent Attitude Scale
Patients' Aid Society
periodic acid-Schiff
peripheral anterior synechia
personality assessment system
physicians' activities system
pregnancy advisory service
Professional Activity Study
pseudoachievement syndrome
pulmonary artery stenosis
PASA See PAS (para-aminosalicylic acid)
PAS-C para-aminosalicylic acid crystallized
PASD after diastase digestion
Pase alkaline phosphatase
PASH periodic acid-Schiff hematoxylin
PASM periodic acid-silver methenamine
Past See P (Pasteurella)
past paste
PAT paroxysmal atrial tachycardia
physical abilities test
platelet aggregation test
preadmission testing
pulmonary artery trunk
PATCO periodic acid-thiosemicarbazide-osmium tetroxide
prednisone, cytosine arabinoside, 6-thioguanine, cyclophosphamide, vincristine (Oncovin)
PATE pulmonary artery thromboendarterectomy
PATH phosphotungstic acid hematoxylin
Path pathology (also Pth)
p aur behind the ear (post aurem)
PAV partial atrioventricular
poikiloderma atrophicans vasculare
posterior arch vein
PAVN paraventricular nucleus
PAW peripheral airways
pulmonary arterial wedge

PAWP pulmonary artery wedge pressure
PB blood pressure (also BP)
pancreaticobiliary
paraffin bath
pentobarbital
perineal body
periodic breathing
peripherial blood
Pharmacopoeia Britannica
phenobarbital
phonetically balanced
pinealoblastoma
piperonyl butoxide
polymyxin B
posterior baffle
premature beat
pressure balanced
pressure breathing
protein bound
P_B barometric pressure
Pb lead (plumbum) (also plumb)
presbyopia
^{210}Pb radioactive isotope of lead
PBA polyclonal B cell activator
pressure breathing assister
pulpobuccoaxial
PBB polybrominated biphenyl
Pb-B lead level in blood
PBC point of basal convergence
prebed care
pregnancy and birth complications
primary biliary cirrhosis
progestin-binding component
PBCV Paramecium bursaria Chlorella virus
PBD percutaneous biliary drainage
PBE Perlsucht bacillen emulsion
PBF peripheral blood flow
phosphate-buffered formalin
placental blood flow
pulmonary blood flow
PBG Penassay broth plus glucose
porphobilinogen
PBGI Physician-Based Group Insurance
PBGM Penassay broth plus glucose plus menadione
PBI Parental Bonding Instrument
protein-bound iodine
PbI lead intoxication
PBL peripheral blood leukocyte
peripheral blood lymphocyte
PBLT peripheral blood lymphocyte transformation
PBM peripheral basement membrane
peripheral blood mononuclear
PBMC peripheral blood mononuclear cell
PBMV pulmonary blood mixing volume
PBN paralytic brachial neuritis
peripheral benign neoplasm
phenoxybenzamine
PBO placebo (also PL, PLBO)
PBOI Public Board of Inquiry
PBP penicillin-binding protein
prostate-binding protein
pseudobulbar palsy
PBPP Philadelphia Blood Pressure Project
PBQ phenylbenzoquinone
PBRT Phonetically Balanced Rhyme Test
PBS phenabarbital sodium
phosphate-buffered saline
pulmonary branch stenosis
PBSP prognostically bad signs during pregnancy
PBT Paul Bunnell test
phenacetin breath test
PBT_4 protein-bound thyroxine
PBV cisplatin, bleomycin, vinblastine
predicted blood volume
pulmonary blood volume
PBW posterior bite wing
PBZ phenylbutazone
Pyribenzamine
PC palmitoyl carnitine
paper chromatography
parent cell
parent to child
particulate component
phosphate cycle
phosphatidylcholine
phosphocholine
phosphocreatine
photoconductive
Phrase Construction
picryl chloride
picture completion
piriform cortex
plasma concentration
plasma cortisol
platelet concentration
platelet count
poor condition
popliteal cyst
portacaval
portal cirrhosis
posterior chamber
posterior column
posterior commissure
prepyriform cortex
present complaint
primary cleavage
primary closure
producing cell
Professional Corporation
proliferative capacity
prostatic carcinoma (also PCA)
provisional cortex
proximal colon
pseudocyst
pubococcygeus
pulmonary capillary
pulmonic closure
Purkinje cell
pyloric canal
pyruvate carboxylase
weight (pondus civile)
Pc penicillin (also PCN, Pen)
pC picocurie (also pCi)
pc after meals (post cibum)
percent (also pct)
PCA para-chloramphetamine
parietal cell antibody
passive cutaneous anaphylaxis
patient care area
patient care assistant
patient care audit
patient-controlled analgesia
perchloric acid
Personal Care Aide
photocontact allergic
plasma catecholamine concentration
portocaval anastomosis
posterior cerebral artery
posterior communicating artery
posterior cricoarytenoid
precoronary care area

prostatic carcinoma (also PC)
pyrrolidone carboxilic acid
PCAS Psychotherapy Competence Assessment Schedule
PCB paracervical block
polychlorinated biphenyl
procarbazine
PcB near point of convergence
PCC Pasteur Culture Collection
phosphate carrier compound
precoronary care
primary care curriculum
propionyl CoA carboxylase
prothrombin complex concentrate
PCc periscopic concave
PCCP percutaneous cord cyst puncture
PCCS parent-child communication schedule
PCD phosphate-citrate-dextrose
polycystic disease
posterior corneal deposits
prolonged contractile duration
PCDD polychlorinated dibenzo-para-dioxin
PCDF polychlorinated dibenzofuran
PCF pharyngoconjunctival fever
posterior cranial fossa
prothrombin conversion factor
PCFS Pacific Coast Fertility Society
PCFT platelet complement fixation test
PCG phonocardiogram
PCH paroxysmal cold hemoglobinuria
PCHRG Public Citizen Health Research Group
PCI pneumatosis cystoides intestinalis
pCi picocurie (also pC)
PCIS postcardiac injury syndrome
PCK polycystic kidney
PCM protein-calorie malnutrition
protein carboxyl methylase
pulse code modulation
PCMB para-chloromercuribenzoate (also PCMBA)
PCMBA para-chloromercuribenzoate (also PCMB)
PCMBSA
para-chloromercuribenzine sulfonic acid
PCMF perceptual cognitive motor function
PCMH Postgraduate Center for Mental Health
PCMO Prinicpal Colonial Medical Officer
PCMP 1-(1-phenylcyclohexyl)-3-methylpiperidine
PCMX para-chloro-m-xylenol
PCN penicillin (also Pc, Pen)
primary care network
PCNA proliferating cell nuclear antigen
PCNB pentachloronitrobenzene
PCO polycystic ovary
predicted cardiac output
procytoxid
pCO_2 partial carbon dioxide pressure (or tension)
PCoA posterior communicating artery
PCOD polycystic ovarian disease
PCOS polycystic ovarian syndrome
PCP para-chlorophenol
para-chlorophenylalanine (also PCPA)
pentachlorophenol
peripheral coronary pressure
phencyclidine 1-(1-phenylcyclohexyl) piperidine
Pneumocystis carinii pneumonia
primary care physician
prochlorperazine
pulmonary capillary pressure
PCPA para-chlorophenylalanine (also PCP)
primary care physician's assistant
PCPFS President's Council on Physical Fitness and Sports
PCPS phosphatidylcholine-phosphatidylserine
Pcpt perception
PCR patient contact record
phosphocreatine
plasma clearance rate
protein catabolic rate
PCS portacaval shunt
postcardiac surgery
postcholecystectomy syndrome
proximal coronary sinus
pseudomotor cerebri syndrome
Pcs preconscious
PCSM percutaneous stone manipulation
PCT plasma clotting time
plasmacrit
polychlorinated triphenyl
porphyria cutanea tarda
portacaval transposition
positron computed tomography (see also PECT, PET, PETT)
postcoital test
progestogen challenge test
proximal convoluted tubule
pulmonary care team
pct percent (also pc)
PCU patient care unit
primary care unit
protein-calorie undernutrition
PCV packed cell volume
parietal cell vagotomy
polycythemia vera
postcapillary venule
premature ventricular contraction
PCV-M myeloid metaplasia with polycythemia vera
PCWP pulmonary capillary wedge pressure
PCx periscopic convex
PCZ pancreozymin
PD by the day (per diem)
Paget's disease
pancreatic duct
paralytic dose
Parkinsonism dementia
Parkinson's disease
paroxysmal discharge
pars distalis
patent ductus
patient day
patient demonstration
pediatrics (also Ped)
peritoneal dialysis
personality disorder
pharmacodynamics
phosphate dehydrogenase
Pick's disease
Pilot Dogs
plasma defect
poorly differentiated
posterior division
postural drainage
potential differential
pressor dose
primary dendrite
prism diopter
problem drinker
progression of disease
protein degradation
protein deprived
psychopathic deviate
psychotic depression

pupillary distance
P.D. Doctor of Pharmacy (also Pharm. D.)
P(D+) probability of having disease
P(D-) probability of not having disease
Pd palladium
^{103}Pd radioactive isotope of palladium
^{109}Pd radioactive isotope of palladium
pd papilla diameter
PDA paraphenylamine diamine
patent ductus arteriosus
patient distress alarm
pediatric allergy
Private Doctors of America
pulmonary disease anemia
PDAB para-dimethylaminobenzaldahyde
PDB Paget's disease of bone
para-dichlorobenzene (also PDCB)
PDC pediatric cardiology
pentadecylcatechol
plasma cell dyscrasia
plasma digoxin concentration
plasma disappearance curve
postdecapitation convulsion
preliminary diagnostic clinic
private diagnostic clinic
PDCB para-dichlorobenzene (also PDB)
PDCD primary degenerative cerebral disease
PDD pervasive developmental disorder
phorbol-12,13-didecanoate
primary degenerative dementia
pyridoxine-deficient diet
PDDB phenododecinium bromide
PDE paroxysmal dyspnea on exertion
phosphodiesterase (also PDIE)
pulsed Doppler echocardiography
PDF Paget's Disease Foundation
Parkinson's Disease Foundation
peritoneal dialysis fluid
PDG phosphate-dependent glutaminase
PDGA pteroyldiglutamic acid
PDGF platelet-derived growth factor
PDH packaged disaster hospital
phosphate dehydrogenase
postdental history
pyruvate dehydrogenase
PDHC pyruvate dehydrogenase complex
PDI Periodontal Disease Index
Pdi transdiaphragmatic pressure
PDIE phosphodiesterase (also PDE)
PDL poorly differentiated lymphocyte
population doubling level
primary dysfunctional labor
Pdl pudendal
PDLL poorly differentiated lymphocytic lymphoma
PDLP predigested liquid protein
PDMEA phosphoryldimethylethanolamine
PDMS pharmacokinetic drug monitoring service
PDN private duty nurse
PDP piperidino-pyrimidine
platelet-depleted plasma
PDPD prolonged dwell peritoneal dialysis
PDQ prescreening developmental questionnaire
Protocol Data Query
PDR pandevelopmental retardation
pediatric radiology
primary drug resistance
proliferative diabetic retinopathy
pdr powder
PDS paroxysmal depolarizing shift
pediatric surgery
primary dependence study
PDUF pulsed Doppler ultrasonic flowmeter
PDV peak diastolic velocity
PE pancreatic extract
partial epilepsy
penile erection
pericardial effusion
peritoneal exudate
pharyngoesophageal
phenylephrine (also PHE)
2-phenylethylamine
phosphatidyl ethanolamine
physical evaluation
physical examination (also PX)
pilocarpine hydrochloride with epinephrine
plasma exchange
plating efficiency
pleural effusion
polyethylene
potential energy
powdered extract
preeclampsia
pressure equalization
prior to exposure
probable error
protein excretion
pulmonary edema
pulmonary embolus
pyramidal eminence
pyroelectric
PE2 secondary plating efficiency
Pe pregnenolone
pressure on expiration
PEA phenylether alcohol agar
phenylethylamine
polysaccharide egg antigen
PEACH Preschool Evaluation and Assessment for Children with Handicaps
PEAO phenylethylamine oxidase
PEAQ Personal Experience and Attitude Questionnaire
PEBC propyl ethyl-n-butylthiolcarbamate
PEBG phenethylbiguanide (also PEDG)
PEC parallel elastic component
peritoneal exudate cell
pyrogenic exotoxin C
$PeCO_2$ mixed expired carbon dioxide
PECT positron emission computed tomography (see also PCT, PET, PETT)
PED pharyngoesophageal diverticulum
pollution and environmental degradation
P Ed physical education
Ped pediatrics (also PD)
PEDG phenethyldiguanide (also PEBG)
PEE parallel elastic element
PEEP positive end-expiratory pressure
PEER Pediatric Examination of Educational Readiness
PEF peak expiratory flow
pharyngoepiglottic fold
Psychiatric Evaluation Form
pulmonary edema fluid
PEFR peak expiratory flow rate
$PEFR_n$ peak expiratory flow rate through the nose
PEFT Preschool Embedded Figures Test
PEFV partial expiratory flow volume
PEG pneumoencephalography
polyethylene glycol
PEI phosphate excretion index
physical efficiency index
polyethyleneimine

PELISA
paper enzyme-linked immunosorbent assay
PELS propionylerythromycin lauryl sulfate
PEM precordial electrocardiographic mapping
prescription-event monitoring
protein-energy malnutrition
pulmonary endothelial membrane
PEMA phenyethylmalonamide
PEMF pulsating electromagnetic field
Pen penicillin (also Pc, PCN)
Pent pentothal
PEO progressive external ophthalmoplegia
PEP performance evaluation procedure
phosphoenolpyruvate
polyestradiol phosphate
positive expiratory pressure
preejection period
PEPA protected environment units and prophylactic antibiotics
Pep A peptidase A
Pep B peptidase B
Pep C peptidase C
PEP_c preejection period corrected
PEPCK phosphoenolpyruvate carboxykinase (also PEPK)
Pep D peptidase D
PEPK phosphoenolpyruvate carboxykinase (also PEPCK)
PEPP positive expiratory pressure plateau
Pep S peptidase S
PER pediatric emergency room
Periodic Evaluation Record
protein efficiency ratio
pudental evoked response
per bid
for a period of two days (per biduum)
PERC potential erythropoietin-responsive cell
percus
percussion (also P)
PERD photoelectric registration device
perf perforation
PERI Psychiatric Epidemiology Research Interview
PERLA pupils equal, react to light and accommodation
perm permutation
per op emet
when action of the emetic is over (peracta operatione emetici)
Per pad
perineal pad
PERRLA
pupils equal, round, regular, react to light and accommodation
PERS patient evaluation rating scale
PES polyethylene sodium sulforate
preepiglottic space
programmed electrical stimulation
PESP postextrasystolic potentiation
pess pessary (pessus)
PEST point estimation by sequential testing
PET parent effectiveness training
peak ejection time
pear-shaped extension tube
polyethylene tube
poor exercise tolerance
positron emission tomography (see also PCT, PECT, PETT)
preeclamptic toxemia
progressive exercise test
PETA pentaerythritol triacrylate
PETN pentaerythritol tetranitrate (also PTEN)
PETT positron-emission transaxial tomography (see also PCT, PECT, PET)
PEU plasma equivalent unit
polyether urethane
PEV pulmonary extravascular fluid volume
PeV peripheral vein (also PV)
PEVN periventricular nucleus
PEWV pulmonary extravascular water volume
PF L-phenylalanine mustard, 5-fluorouracil
pair fed
parallel fiber
parotid fluid
partially follicular
peak flow
perfusion fluid
pericardial fluid
peritoneal fluid
permeability factor
personality factor
phenol formaldehyde
Physicians Forum
picture-frustration
plasma fibronectin
Plasmodium falciparum
platelet factor
pleural fluid
power factor
proflavin
prostatic fluid
protection factor
pterygoid fossa
pulmonary factor
pulmonary function
Purkinje fiber
purpura fulminans
push fluids
P/F pass-fail
16PF Sixteen Personality Factor Questionnaire
PF3 platelet factor 3
PF4 platelet factor 4
Pf See P (Pfeifferella)
pf picofarad
PFA para-flurophenylalanine
phosphonoformate
Pierre Fauchard Academy
PFAGH penalty, frustration, anxiety, guilt, hostility
PFB properdin factor B
pseudofolliculitis barbae
PFC pericardial fluid culture
persistence of fetal circulation
plaque-forming cells
PFFD proximal femoral focal deficiency
PFIB perfluoroisobutylene
PFK phosphofructokinase
PFL profibrinolysin
PFM peak flow meter
PFN partially functional neutrophil
PFO patent foramen ovale
PFP pentafluoropropionyl
preceding foreperiod
PFQ Personality Factor Questionnaire
PFR peak filling rate
peak flow rate
PFRC predicted functional residual capacity
PFST positional feedback stimulation trainer
PFT L-phenylalanine mustard, 5-fluorouracil, tamoxifen
posterior fossa tumor

pulmonary function test
PFT_4 proportion free thyroxin
PFU plaque-forming unit
pock-forming unit
PFUO prolonged fever of unknown origin
PFW peak flow whistle
PG parapsoriasis guttata
paregoric
parotid gland
pentagastrin
pepsinogen
peptidoglycan
pergolide
Pharmacopoeia germanica (also PhG)
phosphatidyl glycerol
phosphoglycerate
pigment granule
plasma gastrin
plasma glucose
postgraduate
postgraft
pregnanediol glucuronide
pregnant (also Preg)
propyl gallate
prostaglandin
proteoglycan
pyoderma gangrenosum
P_G plasma glucose
6PG 6-phosphogluconate
Pg gastric pressure
pregnenolone
pg picogram
PGA polyglycolic acid
prostaglandin A
pteroylglutamic acid
PGA_2 prostaglandin A_2
PG-AC phenylglycine-acid chloride
PGB prostaglandin B
Protestant Guild for the Blind
PGC percentage of goblet cells
primordial germ cell
prostaglandin C
PGD phosphogluconate dehydrogenase (also PGDH)
phosphoglyceraldehyde dehydrogenase
prostaglandin D
PGDF Pilot Guide Dog Foundation
PGDH 15-hydroxy-prostaglandin dehydrogenase
phosphogluconate dehydrogenase (also PGD)
PGDR plasma-glucose disappearance rate
PGE posterior gastroenterostomy
primary generalized epilepsy
prostaglandin E
PGE_1 prostaglandin E_1
PGE_2 prostaglandin E_2
PGEM prostaglandin E metabolite
PGF paternal grandfather
prostaglandin F
PGG polyclonal gamma globulin
prostaglandin G
PGH pituitary growth hormone
porcine growth hormone
prostaglandin H
PGHS Public-General Hospital Section
PGI pepsinogen I
phosphoglucoisomerase
potassium, glucose, and insulin
PGI_2 prostacyclin (prostaglandin I_2)
PGK phosphoglycerate kinase
PGM paternal grandmother
phosphoglucomutase
PGMA polyglycerol methacrylate
PGN proliferative glomerulonephritis
PGO pontogeniculo-occipital
PGP postgamma proteinuria
prepaid group practice plan
PGR psychogalvanic response
PgR progesterone
PGS pineal gonadal syndrome
prostaglandin synthetase
proteoglycan subunit
PGSI prostaglandin synthetase inhibitor
PGSR psychogalvanic skin response
PGT play group therapy
PGTR plasma glucose tolerance rate
PGTT prednisolone glucose tolerance test
PGU peripheral glucose uptake
postgonococcal urethritis
PGUT phospho-galactose-uridyl transferase
PGV proximal gastric vagotomy
PGY postgraduate year
PH parathyroid hormone (also PTH)
passive hemagglutination
past (or previous) history (also PX)
pellosis hepatis
persistent hepatitis
personal history
phenethicillin
phenylalanine hydroxylase
polycythemia hypertonica
porphyria hepatica
posterior hypothalamus
post history
prolyl hydroxylase
proproxyphene hydrochloride
prostatic hypertrophy
pseudohermaphroditism
pubic hair
public health
pulmonary hypertension (also PHT)
punctate hemorrhage
Ph pharmacopoeia
phenyl
phosphate
Ph^1 Philadelphia chromosome
pH hydrogen ion concentration
ph phote
PHA passive hemagglutination
phenylalanine
phytohemagglutinin
public health administrator
pulse height analyzer
pHa arterial pH
PHAlb polymerized human albumin
PHA-m phytohemagglutinin-mucopolysaccharide fraction
PHA-P phytohemagglutinin-protein fraction
Phar.B.
Bachelor of Pharmacy (also Pharm.B.)
Phar.C.
Pharmaceutical Chemist (also Pharm.C.)
Phar.D.
Doctor of Pharmacy (also P.D., Pharm.D.)
Phar.G.
Graduate in Pharmacy (also Pharm.G, Ph.G.)
Phar.M.
Master of Pharmacy (also Pharm.M.)
Pharm pharmaceutical
pharmacy
Pharm.B.
Bachelor of Pharmacy (also Phar.B.)

Pharm.C.
Pharmaceutical Chemist (also Phar.C.)
Pharm.D.
Doctor of Pharmacy (also P.D., Phar.D.)
Pharm.G.
Graduate in Pharmacy (also Phar.G, Ph.G.)
Pharm.M.
Master of Pharmacy (also Phar.M.)
PhB See BP (British Pharmacopoeia)
PHBB propylhydroxybenzyl benzimidazole
PHC posthospital care
premolar aplasia, hyperhidrosis, cavities
primary health care
primary hepatic carcinoma
primary hepatocellular carcinoma (also PHCC)
PHCC primary hepatocellular carcinoma (also PHC)
PHCP Physically Handicapped Children's Program
PHD pulmonary heart disease
Ph.D. Doctor of Philosophy
PHDPE porous high density polyethylene
PHE periodic health examination
phenylephrine (also PE)
proliferative hemorrhagic enteropathy
Phe phenylalanine
PHEMA poly-2-hydroxyethyl-methacrylate
Phen phenformin
PHF paired helical filaments
PHFG primary culture of human fetal glial
PhG Pharmacopoeia germanica (also PG)
Ph.G. Graduate in Pharmacy (also Phar.G, Pharm.G.)
Phgly phenylglycine
PHI peptide histidine isoleucine
phosphohexoisomerase
PhI International Pharmacopoeia
PHK platelet phosphohexokinase
postmortem human kidney
PHLA postheparin lipolytic activity
PHLS Public Health Laboratory Service
PHM psyllium hydrophilic mucilloid
PhM pharyngeal musculature
PHMA postheparin monoglycerdase
PHN Public Health Nurse
PhNCS phenylisothiocyanate
PHO Public Health Official
PHP passive hyperpolarizing potential
peritertiarybutylphenol
prehospital program
prepaid health plan
primary hyperparathyroidism
pseudohypoparathyroidism
PHPP para-hydroxyphenyl pyruvate
PHPT See PHP (pseudohypoparathyroidism)
PHR photoreactivity
PHRG Public Health Research Group
PHRI Public Health Research Institute
PHS patient-heated serum
phenylalanine hydroxylase stimulator
pooled human serum
Public Health Service
PHSC pluripotent hemopoietic stem cell
PHSQ Psychosocial History Screening Questionnaire
PHT phentolamine
phenytoin (also PT)
portal hypertension
primary hyperthyroidism
pulmonary hypertension (also PT)
PHV peak height velocity
pHv mixed venous pH
PHX pulmonary histiocytosis X
PHY phytohemagglutination
Phys physiology
PI international protocol
pacing impulse
pancreatic insufficiency
pars intermedia
performance index
performance intensity
Peridontal Index
permanent incidence
permeability index
phagocytic index
Pharmacopoeia Internationalis
phosphatidylinositol
pipemidic acid
pneumatosis intestinalis
ponderal index
postinoculation
preinduction
premature infant
prematurity index
preparatory interval
present illness
proactive interference
programmed instruction
proinsulin
propidium iodide
protamine insulin
protease inhibitor
proximal intestine
pulmonary incompetence
pulmonary infarction
pyritization index
Pi inorganic phosphate
pressure of inspiration
protease inhibitor
serum inorganic phosphorus
P_i inorganic orthophosphate
pI isoelectric pH value
PIA peripheral interface adapter
phenylisopropyladenosine
photoelectronic intravenous angiography
plasma insulin activity
porcine intestinal adenomatosis
preinfarct angina
Psychiatric Institute of America
PIAT Peabody Individual Achievement Test
PIB psi-interactive biomolecules
PIC postintercourse
PICA Porch Index of Communicative Ability
posterior inferior cerebellar artery
PICD primary irritant contact dermatitis
PICLC polyinosinic acid, polycytidilic acid, poly-l-lysine carboxymethyl cellulose
PICSI Picture Identification for Children-Standardized Index
PICU pediatric intensive care unit
pulmonary intensive care unit
PID pain intensity difference
pelvic inflammatory disease
plasma-iron disappearance
prolapsed intervertebral disease
prolapsed intervertebral disk
proportional-integral-derivative
protruded intervertebral disk
PIDT plasma-iron disappearance time
PIE postinfectious encephalomyelitis
pulmonary infiltration and eosinophilia

pulmonary interstitial edema
pulmonary interstitial emphysema
PIEF isoelectric focusing in polyarylamide
PIF peak inspiratory flow
pigment-inducing factor
point of identical flow
premorbid inferiority feeling
prolactin-inhibiting factor
proliferation-inhibiting factor
prostatic interstitial fluid
PIFG poor intrauterine fetal growth
PIFR peak inspiratory flow rate
PIFT platelet immunofluorescence test
Pig pigmentation
PIGP pyruvate inosine glucose phosphate
PIGPA pyruvate inosine glucose phosphate adenine
PIH pregnancy-induced hypertension
prolactin-inhibiting hormone
PIHH postinfluenza-like hyposmia and hypogeusia
PII plasma inorganic iodine
PIIP portable insulin infusion pump
PIIS posterior inferior iliac spine
pil pill (pilula)
PIM penicillamine-induced myasthenia
PINS person in need of supervision
PIO_2 inspired oxygen tension
intra-alveolar oxygen tension
PIP peak inspiratory pressure
proximal interphalangeal
PIPA platelet ^{125}I-labeled staphylococcal protein A
PIPADA
paraisopropyl acetanilideamino acetate
PIPES 1,4-piperazine(ethane sulfonic acid)
PIPIDA
paraisopropyl iminodiacetic acid
PIPJ proximal interphalangeal joint
PIQ performance intelligence quotient
PIR piriform
piromidic acid
PIT pacing-induced tachycardia
perceived illness threat
plasma iron turnover
PITC See PhNCS
PITR plasma iron turnover rate
PIV parainfluenza virus
PIVH peripheral intravenous hyperalimentation
PIXIE proton-induced x-ray emission
PJ pancreatic juice
PJC premature junctional contraction
PJP pancreatic juice protein
PJS peritoneojugular shunt
PJT paroxysmal junctional tachycardia
PK pericardial knock
pharmacokinetic
protein kinase
psychokinesis
pyruvate kinase
P-K Prausnitz-Kuestner
pK ionization constant of an acid
PKA prekallikrein activator
PKD polycystic kidney disease
PKF phagocytosis and killing function
PKK prekallikrein
PKN parkinsonism
PKR phased knee rehabilitation
PKSAP Psychiatric Knowledge and Skills Self-Assessment Program
PKU phenylketonuria
PKV killed poliomyelitis vaccine
peak kilovolt
PL light perception
palmaris longus
pancreatic lipase
phospholipid
placebo (also PBO, PLBO)
placental lactogen
plantar
plasma lemma
preleukemia platelet
problem list
prolymphocytic leukemia
psychosocial-labile
pulpolingual
Purkinje layer
Pl place
plate
plural
PLA phospholipase
platelet antigen
polyactic acid
polymer of lactic acid
posterior lip of the acetabulum
procaine and lactic acid
pulpolinguoaxial
PLa pulpolabial
Pla left atrial pressure
PLAP placental alkaline phosphatase
PLBO placebo (also PBO, PL)
PLC Personal Locus of Control
phospholipase C
primary liver cell cancer (also PLCC)
proinsulin-like component
protein-lipid complex
PLCC primary liver cell cancer (also PLC)
PLD peripheral light detection
platelet defect
posterior latissimus dorsi
postlaser day
PLDH plasma lactic dehydrogenase
PLE panlobular emphysema
pleura
polymorphic light eruption
protein-losing enteropathy
pseudolupus erythematosus syndrome
PLED periodic lateralized epileptiform discharge
PLF posterior long fiber
PLG Pro-Leu-Gly-NH_2 (also PAG)
PLH palaemontes lightening hormone
PLM percentage of labeled mitoses
plasma level monitoring
polarized light microscopy
PLMV posterior-leaf mitral valve
PLN popliteal lymph node
posterior lip nerve
PLND pelvic lymph node dissection
PLP paraformaldehyde-lysine-periodate
plasma leukopheresis
pyridoxal-5'-phosphate
PLPD pseudoperiodic lateralized paroxysmal discharge
PLR pupillary light reflex
PLRF Pediatric Liver Research Foundation
PLS prostaglandin-like substance
PLT primed lymphocyte test
primed lymphocyte typing
psittacosis, lymphogranuloma, trachoma
PLTS platelets
plumb lead (plumbum) (also Pb)
PLV live poliomyelitis vaccine

panleukopenia virus
phenylalanine-lysin-vasopressin
posterior left ventricle

PLVW See LVPW

PM after death (post mortem)
afternoon (post meridiem)
pacemaker
papilla mammae
papillary muscle
papular mucinosis
paromomycin
partially muscular
partial menisiectomy
peritoneal macrophage
petit mal
photomultiplier
physical medicine
plasma membrane
platelet membrane
pneumomediastinum
polymorphonuclear
polymyositis
posterior mitral
postmortem (also Post)
premamillary nucleus
presystolic murmur
pretibial myxedema
preventive medicine
pterygoid muscle
pulmonary macrophage
pulpomesial

Pm promethium

^{147}Pm radioactive isotope of promethium

^{149}Pm radioactive isotope of promethium

^{151}Pm radioactive isotope of promethium

pm picometer

PMA papillary, marginal, attached
Pharmaceutical Manufacturers Association
phenylmercuric acetate (also PMAC, PMAS)
phorbol myristate acetate
p-methoxyamphetamine
Primary Mental Abilities
progressive muscular atrophy

PMAA Premarket Approval Application

PMAC phenylmercuric acetate (also PMA, PMAS)

PMAS phenylmercuric acetate (also PMA, PMAC)

PMB papillomacular bundle
para-hydroxymercuribenzoate
polychrome methylene blue
polymorphonuclear basophil
polymyxin B
postmenopausal bleeding

PMC phenylmercuric chloride
pleural mesothelial cell
premature mitral closure
pseudomembranous colitis

PMD posterior mandibular depth
primary myocardial disease
private medical doctor
progressive muscular dystrophy

P.M.D. Doctor of Primary Medicine

PME phosphatidyl-N-methylethanolamine
polymorphonuclear eosinophil
progressive myoclonus epilepsy

PMF L-phenylalanine mustard, methotrexate, 5-fluorouracil
phenylmercuric Fixtan
progressive massive fibrosis
pterygomaxillary fossa

PMH past (or previous) medical history
programmed medical history
Public Mental Hospital

PMI patient medical instructions
patient medication instructions
point of maximal impulse
point of maximal intensity
posterior myocardial infarction
previous medical illness

PMK primary monkey kidney

PML posterior mitral leaflet
progressive multifocal leukoencephalopathy
pulmonary microlithiasis

PMLE polymorphous light eruption

PMMA polymethyl methacrylate

PMN polymorphonuclear neutrophil

PMNC percentage of multinucleated cells

PMNG polymorphonuclear granulocyte

PMNL polymorphonuclear leukocyte

PMNR periadenitis mucosa necrotica recurrens

PMO phenylmethyloxadiazole
principal medical officer

PMP past (or previous) menstrual period
patient management problem
patient medication profile
persistent mentoposterior
phenoxymethyl penicillin

PMPO postmenopausal palpable ovary syndrome

PMR perinatal morbidity rate
perinatal mortality rate
periodic medical review
physical medicine and rehabilitation (also PM&R)
polymyalgia rheumatica
proportional morbidity ratio
proportional mortality ratio

PM&R physical medicine and rehabilitation (also PMR)

PMRS Physical Medicine and Rehabilitation Service

PMS phenazine methosulfate
postmarketing surveillance
postmenopausal syndrome
postmitochondrial supernatant
pregnant mare serum
premenstrual syndrome

PMSF phenylmethyl sulfonyl fluoride

PMSG pregnant mare serum gonadotropin

PMT photoelectric multiplier tube
photomultiplier tube
Porteus maze test
premenstrual tension

PMTT pulmonary mean transit time

PMV paralyzed mechanically ventilated

pMVL posterior mitral valve leaflet

PMZ pentamethylenetetrazol

PN nightmare (pavor nocturnus)
papillary necrosis
parenteral nutrition
perceived noise
percussion note
periateritis nodosa (also PAN)
peripheral nerve
peripheral neuropathy
peripheral nodes
phrenic nerve
pneumonia
pontine nucleus
positional nystagmus
posterior nares
practical nurse

predicted normal
propoxyphene napsylate
psychoneurotic
pyelonephritis
pyridine nucleotide
pyrrolnitrin
P/N positive to negative ratio
P&N Psychiatry and Neurology
PN_2 partial pressure of nitrogen
PNA Paris Nomina Anatomica
peanut agglutinin
pediatric nurse associate
pentose nucleic acid (see RNA--ribonucleic acid)
P_{NA} plasma sodium
PNAH polynuclear aromatic hydrocarbon
PNB polymyxin, neomycin, bacitracin
PNBT paranitroblue tetrazoleum
PNC postnecrotic cirrhosis
purine nucleotide cycle
PND paroxysmal nocturnal dyspnea
postnasal drainage
postnasal drip
postneonatal death
See lb
PNdB perceived noise decibel
PNE plasma norepinephrine
PNed Nederlandsche Pharmacopee
PNF prenatatl fluoride
proprioceptive neuromuscular facilitation
PNG pencillin G
pneumogram
PNH paroxysmal nocturnal hemoglobinuria
PNHA Physicians National Housestaff Association
PNI peripheral nerve injury
pseudoneointimal
psychoneuroimmunology
PNL peripheral nerve lesion
polymorphonuclear neutrophilic leukocyte
PNM perinatal mortality
postneonatal mortality
PNMT phenylethanolamine N-methyltransferase
PNNG N-propyl-N'-nitro-N-nitrosoguanidine
PNP para-nitrophenol
pediatric nurse practitioner
polyneuropathy
psychogenic nocturnal polydipsia
purine nucleoside phosphorylase
PNPB positive-negative pressure breathing
PNPP para-nitrophenylphosphate
PNPR positive-negative pressure respiration
PNPS para-nitrophenylsulfate
PNS parasympathetic nervous system
peripheral nervous system
PNT partial nodular transformation
PNU protein nitrogen unit
PNV penicillin phenoxymethyl
PNX pneumonectomy
PNZ posterior necrotic zone
PO parapineal organ
parietal operculum
parieto-occipital
perceptual organization
period of onset
phone order
physician only
posterior
postoperative (also POp, Postop)
predominant organism
P/O oxidative phosphorylation ratio
protein to osmolar ratio
PO_2 oxygen partial pressure (or tension)
Po polonium
position response
progesterone
^{208}Po radioactive isotope of polonium
^{210}Po radioactive isotope of polonium
po by mouth (per os)
POA pancreatic oncofetal antigen
point of application
preoptic area
primary optic atrophy
POAH preoptic anterior hypothalamic
POB phenoxybenzamine
place of birth
POBE Profile of Out-of-Body Experiences
POC postoperative care
procarbazine, vincristine (Oncovin), lomustine (CCNU)
Po/C ocular pressure
POCA Psychiatric Outpatient Centers of America (see also APOCA)
pocill
a small cup (pocillum)
pocul cup (poculum)
POCY postoperative chronologic year
POD peroxidase
place of death
polycystic ovarian disease
postoperative day
PODQ Perceptual Organization Deviation Quotient
PODx preoperative diagnosis
POE port of entry
POF pyruvate oxidation factor
pOH hydroxyl concentration
POHI physically or otherwise health impaired
POHS presumed ocular histoplasmosis syndrome
POI Personal Orientation Inventory
Poik poikilocyte
pois poison
Polio poliomyelitis
Poly polymorphonuclear leukocyte
Poly-IC
polyinosinic-polycytidylic
Poly-ICLC
polyriboinosinic-polyribocytidylic acid stabilized with poly-l-lysine in carboxymethyl
POM pain on motion
POMP 6-mercaptopurine (Purinethol), vincristine (Oncovin), methotrexate, prednisone
POMR problem-oriented medical record
POMS Profile of Mood States
POMS-V
Profile of Mood States, Vigor
pond by weight (pondere)
PONS Profile of Nonverbal Sensitivity
POP paraoxypropione
persistent occipitoposterior
pituitary opioid peptide
plasma oncotic pressure
plaster of Paris
POp postoperative (also PO, Postop)
POPOP 1,4-bis(5-phenyloxazol-2-yl)benzene
POR problem-oriented record
PORH postocclusive reactive hyperemia
PORP partial ossicular replacement prosthesis
Pos positive (also P)

POSCH Program on Surgical Control of Hyperlipidemia
POSM patient-operated sensing mechanism
Pos pr
positive pressure
POSS percutaneous on-surface stimulation
proximal over-shoulder strap
Poss possible
Post posterior (also P)
postmortem (also PM)
Postinoc
postinoculation
Postop
postoperative (also PO, POp)
post prand
after dinner (post prandium)
pot a drink (potus)
potash
potion
POTAGT
potential abnormality of glucose tolerance
PoV portal vein (also PV)
POVT puerperal ovarian vein thrombophlebitis
POW Powassan
prisoner of war
PP pacesetter potential
pancreatic polypeptide
paradoxical pulse
parietal pleura
partial pressure
pathology point
pellagra preventive
pentose pathway
perfusion pressure
permanent partial
Peyer's patch
phosphorylase phosphatase
pink puffer
pinpoint
plane polarization
Planned Parenthood
plasma pepsinogen
plasmapheresis
plasma protein
porcine pancreatic
posterior papillary
postpartum (also P)
postprandial (also p prand)
private patient
private practice
protoporphyrin (also PROTO)
pterygoid process
pulse pressure
pulsus paradoxus
purulent pericarditis
pyrophosphate
P&P prothrombin and proconvertin
PP5 placental protein 5
pp after meals (post prandial)
near point (punctum proximum)
PPA phenylpropanolamine
phenylpyruvic acid
Pittsburgh pneumonia agent
postpill amenorrhea
PP&A palpation, percussion, and ascultation
ppa shake well (phiala prius agitata)
PPAS peripheral pulmonary artery stenosis
PPB platelet-poor blood
positive-pressure breathing
ppb parts per billion
PPBE proteose-peptone-beef extract
PPBS postprandial blood sugar
PPC pentose phosphate cycle
progressive patient care
PPCA plasma prothrombin conversion accelerator
proserum prothrombin conversion accelerator
PPCF peripartum cardiac failure
plasma prothrombin conversion factor
PPCH piperazinylmethyl cyclohexanone
PPCM postpartum cardiomyopathy
PPD packs per day
para-phenylenediamine
permanent partial disability
postpartum day
primary physical dependence
purified protein derivative
PPD-B purified protein derivative-Battey
PPDR preproliferative diabetic retinopathy
PPDS purified protein derivative of Seibert
purified protein derivative-standard
PPE permeability pulmonary edema
programmed physical examination
PPF pellagra-preventive factor
plasma protein fraction
PPFA Planned Parenthood Federation of America
PPG photoplethysmography
polymorphonuclear cells per glomerulus
polyurethane-polyvinyl graphite
pretragal parotid gland
ppg picopicogram
PPGA postpill galactorrhea amenorrhea
PPGP prepaid group practice
PPH persistent pulmonary hypertension
primary pulmonary hypertension
postpartum hemorrhage
protocollagen proline hydroxylase
PPHN persistent pulmonary hypertension of the newborn
PPHP pseudo-pseudohypoparathyroidism
PPI partial permanent impairment
patient package insert
Physician Performance Index
preceding preparatory interval
Present Pain Intensity
purified porcine insulin
PPi inorganic pyrophosphate
PPIM postperinatal infant mortality
PPK palmo-plantar keratosis
PPL penicilloyl polylysine
phospholipid
Ppl pleural pressure
PPLF postperfusion low flow
PPLO pleuropneumonia-like organism
PPM posterior papillary muscle
ppm parts per million
pulses per minute
PPMM postpolycythemia myeloid metaplasia
PPN pedunculopontine nucleus
PPNG penicillinase-producing Neisseria gonorrhoea
PPO 2,5-diphenyloxazole
peak pepsin output
Preferred Provider Organization
prepatient periods to oocyst
PPP pentose phosphate pathway
plasma protamine precipitating
platelet-poor plasma
polyphloretin phosphate
porcine pancreatic polypeptide
portal perfusion pressure

purified placental protein
pustulosis palmaris et plantaris
PPPA Poison Prevention Packaging Act
PPPH purified placental protein, human
PPPI primary private practice income
PPR patient-physician relationship
photopalpebral reflex
poor partial response
Price precipitation reaction
p prand
postprandial (also PP)
PPRF paramedian pontine reticular formation
postpartum renal failure
PPRP phosphoribosylpyrophosphate (also PRPP)
PPS phosphoribosylpyrophosphate synthetase
postperfusion syndrome
postpericardiotomy syndrome
PPSA Pan-Pacific Surgical Association
PPT plant protease test
potassium phosphotungstate
ppt precipitate
prepared (also praep)
PPTT postpartum painless thyroiditis with transient thyrotoxicosis
PPV positive pressure ventilation
progressive pneumonia virus
PPVT Peabody Picture Vocabulary Test
PPZ perphenazine
PPZSO perphenazine sulfoxide
PQ paraquat
permeability quotient
plastoquinone
pyrimethamine-quinine
PQ9 plastoquinone-9
PQD Protocol Data Query
PR Panama red
pars recta
partial reinforcement
partial remission
partial response
patient relations
peer review
percentile rank
peripheral resistance
phenol red
phosphorylase rupturing
photoreaction
physical rehabilitation
piperylon
polymyalgia rheumatica
postural reflex
potential relation
pregnancy rate
presbyopia (also P)
pressoreceptor
production rate
professional relations
progesterone receptor
progressive relaxation
progressive resistance
prolonged remission
propicillin
propranolol
prosthion
psychotherapy responder
Puerto Rican
pulmonary regurgitation
pulse rate
P/R productivity to respiration ratio
P&R pulse and respirations
Pr praseodymium
premature
prism
proctologist
prolactin (also PRL)
protein (also P, Prot)
See P (Propionibacterium, Proteus)
^{142}Pr radioactive isotope of praseodymium
^{143}Pr radioactive isotope of praseodymium
pr far point (punctum remotum)
pair
through the rectum (per rectum)
PRA phonation, respiration, articulation-resonance
phosphoribosylamine
Physician's Recognition Award
plasma renin activity
Psoriasis Research Association
praep prepared (praeparatus) (also ppt)
prand dinner (prandium)
PRAS prereduced anaerobically sterilized
p rat aetat
in proportion to age (pro ratione aetatis)
PRAVD prednisone, Ara-C, asparaginase, vincristine, daunorubicin
PRB Population Reference Bureau
PRBC packed red blood cells
PRBS pseudorandom binary signal
PRBV placental residual blood volume
PRC packed red cells
peer review committee
physician's review committee
plasma renin concentration
professional review committee
PRCA pure red cell agenesis
pure red cell aplasia
PRD partial reaction of degeneration
phosphate restricted diet
polycystic renal disease
postradiation dysplasia
PRE photoreacting enzyme
pigmented retina epithelial
progressive resistive exercise
Pre preliminary
PREE partial reinforcement extinction effect
Preg pregnant (also PG)
Preinoc
preinoculation
Preop preoperative
PREP Pediatric Review and Education Program
Prep prepare
PREVAGT
previous abnormality of glucose tolerance
PRF Personality Research Form
prolactin-releasing factor
pyrogen-releasing factor
pRF polyclonal rheumatoid factor
PRFA plasma recognition factor activity
PRFM prolonged rupture of fetal membranes
PRFR pressure-retaining flow-relieving
PRG phleborheography
PRGI percutaneous retrogasserian glycerol injection
PRH preretinal hemorrhage
prolactin-releasing hormone
PRHBF peak reactive hyperemia blood flow
PRI phosphate reabsorption index
phosphoribose isomerase
plexus rectales inferiores
PRIM&R
Public Responsibility in Medicine and Research

PRIND prolonged reversible ischemic neurologic deficit
PRIST paper radioimmunosorbent technique
paper radioimmunosorbent test
PRK primary rabbit kidney
PRL prolactin (also Pr)
PRM phosphoribomutase
photoreceptor membrane
prematurely ruptured membrane
preventive medicine
primidone
PRM-SOX
pyrimethamine sulfadoxine
PRN principalization
prn as needed (pro re nata)
PRNT plaque reduction neutralization test
PRO Professional Review Organization
projection
Pro proline
prothrombin
Prob probability (also p)
Proct proctology
pro dos
for a dose (pro dose)
Prog prognosis (also PX)
PROM passive range of motion
premature rupture of membranes
prolonged rupture of membranes
ProMace
prednisone, doxorubicin, cyclophosphamide, etoposide, methotrexate, leucovorin
PROMIN
programmable multiple ion monitor
PROMIS
Problem-Oriented Medical Information System
prop propranolol (also P)
PROPLA
prophospholipase A
pro rat aet
according to age (pro ratione aetatis)
Prot protein (also P, Pr)
PROTO protoporphyrin (also PP)
pro us ext
for external use (pro usum externum)
Prox proximal
prox luc
the day before (proxima luce)
PRP panretinal photocoagulation
penicillinase-resistant penicillin
pityriasis rubra pilaris
platelet-rich plasma
polyribophosphate
postreplication repair
pressure rate product
Problem Reporting Program
progressive rubella panencephalitis
Psychotic Reaction Profile
PRPP phosphoribosylpyrophosphate (also PPRP)
PRR proton relaxation rate
PRRP phosphoribosylribitol
PRS Parent's Rating Scale
plasma renin substrate
positive rolandic sharp
Pupil Rating Scale
PRSA plasma renin substrate activity
PRT phosphoribosyltransferase
photoradiation therapy
postoperative respiratory treatment
PRU peripheral resistance unit
PRV polycythemia rubra vera
PRVA peripheral vein renin activity
PRVEP pattern reversed visual evoked potential
PrVS prevesicle space
PRW polymerized ragweed
PRZ prazepam
PS chloropicrin
paired stimulation
paradoxical sleep
paralaryngeal space
parasternal
parasympathetic
partial shoulder
pathologic stage
patient serum
performing scale
periodic syndrome
peripheral smear
permeability surface
phosphatidyl serine
phrenic nerve stimulation
physical status
pigeon serum
plastic surgery
point of symmetry
polysaccharide
population sample
postmaturity syndrome
pregnant serum
prescription
prestimulus
principal sulcus
prostatic secretion
protamine sulfate
protective service
protein synthesis
pulmonic stenosis
pyloric stenosis
P-S pancreozymin-secretin
Porter-Silber
pyramid-surface
P/S polyunsaturated to saturated ratio
P&S paracentesis and suction
Ps pseudocyst
See P (Pseudomonas)
ps per second
PSA picryl sulfonic acid
polyethylene sulfonic acid
prolonged sleep apnea
public service announcement
PSAGN poststreptococcal acute glomerulonephritis
PsAn psychoanalysis
PSC partial subligamentous calcification
physiologic squamocolumnar
pluripotential stem cell
Porter-Silber chromogen
posterior semicircular canal
posterior subcapsular cataract
primary sclerosing cholangitis
PSCC posterior subcapsular cataract
PSCM pokeweed activated spleen conditioned medium
PSD particle size distribution
periodic synchronous discharge
phosphate supplemented diet
photon-stimulated desorption
poststenotic dilation
postsynaptic density
PSDES primary symptomatic diffuse esophageal spasm
PSE paradoxical systolic expansion

partial splenic embolization
point of subjective equality
portal systemic encephalopathy
postshunt encephalopathy
Present State Examination

PSEC poststress ethanol consumption

PSF peak scatter factor
point spread function
prostacycline production stimulating factor

psf pounds per square foot

PSG peak systolic gradient
polysomnogram
presystolic gallop

PSGBI Pathological Society of Great Britain and Ireland

PSGN poststreptococcal glomerulonephritis

PSH postspinal headache

PSI posterior sagittal index
Problem Solving Information
prostaglandin synthetic inhibitor
Psychological Screening Inventory

psi pounds per square inch

psia pounds per square inch, absolute

PSIFT platelet suspension immunofluorescence test

psig pounds per square inch gauge

PSIS posterior superior iliac spine

PSL percent stroke length

PSLI physalaemin-like immunoreactivity

PSM presystolic murmur

PSMA progressive spinal muscular atrophy

PSMF protein-sparing modified fast

PSNS parasympathetic nervous system

PSO physostigmine salicylate ophthalmic
proximal subungual onychomycosis

Psol partly soluble

PSOR psoralen

PSP pacesetter potential
paralytic shellfish poisoning
parathyroid secretory protein
periodic short pulse
phenolsulfonphthalein
positive spike pattern
postsynaptic potential
professional simulated patient
progressive supranuclear palsy

PSPF prostacyclin synthesis stimulating plasma factor

PSPLV posterior superior process of the left ventricle

PSQ Patient Satisfaction Questionnaire

PSR Physicians for Social Responsibility
proliferative sickle retinopathy

PSRC Plastic Surgery Research Council

PSRI Professional Sexual Role Inventory

PSRO Professional Standards Review Organization

PSS painful shoulder syndrome
physiologic saline solution
progressive systemic sclerosis
psoriasis severity scale
Psychiatric Services Section
Psychiatric Status Schedule

PST pancreatic suppression test
paroxysmal supraventricular tachycardia
penicillin, streptomycin, and tetracycline
perceptual span time
phenol sulfotransferase
phonemic segmentation test
platelet survival time
prefrontal sonic treatment
protein-sparing therapy
proximal straight tubule

PSTA Predictive Screening Test of Articulation

PSTH poststimulus time histograph

PSTP pentasodium triphosphate

PSTV potato spindle tuber viroid

PSU primary sampling unit

PSVER pattern-shift visual-evoked response

PSVT paroxysmal supraventricular tachycardia

PSW past sleepwalker
primary surgical ward
psychiatric social worker

Psy psychiatry (also P, Psych)
psychology (also Psych)

PT parathyroid
paroxysmal tachycardia
permanent and total
pharmacy and therapeutics
phenytoin (also PHT)
phonation time
photophobia
physical therapist
physical therapy
physical training
plasma thromboplastin
pneumothorax (also PX)
posterior tibial
postgraduate training
premature termination
preterm
pristinamycin
prothrombin time
protriptyline
pulmonary thrombosis
pulmonary trunk
pure tone
pyramidal tract

Pt patient
platinum
psychoasthenia

^{193}Pt radioactive isotope of platinum

^{197}Pt radioactive isotope of platinum

pt let it be continued (perstetur)
part
pint
point

PTA parathyroid adenoma
percutaneous transluminal angioplasty
persistent trigeminal artery
persistent truncus arteriosus
phosphotungstic acid
plasma thromboplastin antecedent
post-traumatic amnesia
prior to admission
prior to arrival
pure tone acuity
pure tone average

PTAH phosphotungstic acid-hematoxylin

PTAP purified toxoid precipitated by aluminum phosphate

PTB patellar tendon bearing
prior to birth

PTBA percutaneous transluminal balloon angioplasty

PTBD percutaneous transhepatic biliary drainage

PTBP para-tertiary butylphenol

PTBS post-traumatic brain syndrome

PTC percutaneous transhepatic cholangiography

phenylthiocarbamide
pheochromocytoma with thyroid carcinoma
plasma thromboplastin component
premature tricuspid closure
prior to conception
pseudotumor cerebri

PTCA percutaneous transluminal coronary angioplasty

$PtcCO_2$ transcutaneous carbon dioxide tension

$PtcO_2$ transcutaneous oxygen tension

PTCP pseudothrombocytopenia

PTCR percutaneous transluminal coronary recanalization

PTD para-toluenediamine
permanent and total disability

Ptd phosphatidyl

PtdCho phosphatidylcholine

PtdEtn phosphatidylethanolamine

PtdIns phosphatidylinositol

PtdSer phosphatidylserine

PTE parathyroid extract
pulmonary thromboembolism

PTED pulmonary thromboembolic disease

PTEN pentaerythritol tetranitrate (also PETN)

PTF plasma thromboplastin factor

PTFA prothrombin time fixing agent

PTFE polytetrafluoroethylene

PTG parathyroid gland

PTGA pteroyltriglutamic acid

PTH parathormone (parathyroid hormone) (also PH)
phenythiohydantoin
post-transfusion hepatitis

PTh primary thrombocythemia

Pth pathology (also Path)

PTHS parathyroid hormone secretion

PTI persistent tolerant infection
Poetry Therapy Institute
pressure time index

PTL pharyngeotracheal lumen
posterior tricuspid leaflet
protriptyline

PTM post-transfusion mononucleosis
post-traumatic meningitis
pressure time per minute
preterm milk

PTMA phenyltrimethylammonium

PTMD pupil, tension, media, disk

PTMDF pupil, tension, media, disk, fundus

PTN pain transmission neuron

PTNA Provincial Territorial Nurses' Association

PTO percutaneous transhepatic obliteration
Perlsucht Tuberculin Original
2-pyridinethiol 1-oxide

PTP percutaneous transhepatic portography
post-tetanic potentiation
post-transfusion purpura
prior to program

PTPI post-traumatic pulmonary insufficiency

PTQ Parent Teacher Questionnaire

PTR peripheral total resistance
Perlsucht Tuberculin Reaction
psychotic trigger reaction

PTRA percutaneous transluminal renal angioplasty

PTS painful tonic seizure
para-toluenesulfonic acid
patella tendon socket
permanent threshold shift
phosphotransferase system

PTSD post-traumatic stress disorder

PTT partial thromboplastin time
particle transport time
posterior tibial transfer
pulmonary transit time
pulse transmission time

PTU propylthiouracil

PTX parathyroidectomy
phototoxic reaction

PTX-B pumiliotoxin B

PTZ pentamethylenetetrazole

PU pass urine
paternal uncle
pepsin unit
peptic ulcer
posterior urethra
precursor uptake
pregnancy urine

Pu plutonium
putrescine (also PUT)

^{237}Pu radioactive isotope of plutonium

^{239}Pu radioactive isotope of plutonium

^{240}Pu radioactive isotope of plutonium

PUD peptic ulcer disease
pulmonary disease

PUE pyrexia of unknown etiology

PUFA polyunsaturated fatty acid

PUL pubourethral ligament

Pul pulmonary (also pulm)

pulm gruel (pulmentum)
pulmonary (also Pul)

pulv powder (pulvis)

pulv subtil smooth powder (pulvis subtilis)

PUN plasma urea nitrogen

PUO pyrexia of unknown origin

PU-PC polyunsaturated phosphatidylcholine

PUPP prurilic urticarial papules and plaques of pregnancy

PUT putamen
putrescine (also Pu)

PUVA 8-methoxypsoralen and ultraviolet A irradiation
pulsed ultraviolet actinotherapy

PUVD pulsed ultrasonic blood velocity detector

PV pancreatic vein
papillomavirus
paraventricular
pemphigus vulgaris
peripheral vascular
peripheral vein (also PeV)
peripheral vessel
phenoxymethylpenicillin
phonation volume
photovoltaic
pinocytotic vesicle
plasma viscosity
plasma volume
pneumococcus vaccine
polycythemia vera
polyoma virus
polyvinyl
portal vein (also PoV)
postvasectomy
postvoiding
pressure-volume

pure vegetarian
P/V pressure to volume ratio
P&V pyloroplasty and vagotomy (also V&P)
pv through the vagina (per vaginam)
PVA partial villous atrophy
polyvinyl alcohol
Prinzmetal's variant angina
propyl valeric acid
PVB cisplatin, vinblastine, bleomycin
premature ventricular beat
PVC polyvinyl chloride
predicted vital capacity
premature ventricular complex (also VPC)
premature ventricular contraction (also VPC)
pulmonary venous capillary
pulmonary venous congestion
$PvCO_2$ mixed venous carbon dioxide tension
PVD patient very disturbed
peripheral vascular disease
portal vein dilation
posterior vitreous detachmant
postvagotomy diarrhea
pulmonary vascular disease
PVE prosthetic valve endocarditis
PVF portal venous flow
primary ventricular fibrillation
PVH periventricular hemorrhage
PVI periventricular inhibitor
PVM pneumonia virus of mice
PVN paraventricular nucleus
predictive value of a negative test
PVNO polyvinyl pyridine-N-oxide
PvO_2 mixed venous oxygen pressure
PVOD pulmonary vascular obstructive disease
PVP penicillin V potassium
peripheral venous pressure
polyvinyl prolidone
polyvinyl pyrrolidone
portal venous pressure
predictive value of a positive test
pulmonary venous pressure
PVP-I polyvinyl pyrrolidone iodine
PVR peripheral vascular resistance
pulmonary vascular resistance
pulse volume recording
PVRI pulmonary vascular resistance index
PVS paravesicle space
persistent vegetative state
pigmented villonodular synovitis
poliovirus sensitivity
polyvinyl sponge
premature ventricular systole
pulmonary valvular stenosis
pulmonary vein stenosis
PVSG Polycythemia Vera Study Group
PVT paroxysmal ventricular tachycardia
physical volume test
portal vein thrombosis
pressure, volume, temperature
Pvt private
PVW posterior vaginal wall
PW peristaltic wave
posterior wall
Prades-Willi
pulsed wave
PWB partial weight bearing
PWBRT prophylactic whole brain radiation therapy
PWC physical work capacity
PWD precipitated withdrawal diarrhea
PWE posterior wall excursion
PWI posterior wall infarct
PWM pokeweed mitogen
PWP pulmonary wedge pressure
PWS port wine stain
Prader-Willi Syndrome Association
pulse-wave speed
PWV peak weight velocity
posterior wall velocity
pulse wave speed
pulse wave velocity
PX past (or previous) history (also PH)
peroxidase
physical examination (also PE)
pneumothorax (also PT)
prognosis (also Prog)
PXE pseudoxanthoma elasticum
PY person year
Py phosphopyridoxal
PYC proteose-yeast, castione
PyC pyrogenic culture
PYG peptone, yeast, glucose
PYP pyrophosphate
PYR person year rad
Pyr pyridine
Pyro pyrophosphate
PYS pyriform sinus
PZ pancreozymin
prazosin
pregnancy zone
proliferative zone
sulfaphenazole
PZA pyrazinamide
PzB parenzymes buccal
PZC chlorpiprazine
PZ-CKK
pancreozymin-cholecystokinin (also CKK-PZ)
PZD piperazinedione
PZE piezoelectric
PZI protamine zinc insulin

Q

Q cardiac output (also CO, QT)
electric quantity
perfusion (volume flow of blood)
quart (also qt)
quartile
quinidine
quotient
See C (coulomb)
Q_6 ubiquinone-6
Q_{10} temperature coefficient
ubiquinone-10
q every (quaque) (also qq)
frequency of the rarer allele of a gene pair
long arm of a chromosome
quantity (also quant)
quarter
QA quality assurance
quinaldic acid
quisqualic acid
QAC quanternary ammonium compound
QAM every morning (quaque mane) (also qm)
quality assurance monitor

QAP quinine, atabrine, plasmoquine
QAR quality assurance reagent
quantitative autoradiographic
QAS quality assurance standards
QAT quality assurance technical material
QB Quantitative Electrophysiological Battery
Q_B blood flow
QC quality control
quinine chloroquine
quinine colchicine
QCD quantum chromodynamics
Q_{CO2} microliters of carbon dioxide per milligram per hour
Q d See A b
qd every day (quaque die)
qds four times a day (quater die sumendum) (also qid)
QED quantum electrodynamics
qed which was (quod erat demonstrandum)
QET Quality Extinction Test
QF quality factor
Query fever
Q fract
quick fraction
qh every hour (quaque hora) (also qqhor)
q2h every two hours (quaque secunda hora)
q3h every three hours (quaque tertia hora)
q4h every four hours (quaque quarta hora) (also qqh)
qhs every hour of sleep (quaque hora somno)
qid four times a day (quater in die) (also qds)
ql as much as desired (quantum libet)
qm every morning (quaque mane) (also QAM)
qn every night (quaque nocte) (also QPM)
QNB quinuclidinyl benzilate
quinuclidinyl bromide
QNS quantity not sufficient
Queens Nursing Sister
QO_2 oxygen consumption
oxygen quotient
QOC Quality of Contact
QOD every other day
QON every other night
QP quanti-Pirquet
Qp pulmonary blood flow
qp give at will (quantum placeat)
QPC quality of patient care
Qpc pulmonary capillary blood flow
QPM every night (also qn)
Qp/Qs left to right shunt ratio
QPVT Quick Picture Vocabulary Test
qq also (quoque)
each (quaque) (also q)
qqh every four hours (quaque quarta hora) (also q4h)
qqhor every hour (quaque hora) (also qh)
QR quadriradial
Quieting Reflex
qr the quantity is correct (quantum rectum)
QRN quasiresonant nucleus
QRZ wheal reaction time (Quaddel Reaktion Zeit)
QS quiet sleep
Qs systemic blood flow
qs quantity required (quantum satis)
QSAR quantitative structure activity relationship
QSC quasistatic compliance
QS_2I shortened electrochemical systole
QSL communication understood
QSM please repeat message
QSPV quasistatic pressure volume
Qs/Qt intrapulmonary shunt fraction
right to left shunt ratio
QSS quantitative sacroiliac scintigraphy
q-suff
as much as suffices (quantum sufficit)
QT cardiac output (also Q)
Queckenstedt's test
Quick's test
Quick Tan
quinine tetracycline
Qt quiet
qt quart (also Q)
quad quadriplegia
quant quantity (also q)
quart fourth (quartus)
quat four (quattuor)
QUICH quantitative inhalation challenge apparatus
quinq five (quinque)
quint fifth (quintus)
quor of which (quorum)
quot as often as needed (quoties)
quotid
daily (quotidie)
qv as much as desired (quantum vis)
which see (quod vide)
QWL quality of working life

R

R Behnken's unit
metabolic respiratory quotient
organic radical
radioactive
radiology
ramus
Rankine
ratio
rationale
raw
Reaumur
recessive
rectal
rectified average
regression coefficient
regulator gene
rejection factor
remission
remote
resistance
respirations
respiratory exchange ratio
response
resting
Rhabdomonas
Rhinosporidium
Rhipicephalus
Rhizobium
Rhizopus
Rhodomicrobium
Rhodopseudomonas
Rhodospirillum
Rhodotorula
Rhus

rib
Rickettsia
right
right eye
Rinne
roentgen
rough
rub (also ter)
stimulus (Reiz)
take (recipe) (also Rx)
total responses
+R Rinne's test positive
-R Rinne's test negative
r correlation coefficient
radius
ring chromosome
RA radioactivity
Radionic Association
radionuclide angiography
reading age (also RdA)
renal artery
renin activity
renin-angiotensin
repeat action
residual air
retinoic acid
rheumatoid arthritis
rifampicin
right arm
right atrium
right auricle
robustus archistriatalis
room air
Ra radium
^{224}Ra radioactive isotope of radium
^{226}Ra radioactive isotope of radium
R_a airflow resistance
RAA renin angiotensin aldosterone
right atrial appendage
RAAS renin-angiotensin-aldosterone system
RABA rabbit antibladder antibody
RABCa rabbit antibladder cancer
rac racemic
RAD radical
right atrial diameter
right axis deviation
Rad radiotherapy
rad radial
radiation absorbed dose
root (radix)
RADA rosin amine D acetate
RADS reactive airways disease syndrome
RADTS rabbit antidog thymus serum
RAE right atrial enlargement
RaE rabbit erythrocyte
RAF rheumatoid arthritis factor
Ra-F radium-F
RAG ragweed (also RW)
RAH regressing atypical histiocytosis
right atrial hypertrophy
RAHTG rabbit antihuman thymocyte globulin
RAI radioactive iodine
resting ankle index
RAID radioimmunodetection (also RID)
RAIU radioactive iodine uptake
RAL resorcylic acid lactone
RAM random access memory
RAMC Royal Army Medical Corps
RAMP radioactive antigen microprecipitin
right atrial mean pressure
RAMT rabbit antimouse thymocyte
RAN resident's admission notes
RANA rheumatoid arthritis nuclear antigen
RANCA Retired Army Nurse Corps Association
RAO right anterior oblique
RAP recurrent abdominal pain
right atrial pressure
RAPE right atrial pressure elevation
RAPM refractory anemia with partial myeloblastosis
RAR right arm recumbent
RARLS rabbit antirat lymphocyte serum
RAS recurrent aphthous stomatitis
reflex-activating stimulus
renal artery stenosis
renin angiotensin system
reticular activating system
ras shavings (rasurae)
RASP rapidly alternating speech
RAST radioallergosorbent technique
radioallergosorbent test
RASV recovered avian sarcoma virus
RAT rat aortic tissue
repeat-action tablet
rheumatoid arthritis test
right anterior thigh
RATA radioimmunologic assay antithyroid antibody
R-ATG rabbit-antithymocyte globulin
RATHAS
rat thymus antiserum
RATS rabbit antithymocyte serum
RAU radioactive uptake
RAUC raw area under the curve
RAV Roux-associated virus
RAW airway resistance
RB rating board
rebreathing
Renaut body
respiratory bronchiole
respiratory burst
reticulate body
retinoblastoma
rice body
right bundle
round body
Rb rubidium
^{81}Rb radioactive isotope of rubidium
^{82}Rb radioactive isotope of rubidium
^{83}Rb radioactive isotope of rubidium
^{84}Rb radioactive isotope of rubidium
^{86}Rb radioactive isotope of rubidium
RBA right basal artery
rose bengal antigen
RBAF rheumatoid biologically active factor
RBAP repetitive bursts of action potential
RBB right bundle branch
RBBB right bundle branch block
RBB_sB right bundle branch system block
RBC red blood cell
red blood count
rubicydamin
RBCM red blood cell mass
RBC/P red blood cell to plasma ratio
RBCV red blood cell volume
RBD right border of dullness
RBE relative biologic effectiveness
RBF regional blood flow
renal blood flow
riboflavin
RBM Raji cell-binding material
regional bone mass
RBME regenerating bone marrow extract
RBP retinol-binding protein

RBR radiation bowel reaction
RBU Raji binding unit
RB-V right bundle ventricular
RBW relative body weight
RBZ Rubidazone
RC radiocarpal
reaction center
recrystallized
red cell
Red Cross
referred care
reflection coefficient
regenerated cellulose
resistance and capacitance
respiration ceased
respiratory center
retrograde cystogram
rib cage
Roman Catholic
routine cholecystectomy
Rc conditioned response
RCA Raji cell assay
red cell adherence
red cell agglutination
relative chemotactic activity
Ricinus communis agglutinin
right coronary artery
retrograde conduction to the atria
rubicydin
rCBF regional cerebral blood flow
rCBV regional cerebral blood volume
RCC red cell cast
red cell concentrate
red cell count
renal cell carcinoma
right common carotid
right coronary cusp
RCCT randomized controlled clinical trial
RCD relative cardiac dullness
RCDHS Rehabilitation and Chronic Disease Hospital Section
RCDR relative corrected death rate
RCE Resource for Cancer Epidemiology
RCF red cell filterability
red cell folate
relative centrifugal force
RCG radioelectrocardiograph
RCGP Royal College of General Practitioners
RCHF right-sided congestive heart failure
RCI rate change induced
RCIA red cell immune adherence
RCIT red cell iron turnover
RCL range of comfortable loudness
renal clearance
RCLAAR
red cell-linked antigen-antiglobulin reaction
RCM radiocontrast material
radiocontrast media
red cell mass
reinforced clostridial medium
rheumatoid cervical myelopathy
right costal margin
Royal College of Midwives
rufochromomycin
$rCMRO_2$
regional cerebral metabolic rate for oxygen
RCN Royal College of Nursing
RCOG Royal College of Obstetricians and Gynecologists
RCP riboflavin carrier protein
Royal College of Physicians
RCPE Royal College of Physicians, Edinburgh
RCPH red cell peroxide hemolysis
RCPI Royal College of Physicians, Ireland
RCPSC Royal College of Physicians and Surgeons of Canada
RCQG right caudal quarter ganglion
RCR respiratory control ratio
RCRC Rabbanic Center for Research and Counseling
RCS rabbit contracting substance
reticulum cell sarcoma
red cell suspension
Royal College of Surgeons
RCSE Royal College of Surgeons, Edinburgh
RCSI Royal College of Surgeons, Ireland
RCT randomized controlled clinical trial
Rorschach Content Test
RCU respiratory care unit
RCV red cell volume
Royal College of Veterinary Surgeons
RD Raynaud's disease
reaction of (or to) degeneration
renal disease
resistance determinant
respiratory disease
respiratory distress
retinal detachment
right deltoid
R.D. Registered Dietician
R&D research and development
Rd reading
rd rutherford
RDA recommended daily allowance
recommended dietary allowance
right dorsoanterior
rubidium dihydrogen arsenate
RdA reading age (also RA)
RDC Research Diagnostic Criteria
RDDA recommended daily dietary allowance
RDDP RNA-directed DNA polymerase
RDE receptor destroying enzyme
RDEB recessive dystrophic epidermolysis bullosa
RDFS ratio of decayed and filled surfaces
RDFT ratio of decayed and filled teeth
RDG Research Discussion Group
RDI recommended daily intake
recommended dietary intake
rupture-delivery interval
RDIH right direct inguinal hernia
RDP right dorsoposterior
RDPase
RNA-dependent DNA polymerase
RDQ respiratory disease questionnaire
RdQ reading quotient (also RQ)
RDRV rhesus diploid rabies vaccine
RDS respiratory distress syndrome
reticuloendothelial depressant substance
RDSI Revised Developmental Screening Inventory
RDT regular hemodialysis treatment
RE racemic epinephrine
radium emanation
readmission
reflux esophagitis
regional enteritis
regular education
renal excretion
resting energy
reticuloendothelial

right ear (also AD)
right eye
ring enhancement
rostral end
R&E research and education
Re rhenium
^{182}Re radioactive isotope of rhenium
^{186}Re radioactive isotope of rhenium
^{188}Re radioactive isotope of rhenium
re regarding
REA radioenzymatic assay
REACH Rural Efforts to Assist Children at Home
REAC/TS
Radiation Emergency Assistance Center-Training Site
READ Reading Evaluation-Adult Diagnosis
REC receptor
right external carotid
rec fresh (recens)
record
recreation
recurrent
RECA right external carotid artery
RECG radioelectrocardiography
Recip reciprocal
rect rectified
RED rapid erythrocyte degeneration
redig in pulv
let it be reduced to powder (redigatur in pulverem)
red in pulv
reduced to powder (reductus in pulverem)
redox reduction-oxidation
REE resting energy expenditure
R-EEG resting electroencephalogram
REELS Receptive-Expressive Emergent Language Scale
REEP right end-expiratory pressure
REF renal erythropoietic factor
REFCD Research and Education Foundation for Chest Disease
ref doc
referring doctor
REFRAD
released from active duty
REG radiation exposure guide
radioencephalogram
reg umb
umbilical region (regio umbilici)
Rehab rehabilitation
REL rate of energy loss
resting expiratory level
reliq remainder (reliquus)
REM rapid eye movement
recent event memory
reticular erythematous mucinosis
Rem removal
rem roentgen equivalent, mammal
roentgen equivalent, man
REMAB radiation equivalent manikin absorption
REMCAL
radiation equivalent manikin calibration
remp roentgen equivalent, man period
REMS rapid eye movement, sleep
ren sem
renew once (renovetur semel)
REP rest-exercise program
retrograde pyelogram (also RGP)
rep let it be repeated (repetatur)
roentgen equivalent, physical
REPC reticuloendothelial phagocytic capacity
REPS reactive extensor postural synergy
RER renal excretion rate
respiratory exchange ratio
rough endoplasmic reticulum
RERF Radiation Effects Research Foundation
RES Reticuloendothelial Society
reticuloendothelial system
Res research
Resp respectively
respiratory
REST regressive electric shock therapy
reticulospinal tract
RET rational-emotive therapy
ret rad equivalent therapeutic
RETC rat embryo tissue culture
Retic reticulocyte
REV reticuloendotheliosis virus
reversal
Rev review
revise
RF radial fiber
radical fiber
receptive field
recognition factor
regurgitant fraction
Reitland-Franklin
relative flow
relative fluorescence
releasing factor
renal failure
replicative form
resistance factor
resorcinol formaldehyde
respiratory failure
respiratory frequency
retardation factor
reticular formation
rheumatic fever
rheumatoid factor
rifamycin
Rockefeller Foundation
root canal filling
Rf rutherfordium
R_f rate of flow
rf radiofrequency
RFA right femoral artery
right frontoanterior
RFB Recording for the Blind
retained foreign body
rhematoid factor binding
RFC retrograde femoral catheter
right frontal craniotomy
rosette-forming cells
RFFIT rapid fluorescent focus inhibition test
RFI recurrence-free interval
RFL right frontolateral
RFLA rheumatoid factorlike activity
RFLC resistant Friend leukemia cell
RFLP restriction fragment length polymorphism
RFLS rheumatoid factorlike substance
RFP request for proposal
right frontoposterior
RFPS Royal Faculty of Physicians and Surgeons
RFR rapid filling rate
refraction
RFS relapse-free survival
renal function study
RFT right fibrous trigone

right frontotransverse
rod-and-frame test
RFTB riboflavin tetrabutyrate
RFTSW right foot switch
RFW rapid filling wave
RG right gluteal
R/G red/green
RGBMT renal glomerular basement membrane thickness
RGC remnant gastric cancer
retinal ganglion cell
RGD range-gated Doppler
RGE relative gas expansion
respiratory gas equation
RGMT reciprocal geometric mean titer
R.G.N.
Registered General Nurse
RGP retrograde pyelogram (also REP)
rural general practitioner
RGT reversed gastric tube
RH radial hemolysis
reactive hyperemia
recurrent herpes
regional heparionization
relative humidity
releasing hormone
retinal hemorrhage
right hand
Rh rhesus factor
rhodium
See R (Rhipicephalus)
^{102}Rh radioactive isotope of rhodium
^{105}Rh radioactive isotope of rhodium
rh rhonchi/rale
RHA right hepatic artery
Rural Health Associates
RhA rheumatoid arthritis (see RA)
RHB right heart bypass
RHBF reactive hyperemia blood flow
RHBV right-heart blood volume
RHC respirations have ceased
right heart catheterization
RHCD Rural Health Care Delivery
RHD radial head dislocation
relative hepatic dullness
renal hypertensive dog
rheumatic heart disease
round heart disease
RhD rhesus hemolytic disease
RHE respiratory heat exchange
Rheum rheumatic
RHF right heart failure
RHG radial hemolysis in gel
Rhi rhinology
RhIG Rh immune globulin
Rhiz See R (Rhizobium)
RHL right hepatic lobe
RHLN right hilar lymph node
rhm roentgen hour meter
RhMK rhesus monkey kidney (also RMK)
RHMV right heart mixing volume
RHPA reverse hemolytic plaque assay
RHR renal hypertensive rat
RHS right-hand side
rough hard sphere
RHT renal homotransplantation
Rhu rheumatology
RI radioisotope
Radix Institute
refractive index
regenerative index
regional ileitis
Rehabilitation International
relative intensity
remission induced
respiratory illness
respiratory index
retroactive inhibition
ribostamycin
Rolf Institute
rosette inhibition
RIA radioimmunoassay
Registry of Interpreters for the Deaf
Research Institute on Alcoholism
reversible ischemic attack
RIA-DA
radioimmunoassay--double-antibody
Rib ribose
RIC renomedullary interstitial cell
right internal carotid
Royal Institute of Chemistry
RICA reverse immune cytoadhesion
RICE rest, ice, compression, elevation
RICM right intercostal margin
RICS right intercostal space
RICU respiratory intensive care unit
RID radial immunodiffusion
radioimmunodetection
radioimmunodiffusion (also RAID)
remission-inducing drug
Remove Intoxicated Driver
right ventricular internal diameter
RIEP rocket immunoelectrophoresis
RIF rifampin
right iliac fossa
rosette inhibitory factor
RIFA radioiodinated fatty acid
RIFC rat intrinsic factor concentrate
RIFM Research Institute for Fragrance Materials
RIG rabies immune globulin
RIH right inguinal hernia
RIHSA radioactive iodinated human serum albumin
RIM relative intensity measure
RIMA right internal mammary artery
RIMN Research Institute of Metabolism and Nutrition
RIMS resonance ionization mass spectrometry
RIND resolving ischemic neurologic deficit
reversible ischemic neurologic deficit
RIP radioimmunoprecipitation
reflex-inhibiting pattern
respiratory inductance plethysmography
RIPH Royal Institute of Public Health
RIPHH Royal Institute of Public Health and Hygiene
RIRB radioiodinated rose bengal
RIS resonance ionization spectroscopy
RISA radioiodinated serum albumin
RISE Research in Science Education
RISF Repeated Stem Short Form
RIST radioimmunosorbent test
RIT radioiodinated triolein
RITC rhodamine isothiocyanate
rhodamine isothiocyanate conjugated
RIU radioactive iodine uptake
RIVS ruptured interventricular septum
RJI radionuclide joint imaging
RK rabbit kidney
right kidney
RKB red kidney bean
RKY roentgenkymography
RL coarse rales

reduction level
resistive load
right lateral
right leg
right lung
Ringer's lactate

R-L right to left
RL_3 numerous coarse rales
R_L pulmonary resistance
Rl medium rales
Rl_2 moderate number of medium rales
rl fine rales
rl_1 few fine rales
RLA radiographic lung area
RLBCD right lower border of cardiac dullness
RLC rectus and longus capitus
residual lung capacity
rhodopsin-lipid complex
RLD related living donor
resistive load detection
RLE Recent Life Events
right lower extremity
RLF retrolental fibroplasia
RLL right liver lobe
right lower lobe
RLM Regional Library of Medicine
RLMD rat liver mitochondria digitonin
RLN recurrent laryngeal nerve
regional lymph node
RLND retroperitoneal lymph node dissection
RLO residual lymphocyte output
RLP radiation-leukemia-protection
RLQ right lower quadrant
RLR right lateral rectus
right lower rectus
RLS rat lung strip
restless legs syndrome
Ringer's lactate solution
stutterer who mispronounces R,L,S
RLT right lateral thigh
RLV Rauscher leukemia virus
RLWD routine laboratory work done
RM radical mastectomy
random migration
repetitions maximum
resistive movement
respiratory movement
rifamide
right median
Rm relative mobility
RMA right mentoanterior
RMB right mainstem bronchus
RMC right middle cerebral
RMCP I
rat mast cell protease I
RMCP II
rat mast cell protease II
RMCT rat mast cell technique
RMD Doctor of Research Medicine
ratio of the midsagittal diameters
retromanubrial dullness
RMDCC Rocky Mountain Drug Consultation Center
RME resting metabolic expenditure
RMI Reading Miscue Inventory
RMK rhesus monkey kidney (also RhMK)
RML right mediolateral
right mentolateral
right middle lobe
RMLB Rauscher murine leukemia virus
right middle lobe bronchus
R.M.N.
Registered Mental Nurse
RMO Regional Medical Officer
Resident Medical Officer
RMP rapidly miscible pool
Regional Medical Program
resting membrane potential
right mentoposterior
RMPA Royal Medico-Psychological Association
RMPS Regional Medical Programs Service
RMR resting metabolic rate
right medial rectus
RMS rheumatic mitral stenosis
rhodomyosarcoma
root mean square
RMSF Rocky Mountain spotted fever
RMT retromolar trigone
right mentotransverse
RMUI relief medication unit index
RMV respiratory minute volume
RN radionuclide
red nucleus
reflux nephropathy
reticular nucleus
R.N. Registered Nurse
Rn radon
^{222}Rn radioactive isotope of radon
RNA radionuclide angiocardiography
ribonucleic acid
rough noncapsulated avirulent
RNase ribonuclease
RNaseA
ribonuclease A
RND radical neck dissection
reactive neurotic depression
RNG radionuclide angiography
R.N.M.S.
Registered Nurse for the Mentally Sub-Normal
RNP ribonucleoprotein
RNT radioassayable neurotensin
RNTC rat nephroma tissue culture
RNV radionuclide ventriculography
RO reality orientation
relative odds
reverse osmosis
Ritter-Oleson
routine order
R/O rule out
R_o resting radium
ROA rat ovarian augmentation
right occipitoanterior
ROAD reversible obstructive airways disease
ROAP rubidazone, vincristine (Oncovin), Ara-C, prednisone
ROATS rabbit ovarian antitumor serum
ROC receiver operating characteristic
relative operating characteristic
Roent roentgenology
ROH rat ovarian hyperemia
ROI region of interest
ROIH right oblique inguinal hernia
ROL right occipitolateral
ROM range of motion (or movement)
read only memory
rupture of membrane
Rom Romberg
ROP retinopathy of prematurity
right occipitoposterior
Ror Rorschach
ROS review of systems
rod outer segment
ROT remedial occupational therapy
right occipitotransverse

rotating
rule of thumb
ROW rat ovarian weight
RP radiographic planimetry
reaction product
reactive protein
rectal prolapse
red pulp
reentrant pathway
refractory period
relapsing polychondritis
relative potency
resting potential
resting pressure
rest pain
retinitis pigmentosa
retinitis proliferans
rheumatoid polyarthritis
R-5-P ribose-5-phosphate
Rp pulmonary vascular resistance
RPA right pulmonary artery
R.P.A.
Registered Physician's Assistant
RPAR Rural Physician Associate Program
RPAW right pulmonary artery withdrawal
RPB Research to Prevent Blindness
RPC relapsing polychondritis
relative proliferative capacity
reticularis pontis caudalis
RPCF Reiter protein complement fixation
RPCFT Reiter protein complement fixation test
RPE rating of perceived exertion
recurrent pulmonary emboli
retinal pigment epithelium
RPF relaxed pelvic floor
renal plasma flow
retroperitoneal fibrosis
RPF^a arterial renal plasma flow
RPF^v venous renal plasma flow
RPG radiation protection guide
retrograde pyelogram
rheoplethysmography
RPGN rapidly progressive glomerulonephritis
R.Ph. Registered Pharmacist
RPHA reverse passive hemagglutination assay
RPI Racial Perceptions Inventory
Relative Percentage Index
RPLC reverse phase high performance chromatography
RPLD repair of potentially lethal damage
RPM radical pair mechanism
rpm revolutions per minute
RPMI Roswell Park Memorial Institute
R.P.N.
Registered Practical Nurse
RPO right posterior oblique
RPP rate-pressure product
RPPC regional pediatric pulmonary center
RPR rapid plasma reagin
RPRCF rapid plasma reagin complement fixation
RPRCT rapid plasma reagin card test
RPS renal pressor substance
Rps See R (Rhodopseudomonas)
rps revolutions per second
RPT rapid pull-through
R.P.T.
Registered Physical Therapist
RPTA renal percutaneous transluminal angioplasty
RPTC regional poisoning treatment center
RPV right portal vein
right pulmonary vein
RQ reading quotient (also RdQ)
recovery quotient
respiratory quotient
RR radiation reaction
radiation response
rapid radiometric
reading retarded
recovery room
relative risk
renin release
respiratory rate
respiratory reserve
response rate
rheumatoid rosette
roentgenographic pelvimetry
ruthenium red
R&R rest and recuperation
Rr rami
RRA radioreceptor activity
radioreceptor assay
R.R.A.
Registered Records Administrator
RRBC rabbit red blood cell
RRC Risk Reduction Component
RRE radiation-related eosinophilia
regressive resistive exercise
RR&E round, regular, and equal
RRF residual renal function
RR-HPO
rapid recompression--high pressure oxygen
RRI reflex relaxation index
relative response index
R.R.L.
Registered Records Librarian
rRNA ribosomal ribonucleic acid
RRP relative refractory period
RRQG right rostal quarter ganglion
RRR regular rate and rhythm
renin-release rate
risk rescue rating
RRS Radiation Research Society
retrorectal space
Riva-Rocci sphygmomanometer
RRT randomized response technique
resazurin reduction time
R.R.T.
Registered Respiratory Therapist
RRU respiratory resistance unit
RS random sample
rapid smoking
Rating Schedule
Raynaud's syndrome
reading of standard
rectosigmoid
Reed-Sternberg
reinforcement of stimulus
Reiter's syndrome
relative survival
remnant stomach
Repression-Sensitization Scale
reproductive success
resolved sarcoidosis
resorcinol-sulfur
respiratory syncytial
review of systems
Reye's syndrome
right septum
right side
right subclavian
Ringer's solution
Ritchie sedimentation

Rs total systemic resistance
RSA rabbit serum albumin
rat serum albumin
regular spiking activity
Rehabilitation Services Administration
relative specific activity
Research Society on Alcoholism
respiratory sinus arrhythmia
reticulum cell sarcoma
right sacroanterior
right subclavian artery
Rsa total systemic arterial resistance
RSB Regimental Stretcher Bearer
right sternal border
RSBT rhythmic sensory bombardment therapy
RSC rested-state contraction
RScA right scapuloanterior
R.S.C.N.
Registered Sick Children's Nurse
RScP right scapuloposterior
RSD reflex sympathetic dystrophy
relative sagittal depth
relative standard deviation
RSEP right somatosensory evoked potential
RSF raw soybean flour
RSH Royal Society for the Promotion of Health
R-SICU
respiratory-surgical intensive care unit
RSIVP rapid-sequence intravenous pyelogram
RSL right sacrolateral
RSLD repair of sublethal damage
RSM risk-screening model
Royal Society of Medicine
RSMR relative standardized mortality ratio
RSNA Radiological Society of North America
RSO Radiation Safety Officer
RSP recirculating single pass
removable silicone plug
right sacroposterior
RSR regular sinus rhythm
RS response to stimulus
RSSE Russian spring-summer encephalitis
RSSR relatively slow sinus rate
RST radiosensitivity test
right sacrotransverse
rubrospinal tract
RSTMH Royal Society of Tropical Medicine and Hygiene
RSV respiratory syncytial virus
right subclavian vein
Rous sarcoma virus
RSVC right superior vena cava
RSVM ram seminal vesicle microsome
RT rabbit trachia
radiation therapy
radiotelemetry
radiotherapy
radium therapy
random transfusion
raphe transection
reaction time
reading task
reading test
receptor transforming
reciprocative tachycardia
recreational therapy
rectal temperature
red tetrazolium (also TPTZ, TTC)
reduction time
renal transplant
Reporter's Test
reptilase time
resistance transfer
respiratory technology
respiratory therapy
right thigh
room temperature
R.T. Radiologic Technologist
Registered Technician
Registered Therapist
Respiration Therapist
RT_3 resin triiodothyronine
reverse triiodothyronine
RT_4 resin thyroxin
rt right
RTA renal tubular acidosis
renal tubular antigen
road traffic accident
RTC rape treatment center
renal tubular cell
research and training center
return to clinic
ribofuranosyl-triasole-carboxamide
RTD routine test dilution
Rtd retarded
RTE rabbit thymus extract
RTF replication and transfer
resistance transfer factor
respiratory tract fluid
RTI Research Triangle Institute
Rt lat
right lateral
Rtn return
RTOG Radiation Therapy Oncology Group
RTP Regional Transplant Program
renal transplant patient
RTR retention time ratio
return to room
RTRD Registry of Tissue Reactions to Drugs
RTRR return to recovery room
RTS real time scan
relative tumor size
rTSAb rodent thryoid stimulating antibody
RTT radiation therapy technician
RTU relative time unit
RT_3U resin triiodothyronine uptake
RTV room temperature vulcanizing
RU rat unit
reading of unknown
recurrent ulcer
resin uptake
resistance unit
retrograde urogram
right upper
rodent ulcer
roentgen unit
Ru ruthenium
^{97}Ru radioactive isotope of ruthenium
^{103}Ru radioactive isotope of ruthenium
^{106}Ru radioactive isotope of ruthenium
rub red (ruber)
RuBP ribulose bisphosphate
RUE right upper extremity
RUL right upper lobe
RUOQ right upper outer quadrant
RUP right upper pole
Ru-5-P
ribulose-5-phosphate
RUQ right upper quadrant
RUR resin-uptake ratio
RURTI recurrent upper respiratory tract infection

RUS radioulnar synostosis
recurrent ulcerative stomatitis
RUSB right upper sternal border
RUSS recurrent ulcerative scarifying stomatitis
RUV residual urine volume
RV random variable
rat virus
renal venous
reovirus
residual volume
respiratory volume
retinal vasculitis
retroversion
rheumatoid vasculitis
rhinovirus
right ventricle
rubella vaccine
rubella virus
RVA re-entrant ventricular arrhythmia
right ventricular activation
right ventricular apical
right vertebral artery
RVAW right ventricle anterior wall
RVB red venous blood
RVC radioactivity of vegetative cells
responds to verbal commands
RVD rat vas deferens
relative volume decrease
right ventricular dimension
right vertebral density
RVE right ventricular enlargement
RVECP right ventricular endocardial potential
RVEDP right ventricular end-diastolic pressure
RVEDV right ventricular end-diastolic volume
RVEDVI
right ventricular end-diastolic volume index
RVEF right ventricular ejection fraction
right ventricular end flow
RVESVI
right ventricular end-systolic volume index
RVF Rift Valley fever
right ventricular failure
RVFV Rift Valley fever virus
RVG relative value guide
RVH renovascular hypertension
right ventricular hypertrophy
RVI relative value index
RVID right ventricular internal dimension
RVIT right ventricular inflow tract
RVO relaxed vaginal outlet
RVOT right ventricular outflow tract
RVP red veterinary petrolatum
renovascular pressure
resting venous pressure
right ventricular pressure
RVR reduced vascular response
reduced vestibular response
renal vascular resistance
renal vein renin
repetitive ventricular response
resistance to venous return
RVRA renal vein renin activity
RVRC renal vein renin concentration
RVS Relative Value Scale
Relative Value Schedule
Relative Value Study
reported visual sensation
retrovaginal space
RVSO right ventricle stroke output
RVT renal vein thrombosis
RV-TLC
residual volume to total lung capacity
RVU relative value unit
RVV Russell viper venom
RVWD right ventricular wall device
RW radiologic warfare
ragweed (also RAG)
respiratory work
round window
R-W Rideal-Walter
RWP ragweed pollen
RWS ragweed sensitivity
Rx prescription
take (recipe) (also R)
therapy
treatment
Ry Roux-en-Y

S

S relative storage capacity
response to white space
Saccharomyces
sacral
saline (also SAL)
Salmonella
Saprospira
Sarcocystis
Sarcoptes
saturation of hemoglobin
Schistosoma
schizophrenia (also Schiz, SZ)
section (also SEC)
sensation
sensitive
septum (also sept)
sequential analysis
Serratia
Shigella
siemens
silicate
single
Siphunculina
smooth
soft
soil
soluble (also Sol)
son
space (also sp)
spherical (also Sph)
spherical lens (also Sph)
Spirillum
Spirometra
spleen
sporadic
Sporothrix
Sporotrichum
Staphylococcus
stimulus
Stomoxys
storage
Streptobacillus
Streptococcus
Strongyloides
subject

subjective
substrate
sulfur
supravergence
surgery
suture
Svedberg unit
sympathetic
systole
write (signa)

S1...S5
sacral nerve 1 through 5
sacral vertebra 1 through 5

^{35}S radioactive isotope of sulfur

S_1 first heart sound

S_2 second heart sound

S_3 ventricular gallop (third heart sound)

S_4 atrial gallop (fourth heart sound)

s half (semis) (also sem)
left (sinister)
let it be taken (sumat)
label (signa)
second (also sec)
steady state (also SS, ss)

$\bar{s}$ without (sine) (also s)

SA salicylamide (also SAM)
salicylic acid
sarcoma
Scoliosis Association
second antibody
secondary amenorrhea
secondary anemia
secondary arrest
self-agglutinating
seman analysis
senile atrophy
sensitizing antibody
serum albumin (also SAB)
serum aldolase
sialic acid
siblings raised apart
Singh's Aedes albopictus
sinoatrial (also S-A)
sinus arrest
sinus arrhythmia
skeletal age
slightly active
social acquiescence
soluble in alkaline solution
Spanish American
spatial average
specific activity
sperm abnormality
spermagglutinin
Staphylococcus aureus
Stokes-Adams
suicide attempt
surface antigen
surface area
surgeon's assistant
sustained action
sympathetic activity
systemic artery

S-A sinoatrial (also SA)

S&A sugar and acetone

S_2A second heart sound, aortic component

Sa samarium

^{153}Sa radioactive isotope of samarium

sa according to skill (secundum artem)

SAA serum amyloid A
Stokes-Adams attack

SAARD slow-acting antirheumatic drug

SAAST self-administered alcohol screening test

SAB serum albumin (also SA)
significant asymptomatic bacteriuria
sinoatrial block
Society of American Bacteriologists

SAC saccharin
screening and acute care
splenic adherent cell

SACD subacute combined degeneration

SACE serum angiotensive converting enzyme

SACED Self-Assessment and Continuing Education

SACH solid ankle cushion heel

SACHT serum antichromotrypsin

SACS secondary anticoagulation system

SACSF subarachnoid cerebral spinal fluid

SACT sinoatrial conduction time

SAD separation anxiety disorder
small airways dysfunction
social avoidance and distress
source to axis distance
Street Alabama Dufferin
sugar, acetone, diacetic acid
suppressor activating determinant

SADBE dibutylester of squaric acid

SADD Standardized Assessment of Depressive Disorders

SADL simulated activities of daily living

SADR suspected adverse reaction

SADS Schedule for Affective Disorders and Schizophrenia
Shipman Anxiety Depression Scale

SADS-C
Schedule for Affective Disorders and Schizophrenia--Change

SADS-L
Schedule for Affective Disorders and Schizophrenia--Lifetime Version

SAE specific action exercise
supported arm exercise

SAEB sinoatrial entrance block

SAF serum accelerator factor
simultaneous auditory feedback

SAFA Society of Air Force Anesthesiologists
soluble antigen fluorescent antibody

SAFE simulated aircraft fire and emergency

SAG streptavidin gold
Swiss agammaglobulinemia

SAGES Society of American Gastrointestinal Endoscopic Surgeons

SAGN sodium chloride, adenine, glucose, mannitol

SAH S-adenosyl homocystein
subarachnoid hemorrhage

SAHS sleep apnea hypersomnolence syndrome

SAI Social Adequacy Index
systemic active immunotherapy

SAICAR
succino-aminoimidazolecarboxamide ribonucleotide

SAID sexually acquired immunodeficiency syndrome

SAIN Society for Advancement in Nursing

SAL salbutamol
saline (also S)
sensorineural acuity level
specified antilymphocytic

Sal See S (Salmonella)

sal according to the rules of art (secundum artis leges)
salicylate

SAM S-adenosylmethionine (also AdoMet)
salicylamide (also SA)
Society for Adolescent Medicine
surface active material
synthetic, adhesive, moisture vapor permeable
systolic anterior motion (or movement)
sulfated acid mucopolysaccharide
SAMA Scientific Apparatus Makers Association
Student American Medical Association
SAMD S-adenosyl methione decarboxylase
SAMF single antibody millipore filtration
SAMI socially acceptable monitoring instrument
SAMPE Society for the Advancement of Material and Process Engineering
SAMS Society for Advanced Medical Systems
SAN sinoatrial node
sinoauricular node
slept all night
solitary autonomous nodule
SANS Scale for the Assessment of Negative Symptoms
SAO small airway obstruction
SaO_2 arterial oxygen saturation
SAODAP
Specoal Action Office for Drug Abuse Protection
SAP sensory action potential
serum acid phosphatase
serum alkaline phosphatase
serum amyloid P
Staphylococcus aureus protease
systemic arterial pressure
SAPD self-administration of psychoactive drugs
SAPhA Student American Pharmaceutical Association
SAPP sodium acid pyrophosphate
SAQC statistical analysis and quality control
SAR sexual attitude reassessment
sexual attitude restructuring
Sar sulfarsphenamine
SARS Sexual Assault Resource Service
SART sinoatrial recovery time
SAS self-rating anxiety scale
sleep apnea syndrome
small animal surgery
Social Adaptation Status
statistical analysis system
subaortic stenosis
subarachnoid space
sulfasalazine (also SAZ)
supravalvular aortic stenosis
surface-active substance
SASP salazosulfapyridine
SAS-SR
Social Adjustment Self-Report Scale
SAT Scholastic Aptitude Test
serum antitrypsin
Slide Agglutination Test
specified antithymocytic
speech awareness threshold
spermatogenic activity test
spontaneous autoimmune thyroiditis
Stanford Achievement Test
structural atypia
subacute thyroiditis
Sat saturated
SATA spatial average temporal average
SATH Society for the Advancement of Travel for the Handicapped
SATM sodium aurothiomalate
SATP spatial average temporal peak
SAV streptavidin
supra-anular valve
SAZ sulfasalazine (also SAS)
SB sandbag
serum bilirubin
single blind
single breath
sinus bradycardia
small bowel
spina bifida
spontaneous blastogenesis
spontaneously breathing
Stanford-Binet
sternal border
stillbirth (see also Stb)
S-B Sengstaken-Blakemore
Sb antimony (stibium)
strabismus
^{122}Sb radioactive isotope of antimony
^{124}Sb radioactive isotope of antimony
^{125}Sb radioactive isotope of antimony
SBA serum bile acid
soybean agglutinin
spina bifida aperta
Spina Bifida Association
SBAA Spina Bifida Association of America
SBB simultaneous binaural, bithermal
SBC serum bactericidal concentration
sunburn cell
SBD suggested brain dysfunction
SBDP standard dose beclomethasone dipropionate
SBE self breast examination (also BSE)
subacute bacterial endocarditis
SBET Society for Biomedical Equipment Technicians
SBF serum blocking factor
specific blocking factor
splanchnic blood flow
splenic blood flow
SBFT small bowel follow through
SBG selenite brilliant green
SBIS Stanford-Binet Intelligence Scale
SBN single breath nitrogen
SBNT single breath nitrogen test
SBNW single breath nitrogen washout
SBO small bowel obstruction
spina bifida occulta
SBOM soybean oil meal
SBP School Breakfast Program
serotonin-binding protein
Society of Biological Psychiatry
spontaneous bacterial peritonitis
steroid-binding plasma protein
sulfobromophthalein (also BSP)
systemic blood pressure
systolic blood pressure
SBPC sulfobenzyl penicillin
SBQ Smoking Behavior Questionnaire
SBR spleen to body weight ratio
stillbirth rate
strict bed rest
SBS short bowel syndrome
side to back to side
social-breakdown syndrome
SBT serum bactericidal test
serum bactericidal titer
single breath test
SBTI soybean trypsin inhibitor

SC closure of the semilunar valves
sacrococcygeal
schedule change
Schwann cell
scruple (also Scr)
secondary cleavage
secretory component
self-care
self-control
semicircular
semiclosed
serum creatinine
service connected
short circuit
sick call
sickle cell
single chemical
skin conductance
Smeloff-Cutter
Snellen's chart
Society for Cyrosurgery
Special Care
specific characteristic
spinal cord (also sp cd)
spleen cell
stellate cell
stepped care
sternoclavicular
stimulus, conditioned
stratum corneum
stroke count
subcellular
subclavian
subcortical
subcutaneous
succinylcholine
sugar coated
sulfur colloid
sulfur containing
superior colliculus
superior constrictor
superior cornu
supportive care
supressor cell
surface colony
surgical cone

Sc scandium
scapula
science (also Sci)

^{43}Sc radioactive isotope of scandium

^{44}Sc radioactive isotope of scandium

^{46}Sc radioactive isotope of scandium

^{47}Sc radioactive isotope of scandium

SCA self-care agency
severe congenital anomaly
sickle cell anemia
spleen colony assay
subclavian artery
superior cerebellar artery
supressor cell activity

S_{Ca} serum calcium

SCAb autoantibody to stratum corneum

SCAG Sandoz Clinical Assessment for Geriatrics
single coronary artery graft

SCAN suspected child abuse and neglect
systolic coronary artery narrowing

SCAS semicontinuous activated sludge

SCAT School and College Ability Test
sheep cell agglutination test
sickle cell anemia test

scat box (scatula)

scat orig
original package (scatular originalis)

SCB sedative cabinet bath
stratum corneum basic
strictly confined to bed

SCBH systemic cutaneous basophil hypersensitivity

SCBU special care baby unit

ScBU screening bacteriuria

SCC Sabouraud-cycloheximide-chloramphenicol
sequential combination chemotherapy
short-circuit current
short-course chemotherapy
Sickle Cell Center
small cell cancer
squamous carcinoma of the cervix
squamous cell carcinoma

SCCB small cell carcinoma of the bronchus

SCCHN squamous cell carcinoma of the head and neck

SCCL small cell carcinoma of the lung (see also SCLC)

SCCM Society of Critical Care Medicine

SCD service-connected disability
sickle cell disease
spinocerebellar degeneration
subacute combined degeneration
sudden cardiac death
sudden coronary death
sulfur-carbon drug

5-S-CD
5-S-cysteinyldopa

Sc.D. Doctor of Science (also D.Sc.)

ScDA scapulodextra anterior

SCDFGNY
Sickle Cell Disease Foundation of Greater New York

ScDP scapulodextra posterior

SCE saturated calomel electrode
sister chromatid exchange
Society for Clinical Ecology
subcutaneous emphysema

SCEC S-carboxyethylcysteine

SCEH Society for Clinical and Experimental Hypnosis

SCER sister chromatid exchange rate

SCF Skin Cancer Foundation
supercritical fluid

scf standard cubit foot

SCFA short chain fatty acid

SCFE slipped capital femoral epiphysis

SCFI specific clotting factors and inhibitors

SCG sodium cromoglycate
superior cervical ganglion

SCH Schirmer
succinylcholine
suprachiasmatic

sched schedule

Schiz schizophrenia (also S, SZ)

SCHL subcapsular hematoma of the liver

SCI short crus of incus
spinal cord injury
Stroke Club International
structured clinical interview

Sci science (also Sc)

SCIBTA
stem cell indicated by transplantation assay

SCID severe combined immunodeficiency disease

SCIPP sacrococcygeal to inferior pubic point

Statewide Childhood Injury Prevention Program
SCIS Spinal Cord Injury Service
SCIU Spinal Cord Injury Unit
SCJ sternoclavicular joint
SCK serum creatine kinase
SCL scleroderma
serum copper level
symptom checklist
ScLA scapulolaeva anterior
SCLC small cell lung cancer (see also SCCL)
ScLP scapulolaeva posterior
SCM Society for Computer Medicine
sodium colistimethate
spondylotic caudal myelopathy
State Certified Midwife
steatocystoma multiplex
sternocleidomastoid
structure of the cytoplasmic matrix
surface-connecting membrane
ScM scalene muscle
SCMC S-carboxymethylcysteine
sodium carboxymethylcellulose
spontaneous cell-mediated cytotoxicity
SCMI Society to Conquer Mental Illness
SCMT delta^{24}-sterol-C-methyltransferase
SCN serum thiocyanate
sodium thiocyanate
suprachiasmatic nucleus
SCNS subcutaneous nerve stimulation
SCO Society for Contemporary Ophthalmology
Society for Cryo-Ophthalmology
Scop scopolamine
SCOPE Scientific Committee on Problems of the Environment
SCOR Specialized Centers of Research
SCP single-cell protein
Standardized Care Plan
submucous cleft palate
superior cerebellar peduncle
SCPK serum creatine phosphokinase
SCPV Special Virus Cancer Program
SCR skin conductance response
Society of Cardiovascular Radiology
spondylotic caudal rediculopathy
Scr scruple (also SC)
SCRAM speech controlled respirometer for ambulation measurement
SCRAP simple complex reaction time apparatus
SCRS Short Clinical Rating Scale
SCS Society of Clinical Surgery
SCSP supracondylar, suprapatellar
SCT salmon calcitonin
sentence completion test
sex chromatin test
sickle cell trait
sperm cytotoxic
spinal computed tomography
spinocervicothalamic
staphylococcal clumping test
sugar-coated tablet
SCTAT sex cord tumor with anular tubules
SCU special care unit
SCUBA self-contained underwater breathing apparatus
SCUD septicemic cutaneous ulcerative disease
SCUM secondary carcinoma of the upper mediastinum
SCV sensory conduction velocity
smooth, capsulated, virulent
squamous cell carcinoma of the vulva
subclavian vein
SCV-CPR
simultaneous compression ventilation-cardiopulmonary resuscitation
SD secretion droplet
senile dementia
septal defect
serologically defined
serologically detected
serum defect
severe disability
shoulder dislocation
Shy-Drager
skin dose
socialized delinquency
somadendritic
spontaneous delivery
Sprague-Dawley
standard deviation
Stensen's duct
stimulus drive
streptodornase
succinate dehydrogenase
sudden death
sulfadiazine
systolic discharge
S/D systolic to diastolic ratio
SDA Sabouraud dextrose agar
sacrodextra anterior
sialodacryoadenitis virus
specific dynamic action
State Dental Association
succinic dehydrogenase activity
SDAT senile dementia of the Alzheimer type
SDB sleep disordered breathing
SDBP seated diastolic blood pressure
standing diastolic blood pressure
supine diastolic blood pressure
SDC serum digoxin concentration
sodium deoxycholate
succinyldicholine
sulfodeoxycholate
SDCL symptom distress checklist
SDD sporadic depressive disease
SDE specific dynamic effect
SDES symptomatic diffuse esophageal spasm
SDF stream dilution factor
stress distribution factor
SDG short distance group
succinate dehydrogenase
SDGC sucrose density gradient centrifugation
SDGU sucrose density gradient ultracentrifugation
SDH serine dehydrase
sorbital dehydrogenase
spinal dorsal horn
subdural hematoma
succinate dehydrogenase
SDI Surtees' Difficulties Index
SDL self-directed learning
serum digoxin level
speech discrimination loss
SDM sensory detection method
standard deviation of the mean
sulfadimidine
SDMS Society of Diagnostic Medical Sonographers
SDN sexually dimorphic nucleus
SDNA single-strand deoxyribonucleic acid
SDO sudden-dosage onset
SDP sacrodextra posterior
stomach, duodenum, pancreas

SDPH sodium diphenylhydantoin
SDR spontaneously diabetic rat
SDRT Stanford Diagnostic Reading Test
SDS Self-rating Depression Scale
sensory deprivation syndrome
Shy-Drager syndrome
simple descriptive scale
single dose suppression
sodium dodecyl sulfate
speech discrimination score
standard deviation score
sudden death syndrome
sulfadiazine silver
sustained depolarizing shift
SDT sacrodextra transversa
sensory decision theory
single donor transfusion
speech detection threshold
SDU short double upright
standard deviation unit
SDW separated, divorced, or widowed
SE saline enema
sanitary engineer
Seeing Eye
self-explanatory
sheep erythrocyte (also SRBC)
side effect
smoke exposure
smoke extract
soft exudate
sphenoethmoidal
spherical equivalent
spongiform encephalopathy
squamous epithelium
standard error
Starr-Edwards
status epilepticus
sterol ester
subendothelial
supernormal excitability
sustained engraftment
Se selenium
^{34}Se radioactive isotope of selenium
SEA Science and Education Administration
Sea Education Association
sheep erythrocyte agglutination
shock elicited aggression
soluble egg antigen
spontaneous electrical activity
SEAN State Enrolled Assistant Nurse
SEB Scale for Emotional Blunting
staphylococcal enterotoxin B
SEBL self-emptying blind loop
SEBM Society for Experimental Biology and Medicine
SEC secondary
secretin
section (also S)
series elastic component
size exclusion chromatography
soft elastic capsule
sec second (also s)
SECA Shiatsu Education Center of America
SECRA Southeastern Cancer Research Association
SECSG Southeastern Cancer Study Group
SED skin erythema dose
spondyloepiphyseal dysplasia
standard error of difference
strain energy density
surgeon, emergency department
Sed sedimentation
sed stool (sedes)
SEDD Szondi's Experimental Diagnostics of Drives
SEDR Science Education Development and Research
sed rt
sedimentation rate (also SR)
SEE series elastic element
standard error of the estimate
SEER Surveillance, Epidemiology, and End Result
SEF staphylococcal enterotoxin F
SEG sonoencephalogram
Seg segment
SEGS segmented neutrophils
SEH subependymal hemorrhage
SEI Self-Esteem Inventory
Surtees' Events Index
SEM scanning electron miscroscopy
serum methylguanidine
smoke exposure machine
standard error of the mean
systolic ejection murmur
sem half (semi) (also s)
seed (semen)
semid half a drachm (semidrachma)
semih half an hour (semihora)
sem in d
once a day (semel in die)
Sem ves
seminal vesicle
SENIC Study of the Efficacy of Nosocomial Infection Control
Sens sensorium
SENTAC
Society for Ear, Nose, and Throat Advances in Children
SEP sensory evoked potential
somatosensory evoked potential (also SSEP)
spinal evoked potential
surface epithelium
systolic ejection period
SEPA State Employed Physicians Association
sept septum (also S)
seven (septem)
SEQ side-effects questionnaire
simultaneous equation
Seq sequela
sequential
sequestrum
seq luc
the following day (sequenti luce)
SER sebum excretion rate
sensory evoked response
smooth endoplasmic reticulum
Society for Epidemiologic Research
somatosensory evoked response (also SSER)
systolic ejection rate
Ser serine
SERI Solar Energy Research Institute
Spondee Error Index
serv preserve (serva)
SES Society of Eye Surgeons
socioeconomic status
sodium 2,4-dichlorophenoxyethyl sulfate
SESAP Surgical Education and Self-Assessment Program
sesquih
an hour and a half (sesquihora)
Sess sessile

SET systolic ejection time
Sev severe
severed
SeXO serum xanthine oxidase
SF salt free
scarlet fever
seizure frequency
serum factor
sham feeding
shell fragment
shrapnel fragment
shunt flow
skin fluorescence
slow function
snack food
soft feces
spinal fluid
spontaneous fibrillation
spontaneous fluctuation
spontaneous fracture
stable factor
Streptococcus faecalis
stress formula
sulfonamide
superior facet
suprasternal fossa
supressor factor
survival fraction
synovial fluid
Sf Svedberg flotation
S_f flotation constant
SFA saturated fatty acid
seminal fluid assay
Sigmund Freud Archives
superficial femoral artery
SFBL self-filling blind loop
SFC serum fungicidal
spinal fluid count
SFD sheep factor delta
short food drape
small for date
soy-free diet
SFEMG single fiber electromyography
SFF speaking fundamental frequency
specific-pathogen free
SFFF sedimentation field flow fractionation
SFFV spleen focus forming virus
spleen focus Friend virus
SFG spotted fever group
SFH schizophrenia family history
stroma-free hemoglobin
SFI Sexual Functioning Index
Social Function Index
SFLE Stress from Life Experience
SFM soluble fibrin monomer
SFMC soluble fibrin monomer complex
SFO subfornical organ
SFP screen filtration pressure
spinal fluid pressure
stop flow pressure
SFR screen filtration resistance
SFS serum fungistatic
skin and fascia stapler
split function study
SFT sensory feedback therapy
serum-free thyroxine
skinfold thickness
SFTAA Short Form Test of Academic Aptitude
SFTR sagittal, frontal, transverse, rotation
SFV Semliki Forest virus
SFW shell fragment wound
shrapnel fragment wound
slow filling wave
SG secretory granule
serous granule
serum globulin
serum glucose
sign
skin graft
soluble gelatin
specific gravity (also SPG, sp gr)
substantia gelatinose
Surgeon General
S-G Sachs-Georgi
Swan-Ganz
s-g subgenus
SGA small for gestational age
Society of Gastrointestinal Assistants
SG_a specific conductance
SG_{aw} specific airway conductance
SG-C serum gentamicin concentration
SGE secondary generalized epilepsy
SGF silica gel filtered
skeletal growth factor
SGH subgaleal hematoma
SGI Society for Gynecologic Investigation
SGO Society of Gynecologic Oncologists
Surgeon General's Office
surgery, gynecology, and obstetrics
SGOT serum glutamic oxaloacetic transaminase (see AST--aspartate transaminase)
SGP Society of General Physiologists
SGPT serum glutamic pyruvic transaminase
SGTT standard glucose tolerance test
SGV salivary gland virus
selective gastric vagotomy
small granular vesicle
SH serum hepatitis
service hours
sex hormone
sham operated
shared haptotypes
social history
somatotrophic hormone
spontaneously hypertensive
sulfhydryl
surgical history
symptomatic hypoglycemia
systemic hyperthermia
S&H speech and hearing
Sh short
shoulder
See S (Shigella)
SHA soluble HLA antigen
staphylococcal hemagglutinating anti-body
SHAM salicythydroxamic acid
SHARE Standard Hospital Accounting and Rate Evaluation System
SHAV superior hemiazygos vein
SHB sulfhemoglobin
SHBD serum hydroxybutyrate dehydrogenase
SHBG sex hormone-binding globulin
SHC state health commissioner
state health corporation
SHCC Statewide Health Coordinating Council
SHCO sulfated hydrogenated castor oil
SHEENT
skin, head, eyes, ears, nose, throat
shf superhigh frequency
SHG synthetic human gastrin
Shhh Self-Help for Hard of Hearing People
SHHV Society for Health and Human Values
SHL sensorneual hearing loss

SHML sinus histiocytosis with massive lymphadenopathy
SHMT serine hydroxymethyltransferase
SHN subacute hepatic necrosis
SHNS Society for Head and Neck Surgery
SHO secondary hypertrophic osteoarthropathy
student health organization
SHP secondary hyperparathyroidism
Shoenlein-Henoch purpura
SHR spontaneously hypertensive rat
SHRC shortened, held, resisted, contraction
SHR/HR
streptomycin-isoniazid-rifampicin/isoniazil-rifampicin
SHS super high speed
SHRsp stroke prone spontaneously hypertensive rat (also spSHR)
SHSS Stanford Hypnotic Susceptibility Scale
SI International System of Units (Systeme International d'Unites)
sacroiliac
saturation index
self-inflicted
sensitive index
seriously ill
service index
serum insulin
serum iron
single injection
small intestine
social introversion
soluble insulin
stimulation index
streptozotocin induced
stroke index
sulfated insulin
systolic index
S/I sucrose to isomaltase ratio
Si silicon
venous sinus
^{31}Si radioactive isotope of silicon
SIA serum inhibitory activity
stimulation-induced analgesia
SIADH syndrome of inappropriate secretion of antidiuretic hormone
SIASP Society for Italian-American Scientists and Physicians
Sib sibling
SIBIA Salk Institute Biotechnology/Industrial Associates
SIC serum inhibitory concentration
serum insulin concentration
sic dry (siccus)
SICD Sequenced Inventory of Communication Development
serum isocitric dehydrogenase
SICU spinal intensive care unit
surgical intensive care unit
SID Society for Investigative Dermatology
sucrase-isomaltase deficiency
sudden infant death
systemic inflammatory disease
SIDS sudden infant death syndrome
SIDUO International Symposium on Ultrasonic Diagnostics in Ophthalmology
SIE stroke in evolution
SIF serum inhibitory factor
small, intensely fluorescent
SIFT selected ion flow tube
SIG special interest group
SIg surface immunoglobulin
sig let it be labeled (signetur)
significant
SIgA secretory immunoglobulin A
surface immunoglobulin A
SIGBIO
Special Interest Group on Biomedical Computing
sig n pro
label with the proper name (signa nomine proprio)
SIJ sacroiliac joint
SIL speech interference level
SILD Sequenced Inventory of Language Development
SIM selected ion monitoring
Society of Industrial Medicine
sucrase-isomaltose
sulfine indole motility
SIMS secondary ion mass spectrometry
Simul simultaneous
SIMV synchronized intermittent mandatory ventilation
sing of each (singulorum)
sing aur
every morning (singulis auroris)
sing hor quad
every quarter of an hour (singulis horae quadrantibus)
si non val
if it is not enough (si non valeat)
SIOP International Society of Pediatric Oncology
si op sit
if it is necessary (si opus sit)
SIP segment inertial properties
Sickness Impact Profile
surface inductive plethysmography
SIR specific immune release
standardized incidence ratio
SIRF severely impaired renal function
SIRS soluble immune response suppressor
SIS sisomicin
sterile injectable suspension
SISI short increment sensitivity index
SISO See SIS (sisomicin)
SISS serum inhibitor of streptolysin S
SiSV simian sarcoma virus
SIT-F Sperm Immobilization Test-Fjabrant
SIT-I Sperm Immobilization Test-Isojima
si vir perm
if the strength will permit (si vires permittant)
SIW self-inflicted wound
S-J Stevens-Johnson
SJM St. Jude Medical
SJR Shinawora-Jones-Reinhart
SJS Stevens-Johnson syndrome
SK senile keratosis
skin specific
solar keratosis
streptokinase
SKA supracondylar knee-ankle
SKAP Surgical Knowledge Self-Assessment Program
SKAT Sex Knowledge and Attitude Test
SKI Sister Kenny Institute
skin
SKSD streptokinase-streptodornase
SL salt loser
satellite-like
sensation level
sensory latency
signal level

slit light
small lymphocyte
soda lime
sodium lactate
sound level
streptolysin
sublingual
sulfametrole

S/L sucrase to lactase ratio
Sl slight
sl according to law (secundum legem)
slyke
SLA sacrolaeva anterior
SLB short leg brace
SLC short leg cast
Sociopolitical Locus of Control
sodium lithium countertransport
SLCC sulfated lithocholic conjugate
SLCG sulfolithocholylglycine
SLD serum lactic dehydrogenase
SLDH See SLD
SLE St. Louis encephalitis
systemic lupus erythematosus
SLEA sheep erythrocyte antibody
sheep erythrocyte antigen
SLEV St. Louis encephalitis virus
SLHR sex-linked hypophosphatemic rickets
SLHRP Society for Life History Research in Psychopathology
SLI secretin-like immunoreactivity
selective lymphoid irradiation
somatostatin-like immunoreactivity
speech and language impaired
splenic localization index
SLIP Singer-Loomis Inventory of Personality
SLKC superior limbic keratoconjunctivitis
SLM sound level meter
SLN sublentiform nucleus
superior laryngeal nerve
SLO streptolysin-O
SLP sacrolaeva posterior
speech-language pathologist
subluxation of the patella
SLR single lens reflex
straight leg raising
Streptococcus lactis R
SLS segment long-spacing
single-limb support
Stein-Leventhal syndrome
SLSQ Speech and Language Screening Questionnaire
SLT sacrolaeva transversa
SLUD salivation, lacrimation, urination, defecation
SLZ serum lysozyme
SM self-monitoring
semimembranosus
Shigella mutant
simple mastectomy
skim milk
smoker
smooth muscle
stapedius muscle
streptomycin
submandibular
submucosal
substituted metabolites
substitute for morphine
suction method
sulfamerazine
superior mesenteric
supramamillary nucleus
sustained medication
symptom
synovial membrane
systolic mean
systolic murmur
S.M. Master of Science
S/M sadism/masochism
S&M Sabouraud's and Mycosel
Sm samarium
small
SMA sequential multiple analysis
serial multiple analysis
serum muramidase activity
simultaneous multichannel autoanalyzer
smooth muscle antibody
smooth muscle autoantibody
Southern Medical Association
spinal muscular atrophy
superior mesenteric artery
supplementary motor area
SMABV superior mesenteric artery blood ve-locity
SMAC Sequential Multiple Analyzer Computer
SMAE superior mesenteric artery embolus
SMAF specific macrophage arming factor
superior mesenteric artery blood flow
SMAL serum methyl alcohol level
SMART simultaneous multiple-angle reconstruction technique
SMAS submuscular aponeurotic system
SMAST Short Michigan Alcoholism Screening Test
SMB selected mucosal biopsy
suckling mouse brain
SMBP serum myelin basic protein
SMC smooth muscle cell
special monthly compensation
succinylmonocholine
SMCA smooth muscle contracting agent
SMCAF Society of Medical Consultants to the Armed Forces
SMCD senile macular choroidal degeneration
SMD senile macular degeneration
sternocleidomastoid diameter
SMEDI stillbirth, mummification, embryonic death, infertility
SMEPP subminiature end-plate potential
SMF streptozotocin, mitomycin C, 5-fluorouracil
SMG submandibular gland
SMH state mental hospital
SMI senior medical investigator
severely mentally impaired
supplementary medical insurance
SMJ Society of Medical Jurisprudence
SML single major locus
SMMD specimen mass-measurement device
SMN second malignant neoplasm
SMNB submaximal neuromuscular block
SMO Medical Officer of Schools
Senior Medical Officer
serum monoamine oxidase
slip made out
Society of Military Otolaryngologists
SMON subacute myelo-optic neuropathy
SMP slow-moving protease
special monthly pension
standard medical practice
standard medical procedure
submitochondrial particle
SMR sensorimotor rhythm
somnolent metabolic rate

standard metabolic rate
standard mortality ratio
submucous resection
submucous resection and rhinoplasty

SMS sodium 2-mercaptoethane sulfonate
stiff-man syndrome

SMSA Standard Metropolitan Statistical Area

SMT Sertoli cell/mesenchyme tumor
Snider Match Test
spindle microtubule

SMV slow-moving vehicle
small volume
submentovertical
superior mesenteric vein

SMWD Sep
single, married, widowed, divorced, or separated

SMX sulfamethoxazole (also SMZ)

SMZ sulfamethazine
sulfamethoxazole (also SMX)

SN sensorineural
sensory neuron
seronegative
serum-neutralizing
single nephron
sinus node
spontaneous nystagmus
staff nurse
student nurse
substantia nigra
supernatant
supernormal
suprasternal notch

S/N signal to noise ratio (also SNR)
speech to noise ratio

Sn tin (stannum)

^{113}Sn radioactive isotope of tin

^{121}Sn radioactive isotope of tin

^{119}Sn radioactive isotope of tin

sn according to nature (secundum naturam)

SNA specimen not available
State Nurses' Association
superior nasal artery

SNB scalene node biopsy

SND striatonigral degeneration

SNE sinus node electrogram
subacute necrotizing encephalomyelopathy

SNF skilled nursing facility

SNFH schizoprhenia nonfamily history

SNGBF single nephron glomerular blood flow

SNGFR single nephron glomerular filtration rate

SNGPF single nephron glomerular plasma flow

SNHL sensorineural hearing loss

SNM Society of Nuclear Medicine

SNMA Student National Medical Association

SNMT Society of Nuclear Medical Technologists

SNOP Systematized Nomenclature of Pathology

SNP sodium nitroprusside

S.N.P.
School Nurse Practitioner

SNQ superior nasal quadrant

SNR signal to noise ratio (also S/N)

SNRT sinus node recovery time

SNS Society of Neurological Surgeons
sympathetic nervous system

SNV superior nasal vein

SO salpingo-oophorectomy
sham operated
slow oxidative
spheno-occipital
sphincter of Oddi
supraoptic

$^{35}SO_2$ radioactive labeled sulfur dioxide

SO_4 sulfate radical

So socialization

SOAM stitches out in morning

SOAP Society for Obstetric Anesthesia and Perinatology
subjective, objective, assessment, plan

SOB see order blank
shortness of breath
suboccipitobregmatic

SOC sequential oral contraceptive
standard of care
state of consciousness

SOCD Separation of Circle-Diamond

SOCMA Synthetic Organic Chemical Manufacturers Association

SOD spike occurrence density
superoxide dismutase

SOEH Society for Occupational and Environmental Health

SOFS spontaneous osteoporotic fracture of the sacrum

SOFT Sorting of Figures Test

SOHN supraoptic hypothalmic nucleus

SOL space-occupying lesion

Sol soleus
soluble (also S)
solution (also Soln)

SOLER squarely face person, open posture, lean toward person, eye contact, relaxed

Soln solution (also Sol)

SOLST Stephens Oral Language Screening Test

Solv dissolve (solve)

SOM secretory otitis media
serous otitis media
sulformethoxine

SON supraoptic nucleus

SONP soft organs nonpalpable

SOP standard operating procedure
standing operative procedure

SOPHE Society for Public Health Education

SOPM stitches out in afternoon

SOPO Society of Oral Physiology and Occlusion

SOPP splanchnic occluded portal pressure

s op s
if necessary (si opus sit) (also sos)

SOQ Suicide Opinion Questionnaire

SOR stimulus organism response

SOREMP
sleep-onset rapid eye movement period

SORSI Sacro Occipital Research Society International

SOS self-obtained smear
Society for Occlusal Studies
stimulation of senses

sos if necessary (si opus sit) (also s op s)

SOT Society of Toxicology
stream of thought
systemic oxygen transport

SOTT synthetic medium, old tuberculin, trichloracetic acid

SP sacral promontory
sacrum to pubis
secretory piece
semiprivate
senile plaques

septal pore
serine proteinase
seropositive
shunt pressure
shunt procedure
skin potential
small protein
soft palate
spatial peak
specific glycoprotein
speech pathology
spike potential
spiramycin
spirometry
standard of performance
steady potential
stool preservative
substance P
subtilopeptidase
summating potential
suprapatellar pouch
suprapubic
suprapubic puncture
symphysis pubis
synthase phosphatase
systolic pressure

SP-1 Schwangerschaftsproteine
specific protein 1

S_2P second heart sound, pulmonic component

Sp serum phosphorus
spermine
See S (Spirillum)

sp space (also S)
species (singular) (see also spp)
spine
spirit (spiritus) (also spir)

SPA schizophrenia with premorbid asociality
sperm penetration assay
staphylococcal protein A
State Planning Agency
stimulation produced analgesia
suprapatellar amputation
suprapubic aspiration

SPAC sectionally processed antibody coated

SPAI steroid protein activity index

SPAR sensitivity prediction by acoustic reflex

SPBI serum protein-bound iodine

S-PBIgG serum-platelet bindable immunoglobulin G

SPC salicylamide, phenacetin, and caffeine
serum phenylalanine concentration
sickle-shaped particle cell
single palmar crease
single photoelectron counting
single proton counting
small pyramidal cell
spike-processed contraction

SPCA serum prothrombin conversion accelerator
Society for the Prevention of Cruelty to Animals

sp cd spinal cord (also SC)

SPCK serum creatine phosphokinase

SPCP Society of Professors of Child Psychiatry

SPD salmon poisoning disease
silicon photodiode
Society for Pediatric Dermatology
specific paroxysmal discharge
spectral power distribution
spermidine
standard peak dilution
storage pool deficiency

Spd spermidine

SPE septic pulmonary edema
serum protein electrophoresis (also SPEP)
streptococcal pyrogenic exotoxin
subjective paranormal experience
sucrose polyester

spec specimen

SPECT single photon emission computed tomography

SPEM smooth pursuit eye movement

SPEP serum protein electrophoresis (also SPE)

SPF specific-pathogen free
spectrophotofluorometric
split products of fibrin
streptococcal proliferative factor
Stuart-Prower factor
sun protecting factor
suntan photoprotection factor

SPG specific gravity (also SG, sp gr)
sucrose, phosphate, glutamate
symmetrical peripheral gangrene

sp gr specific gravity (also SG, SPG)

SPH secondary pulmonary hemosiderosis
sphingomyelin

Sph sperical (also S)
spherical lens (also S)
spherocytosis

sp ht specific heat

SPI serum precipitable iodine
somatotyping ponderal index
subclinical papillomavirus infection

SPIA solid-phase immunoabsorbant
solid-phase immunoassay

SPID sum of pain intensity difference

SPIF solid-phase immunoassay fluorescence

SPIH superimposed pregnancy-induced hypertension

spir spirit (spiritus) (also sp)

SPK serum pyruvate kinase
superficial punctate keratitis

SPL sound pressure level
spontaneous lesion
staphlococcal phage lysate

SPLATT split anterior tibial tendon transfer

SPM self-phase modulation
shocks per minute
significance probability mapping
Society of Prospective Medicine
spectinomycin
spermine
suspended particulate matter
syllables per minute
synaptic plasma membrane

SPMA spinal progressive muscular atrophy

SPMB strong partial maternal behavior

SPMR standardized proportionate mortality ratio

SPMSQ Short Portable Mental Status Questionnaire

SPN solitary pulmonary nodule
student practical nurse
supplementary parenteral nutrition

sp n new species (species novum)

Spont spontaneous

SPP suprapubic prostatectomy

spp species (plural) (see also sp)

SPPS stable plasma protein solution
SPR scan projection radiography
serial probe recognition
skin potential reflex
Society of Patient Representatives
Society for Pediatric Radiology
Society for Pediatric Research
Society for Physical Research
solid phase radioimmunoassay
SPRI Social Psychiatry Research Institute
SPRIA solid phase radioimmunoassay
SPROM spontaneous premature rupture of membrane
SPS Society of Pelvic Surgeons
sodium polyanetholesulfonate
special Pap smear
status postsurgery
sulfadiazine
sulfite polymyxin
stimulated protein synthesis
systemic progressive sclerosis
SpS sphenoid sinus
SPSA Society of Philippine Surgeons in America
spSHR stroke prone spontaneous hypertensive rat (also SHRsp)
SPSS Statistical Package for the Social Sciences
SPT slow pull-through
spectinomycin (also SPM)
spinal tap
Spobdee Picture Test
spt spirit
SPTA spatial peak temporal average
SPTI systolic pressure time index
SPTP spatial peak temporal peak
SPU Society for Pediatric Urology
SPUN Society for the Protection of the Unborn Through Nutrition
SPZ secretin pancreozymin
sulfinpyrazone
SQ social quotient
squalene
square
subcutaneous (also Subcu, Subq)
survey question
symptom questionnaire
sq ft square foot
sq in square inch
sqq and following (sequentia)
SQUID superconductivity quantum interference device
SR sacroreticular
sarcoplasmic reticulum
saturation recovery
secretion rate
sedimentation rate (also sed rt)
seizure resistant
self-recording
sensitization response
sentence repetition
service record
sex ratio
sigma reaction
silicone rubber
sinus rhythm
skin resistance
specific resistance
specific response
stimulus response
stomach rumble
stress relaxation
stretch reflex
superior rectus
supply room
systemic reaction
systemic resistance
systems research
systems review
Sr strontium
^{85}Sr radioactive isotope of strontium
^{87}Sr radioactive isotope of strontium
^{89}Sr radioactive isotope of strontium
^{90}Sr radioactive isotope of strontium
SRA segmental renal artery
SRBC sheep red blood cell (also SE--sheep erythrocyte)
SRC sedimented red cell
senitization response cell
sheep red cell
Social Rehabilitation Clinic
SRCA specific red cell adherence
SRCBC serum reserve cholesterol binding capacity
SRCD Society for Research in Child Development
SRD specific reading disability
SRE Schedule of Recent Experience
SREB Southern Regional Education Board
SRF severe renal failure
skin-reactive factor
slow-reacting factor
somatotropin-releasing factor
split renal function
SRFD Society for the Rehabilitation of the Facially Disfigured
SRFOA slow-reacting factor of anaphylaxis (see also SRSA)
SRFS split renal function study
SRG Society of Remedial Gymnasts
SRH signs of recent hemorrhage
single radial hemolysis
somatotropin-releasing hormone
stigmata of recent hemorrhage
SRIC Staff-Resident Interaction Chronograph
SRID single radial immunodiffusion
SRIF somatostatin (somatotropin release-inhibiting factor) (also SS, SST)
SRIP specifications for reagents in the International Pharmacopoeia
SRN State Registered Nurse
SRNA soluble ribonucleic acid
SRNV subretinal neovascularization
SRO single room occupancy
SROM spontaneous rupture of membrane
SRP signal recognition protein
simple response paradigm
SRR slow rotation room
stabilized relative response
surgical recovery room
SRRS Social Readjustment Rating Scale
SRS sex reassignment surgery
Silver-Russell syndrome
slow-reacting substance
Social and Rehabilitation Service
Symptom Rating Scale
SRSA slow-reacting substance of anaphylaxis (see also SRFOA)
SRT sick role tendency
speech reception test
speech reception threshold
spontaneously resolving thyrotoxicosis
sustained release theophylline
Symptom Rating Test

SRV superior radicular vein
SS saline soak
saline solution
saliva sample
Salmonella and Shigella
saturated solution
schizophrenia spectrum
seizure sensitive
Sezary syndrome
Shigella and Salmonella
sickle cell (homozygous)
side to side
signs and symptoms (also S&S)
Sjogren's syndrome
slow wave sleep
soapsuds
social service
sodium salicylate
somatostatin (also SRIF, SST)
special service
stable sarcoidosis
staccato syndrome
standard score
statistically significant
steady state (also s, ss)
sterile solution
steroid sulfurylation
subaortic stenosis
subscapularis
subsegmental
subsequent sibling
substernal
suction socket
sum of squares
supersaturated
systemic sclerosis
S&S signs and symptoms (also SS)
Ss serum soluble antigen
subjects
ss in the strict sense (sensu stricto)
one-half (semis)
steady state (also s, SS)
SSA salicylsalicylic acid
sickle cell anemia
Single State Agency
skin sensitizing antibody
Smith surface antigen
special somatic afferent
subsegmential airway
sulfosalicylic (salicylsulfonic) acid
SSAT Society for Surgery of the Alimentary Tract
SSAV simian sarcoma-associated virus
SSB Society for the Study of Blood
SSC somatosensory cortex
superior semicircular canal
SSCA sensitized sheep cell agglutination
spontaneous suppressor cell activity
SSCF sleep stage change frequency
SSD source to skin distance
source to surface distance
speech sound discrimination
sudden sniffing death
sum of square deviations
SSE saline solution enema
soapsuds enema
steady state exercise
subacute spongiform encephalopathy
SSEP somatosensory evoked potential (also SEP)
SSER somatosensory evoked response (also SER)
SSF soluble suppressor factor
supplementary sensory feedback
SSFIPD
social stress and function-ability inventory
SSHb homozygous for sickle hemoglobin
SSHL severe sensorineural hearing loss
SSI segmental sequestral irradiation
stuttering severity instrument
Supplemental Security Income
synthetic sentence identification
SSKI saturated solution of potassium iodide
SSL skin surface lipid
synthetic sentence list
SSN severely subnormal
SSO Society of Surgical Oncology
SSP Sanarelli-Shwartzman phenomenon
Scientific Subroutine Package
small spherical particle
subacute sclerosing panencephalitis (also SSPE)
SSPE subacute sclerosing panencephalitis (also SSP)
SSPG steady state plasma glucose
SSPI steady state plasma insulin
SSPL saturation sound pressure level
SSR Society for the Study of Reproduction
steady state rest
steroid resistant rejection
surgical supply room
SSS Sensation-Seeking Scale
sick sinus syndrome
specific soluble substance
sterile saline soak
sulfonamides
systemic sicca syndrome
sss layer upon layer (stratum super stratum)
SSSS Society for the Scientific Study of Sex
staphylococcal scalded skin syndrome
SSSV superior sagittal sinus velocity
SSST superior sagittal sinus thrombosis
SST sodium sulfite titration
somatosensory thalamus
somatostatin (also SRIF, SS)
SSTAR Study for Sex Therapy and Research
s str in the strict sense (senso stricto)
SSU Saybolt seconds universal
self-service unit
sterile supply unit
SSV sheep seminal vesicles
simian sacroma virus
ssv under a poison label (sub signo veneni)
SSW staggered spondaic word
ST esotropia
scala tympani
sclerotherapy
sedimentation time
semitendinosus
septal thickness
siblings raised together
similarly tested
sinus tachycardia
sinus tympani
skin temperature
skin test
slight trace
Society for Theriogenology
sodium taurocholate
speech therapy
stable toxin
standardized test

standard treatment
starting time
sternothyroid
stopping
striatum (also Str)
subtalar
subtotal
sulfathiozole
surface tension
surgical therapy
survival time
systolic time

St stomach
subtype

st let it stand (stet)
let them stand (stent)

STA serum thrombotic accelerator
serum tobramycin assay
superficial temporal artery
superior temporal artery

S-Ta atrial S-T segment change

Stab stab neutrophil

STACL Screening Test for Auditory Comprehension of Language

S-TAG slow-binding target-attaching globulin

STAI State-Trait Anxiety Inventory

Staph See S (Staphylococcus)

STAT Suprathreshold Adaptation Test

stat German unit of radium emanation
immediately (statim)

Stb stillborn (see also SB)

STC serum theophylline concentration
sexually transmitted condition
Society for Technical Communication
soft-tissue calcification
Stroke Treatment Center

STD sexually transmitted disease
skin test dose
skin to tumor distance
standard density reference
standard test dose

STDH skin test for delayed-type hypersensitivity

STDT standard tone-decay test

STEM scanning transmission electron microscope
Society of Teachers of Emergency Medicine

STEP Sequential Tests of Educational Progress

STEPS sequential treatment employing pharmacologic supports

STET submaximal treadmill exercise test

STF slow twitch fiber
small third trimester fetus
special tube feeding
sudden transient freezing

STFM Society of Teachers of Family Medicine

STG short-term goal

STGC syncytiotrophoblastic giant cell

STH somatotropic hormone
supplemental thyroid hormone

S-Thal
sickle cell thalassemia

STI serum trypsin inhibitor
soybean trypsin inhibitor
systolic time interval

STIC serum trypsin inhibition capacity

stillat
by drops or in small quantities (stillatim)

STK streptokinase

STL serum theophyllin level

STM short-term memory
streptomycin

StMPM synctiotrophoblast microvillae plasma membrane

STN supratrochlear nucleus

STNR symmetrical tonic neck reflex

STNS sham transcutaneous nerve stimulation

STP dimethoxymethylamphetamine (also DOM)
scientifically treated petroleum
serenity, tranquility, peace
Sibling Training Program
standard temperature and pressure
standard temperature and pulse

STPD standard temperature and pressure, dry

STPI State-Trait Personality Inventory

STPP sodium tripolyphosphate

STQ superior temporal quadrant

STR Society of Therapeutic Radiologists
soft tissue rheumatism

Str striatum (also ST)
See S (Streptococcus)

Strep See S (Streptococcus)

STRT skin temperature recovery time

STS serologic test for syphilis
serum test for syphilis
sexual tubal sterilization
short-term storage
Society of Thoracic Surgeons
sodium tetradecyl sulfate
standard test for syphilis

STSA Southern Thoracic Surgical Association

STSG split thickness skin graft

STT sensitization test
serial thrombin time

STU skin test unit

STV superior temporal vein

STVA subtotal villose atrophy

STX saxitoxin

STZ serum-treated zymosan
streptozotocin

SU sensation unit
solar urticaria
sorbent unit
spectrophotometric unit
strontium unit
sulfonyl urea
supine

Su sulfonamide

su let him take (sumat)

SUA serum uric acid
single umbilical artery
single unit activity

Subcu subcutaneous (also SQ, Subq)

Subling
under the tongue

Subq subcutaneous (also SQ, Subcu)

SUD skin unit dose
sudden unexpected death
sudden unexplained death

suff sufficient

SUI stress urinary incontinence

SUID sudden unexpected infant death
sudden unexplained infant death

sum let him take (sumat)

SUMIT streptokinase urokinase myocardial infarction trial

sum tal
take one this time (sumat talem)

SUN serum urea nitrogen

SUP superficial
superior

supinator
sup above (supra)
supp suppository
SURG surgery
SUS Society of University Surgeons
stained urinary sediment
supressor sensitive
susp suspension
SUTI symptomatic urinary tract infection
SUUD sudden unexpected, unexplained death
SV saphenous vein
sarcoma virus
satellite virus
selective vagotomy
semilunar valve
Sendai virus
severe
simian virus
single ventricle
sinus venosus
snake venom
splenic vein
spontaneous ventilation
stroke volume
subclavian vein
supravital
SV 40 simian virus 40
Sv sievert
sv alcoholic spirit (spiritus vini)
SVA selective vagotomy with antrectomy
selective visceral angiography
spatial voltage at maximun anterior forces
special visceral afferent
subtotal villous atrophy
SVAS subvalvular aortic stenosis
supravalvular aortic stenosis
SVC segmental venous capacitance
slow vital capacity
subclavian vein catheterization
superior vena cava
suprahepatic vena cava
SVCG spatial vectocardiogram
SVCO superior vena cava obstruction
SVC-PA
superior vena cava to pulmonary artery
SVCR segmental venous capacitance ratio
SVC-RPA
superior vena cava to right pulmonary artery
SVCS superior vena cava syndrome
SVD small vessel disease
spontaneous vaginal delivery
spontaneous vertex delivery
SVE special visceral efferent
Streptococcus viridans endocarditis
SVG saphenous vein graft
SVI stroke volume index
SVIB Strong Vocational Interest Blank
SVM seminal vesicle microsome
spatial voltage at maximum posterior forces
syncytiovascular membrane
S_{VO2} venous oxygen saturation
SVP selective vagotomy with pyloroplasty
spatial voltage at maximum posterior forces
standing venous pressure
static volume pressure
superficial vascular plexus
SVR sequential vascular response
systemic vascular resistance
svr rectified spirit of wine (spiritus vini rectificatus)
SVRI systemic vascular resistance index
SVS Society for Vascular Surgery
SVSe supravaginal septum
SVT sinoventricular tachyarrhythemia
sinoventricular tachycardia
supraventricular tachyarrhythemia
supraventricular tachycardia
svt proof spirit (spiritus vini tenuis)
SW shortwave
social worker
spherule wall
spiral wound
stroke work
SWAMP swine-associated mucoprotein
SWC submaximal working capacity
SWD shortwave diathermy
SWFI sterile water for injection
SWI stroke work index
surgical wound infection
SWIM sperm-washing insemination method
SWJ square wave jerk
SWO superficial white onychonycosis
SWOG Southwest Oncology Group
SWR serum Wassermann reaction
SWS slow wave sleep
SWSC Statewide Services Contract
SWT Speech Weber Test
SX sulfamethoxypyridazine
Sx signs
symptoms (also sym)
SXT sulfamethoxazole/trimethoprim
sym symmetrical
symptoms (also Sx)
Syn joint (synchondrosis)
syr syrup
SYS stretching and yawning syndrome
SZ schizophrenia (also S, Schiz)
sulfamethizole
Sz seizure
streptozotocin
SZD streptozotocin diabetes

T

T ribosylthymine (also Thd)
ribothymidine (also Thd)
Tabanus
Taenia
tamoxifen
tanycytes
T-bandage
T-bar
temperature (also temp)
tension, intraocular
tertiary
tesla
testosterone
Tetrahymena
T-fiber
theophylline
thoracic (also Th)
thrombus
thymidine
thymine (also Thy)
thymus

time
tocopherol
total
toxicity
Toxoplasma
trace
transmittance
transverse
tray
Treponema
Triatoma
Trichinella
Trichomonas
Trichophyton
Trichosporon
Trichostrongylus
Trichuris
triggered
Trombicula
Trypanosoma
tuberculum
tuberosity
tumor
Tunga
T-wave
type

2,4,5-T 2,4,5-trichlorophenoxy acetic acid
T1/2 half-life time
T1...T12 thoracic nerve 1 through 12
thoracic vertebra 1 through 12
T_3 triiodothyronine
T_4 thyroxine
T-1824 Evans blue
T+ increased tension
T- decreased tension
t temporal (also temp)
tertiary
test of significance
three times (ter)
ton
translocation
tritium
TA Technical Assistance
teichoic acid
temperature, axillary
temporal arteritis
temporal average
terminal antrum
test age
therapeutic abortion
thyroid antibody
thyroid autoantibody
tibialis anterior
titratable acid
toxin-antitoxin (also TAT)
Transactional Analysis
transaldolase
transantral
trapped air
treatment assignment
tricholomic acid
tricuspid annuloplasty
tricuspid atresia
trophoblast antigen
truncus arteriosus
trytophane acid
tube agglutination
tuberculin, alkaline
tumor antigen
T&A tonsillectomy and adenoidectomy
Ta T-amplifier
tantalum
^{182}Ta radioactive isotope of tantalum
TAA taka-amylase A
transverse aortic arch
tumor-associated antigen
TAAC Technology Assessment Advisory Council
TAB typhoid, paratyphoid A and B
tab tablet
TABC typhoid, paratyphoid A, B, and C
TABT typhoid, paratyphoid A and B, and tetanus toxoid
TABTD typhoid, paratyphoid A and B, tetanus toxoid, and diphtheria toxoid
TAC terminal antrum contraction
tetracaine, epinephrine (Adrenalin), cocaine
total aganglionosis coli
Toxicant Analysis Center
triamcinolone acetonide
TACE chlorotrianisene
tripara-anisylchloroethylene
TAD 6-thioguanine, cytosine arabinoside, daunorubicin
thoracic asphyxiant dystrophy
TAF albumose-free tuberculin
tissue angiogenesis factor
toxin-antitoxin floccule
toxoid-antitoxin floccule
trypsin-aldehyde-fuchsin
tumor angiogenesis factor
TAG target-attaching globulin
triacylglycerol
TAH total abdominal hysterectomy
total artificial heart
transabdominal hysterectomy
TAI tissue antagonist of interferon
TAL tendon Achilles lengthening
tal of such (talis)
TALS The American Lupus Society
TAM teenage mother
thermoacidurans agar modified
toxoid-antitoxin mixture
TAME toluene-sulfotrypsin arginine methyl ester
tosyl arginine methyl esterase
TAMe toxoid-antitoxin mixture esterase
TAN total adenine nucleotides
total ammonia nitrogen
tan tangent
TANI total axial node irradiation
TAO thromboangiitis obliterans
triacetyloleandomycin
troleandomycin
turning against object
TAPA Turkish American Physicians Association
TAPS training and placement service
TAPVC total anomalous pulmonary venous connection
TAPVD total anomalous pulmonary venous drainage
TAPVR total anomalous pulmonary venous return
TAQW transient abnormal Q waves
TAR thrombocytopenia with absent radius
tissue to air ratio
total abortion rate
TAS tetanus antitoxic serum
turning against self
Tyrode albumin solution
TASC Treatment Alternatives to Street Crime
T'ASE tryptophane synthetase

TAT tetanus antitoxin
Thematic Apperception Test
Thematic Aptitude Test
thromboplastin activation test
total antitryptic activity
toxin-antitoxin (also TA)
transaxial tomogram
transverse axial tomography
tray agglutination test
tyrosine aminotransferase
TATA tumor-associated transplantation antigen
TATBA triamcinolone acetomide tert-butyl acetate
TATD thiamine 8-(methyl 6-acetyldihydrothioctate) disulfide
TAV trapped air volume
TB Tapes for the Blind
terminal bronchiole
thymol blue
total base
total bilirubin
total body
tracheobronchitis
tributyrin tumor bearing
tubercle bacillus
tuberculin
tuberculosis (also TBC, Tuberc)
tumor bearing
Tb terbium
^{160}Tb radioactive isotope of terbium
^{161}Tb radioactive isotope of terbium
T_b body temperature
TBA tertiary butylacetate
testosterone-binding affinity
thiobarbituric acid
total bile acid
traditional birth attendant
trenbolone acetate
trypsin-binding activity
TBACA 3,4,5-trimethoxybenzoyl-epsilon-aminocaproic acid (also ATBAC)
TBB transbronchial biopsy
TBBC total B_{12} binding capacity
TBC total body calcium
total body clearance
total body counting
tubercidin
tuberculosis (also TB, Tuberc)
TBD total body density
TBE tick-borne encephalitis
tuberculin bacillus emulsion
TBF total body fat
TBFB tracheobronchial foreign body
TBG testosterone-binding globulin
thyroid-binding globulin
thyroxine-binding globulin
tracheobronchogram
TBGE thyroxine-binding globulin estimate
TBGI thyroxine-binding globulin index
TBGP total blood granulocyte pool
TBI thyroid-binding index
tooth-brushing instruction
total body irradiation
TBK total body potassium
TBLB transbronchial lung biopsy
TBLC term birth, living child
TBM total body mass
tuberculous meningitis
tubular basement membrane
TBN total body nitrogen
See TBE (tuberculin bacillus emulsion)
TBNAA total body neutron activation analysis
TBP bithionol (2,2'-thiobis 4,6-dichlorophenol)
testosterone-binding protein
thyroxine-binding protein
tributyl phosphate
tuberculous peritonitis
TBPA thyroxine-binding prealbumin
TB-RD tuberculosis-respiratory disease
TBRS Timed Behavioral Rating Sheet
TBS 4-tert-butylphenyl salicylate
total body solids
total body surface
total bypass
tracheobronchoscopy
tribromosalicylanilide
tribromsalan
triethanolamine-buffered saline
TBSA total body surface area
tbsp tablespoonful
TBT tolbutamide test
tracheobronchial toilet
tracheobronchial tree
TBTO Bis (tri-n-butyltin) oxide
TBTT tuberculin tine test
TBUT tear break-up time
TBV total blood volume
TBW total body washout
total body water
total body weight
TBX total body irradiation
TBZ tetrabenazine
TC target cell
taurocholate
telephone call
temperature compensation
teratocarcinoma
tertiary cleavage
testosterone cypionate
tetracycline (also TE)
therapeutic community
throat culture
throat tissue
thyrocalcitonin
tissue culture
to contain
total calcium
total capacity
total cholesterol
total correction
transcobalamin
transplant center
transverse colon
tuberculin, contagious
tubocurarine
tumor cell
T&C turn and cough
type and crossmatch
TCI,TCII,...
transcobalamin I, transcobalamin II,...
TC_{50} median toxic concentration
Tc core temperature
T cytolytic
T cytotoxic
technetium
temporal complex
^{99m}Tc technetium-99m
TCA thyrocalcitonin (also TCT)
total circulating albumin
total circulatory arrest
tricalcium aluminate
tricarbolic acid

tricarboxylic acid
trichloroacetic acid
tricyclic antidepressant (also TCAD)
TCAD tetracyclic antidepressant
tricyclic antidepressant (also TCA)
TCAG triple coronary artery graft
TCAP trimethylcetylammonium pentachlorophenate
TCB total cardiopulmonary bypass
transcatheter biopsy
TCBS thiosulfate, citrate, bile salts
thiosulfate, citrate, bile salts, sucrose
TCC thromboplastic cell component
toroidal coil chromatography
transitional cell carcinoma
trichlocarban
trichlorocarbanilide
TCCA transitional cell cancer associated
TCCL T cell chronic lymphocytic leukemia
TCD tissue culture dose
transverse cardiac diameter
TCD_{50} median tissue culture dose
TCDB turn, cough, deep breathe
TCDC taurochenodeoxycholate
TCDD tetrachlorodibenzo-p-dioxin
TcDISIDA
technetium diisopropyliminodiacetic acid
TCE T cell enriched
trichloroethylene
T-cell
thymus-derived lymphocyte
TCF tissue coding factor
total coronary flow
Treacher-Collins-Franceschetti syndrome
TCG time compensation gain
TCGF T cell growth factor
TCH tanned cell hemagglutination
thiophene-2-carboxylic acid
total circulating hemoglobin
TChE total cholinesterase
TCHH tricyclohexyltin hydroxide
TCI to come in
Totman's Change Index
transient cerebral ischemia
TCID tissue culture infective dose
$TCID_{50}$
50 percent (or median) tissue culture infective dose
TcIDA technetium iminodiacetic acid
TCIE transient cerebral ischemic episode
TCIPA tumor cell induced platelet aggregation
TCL chlorguanide triazine
TCLL T-derived chronic lymphocytic leukemia
TCM tanylcypromine
tissue culture medium
TCNE tetracyanoethylene
TCP teacher-child-parent
therapeutic class profile
therapeutic continuous penicillin
total circulating protein
tricalcium phosphate
tricresyl phosphate
TCPA tetrachlorophthalic anhydride
TCPE trichlorophenoxyethanol
$TCP\text{-}O_2$
transcutaneous oxygen monitor
TCPPA trichlorophenoxy propionic acid
TCR T cell reactivity
thalamocortical relay
total cytoplasmic ribosome
TCRP total cellular receptor pool
TCS T cell supernatant
total cellular score
total coronary score
Tcs T cell mediating contact sensitivity
TCSA tetrachlorosalicylanilide
TCT thrombin clotting time
thyrocalcitonin (also TCA)
transmission computed tomography
TD tardive dyskinesia
T cell dependent
teratoma differentiated
terminal device
tetanus-diphtheria
therapeutic dietitian
therapy discontinued
thoracic duct
threshold of detectability
threshold of discomfort
thymus-dependent
timed disintegration
tocopherol deficient
to deliver
tolerance dose
tone decay
torsion dystonia
total disability
toxic dose
tracheal diameter
tracking dye
transdermal
transverse diameter
treatment discontinued
tuberoinfundibular dopaminergic
typhoid dysentery
T_4D serum thyroxine
TD_{50} median toxic dose
td three times a day (ter in die) (also tdd, tid)
TDA thyrotropin displacing activity
TDB tripotassium dicitrato bismuthate
TDC taurodeoxycholate
total dietary calories
TDD thoracic duct drainage
total digitalizing dose
tdd three times a day (ter de die) (also td, tid)
TDE tetrachlorodiphenylethane (also DDD)
time-delayed exponential
triethylene glycol diglycidyl ether
TDF testis determining factor
Thinking Disturbance Factor
thoracic duct fistula
thoracic duct flow
time-dose fractionation factor
tissue-damaging factor
tris-disrupted fraction
TDH total decreased histamine
toxic dose high
TDI Telecommunications for the Deaf
temperature difference integrator
toluene diisocyanate
total dose infusion
TDL thoracic duct lymph
thoracic duct lymphocyte
toxic dose low
TDM tartaric dimalonate
therapeutic drug monitoring
trelialose dimycolate
TDN total digestible nutrients
tDNA transfer deoxyribonucleic acid
TDP ribothymidine 5'-diphosphate

tarsade de pointes
thoracic duct pressure
thymidine diphosphate
TDS temperature, depth, salinity
tds take three times a day (ter die sumendum)
TDT tentative discharge tomorrow
tone decay test
tumor doubling time
TdT terminal deoxynucleotidyl transferase
TE tennis elbow
test ear
tetanus
tetracycline (also TC)
threshold energy
thromboembolism
thyrotoxic exophthalmos
time estimation
tissue equivalent
tooth extracted
total estrogen
trace element
tracheoesophageal
transepithelial elimination terminated
treadmill exercise
T&E testing and evaluation
training and experience
trial and error
Te tellurium
^{125}Te radioactive isotope of tellurium
^{127}Te radioactive isotope of tellurium
^{129}Te radioactive isotope of tellurium
^{132}Te radioactive isotope of tellurium
TEA tetraethylammonium
thermal energy analyzer
thromboendarterectomy
transient emboligenic aortoarteritis
transversely excited atomospheric pressure
TEAB tetraethylammonium bromide
TEAC tetraethylammonium chloride
TEAE triethylaminoethyl
TEBG testosterone-estrogen-binding globulin
TeBG testosterone-binding globulin
TEC total eosinophil count
transient erythroblastopenia of childhood
TED Tasks of Emotional Development
threshold erythema dose
thromboembolytic disease
tracheoesophageal dysraphism (also TOD)
tris-EDTA-dithiothreitol
TEDP tetraethyl dithionopyrophosphate
TEE thermic effect of exercise
tyrosine ethyl ester
TEEM tanned erythrocyte electrophoretic mobility
TEEP tetraethyl pyrophosphate
TEF thermic effect of food
tracheoesophageal fistula
TEG thromboelastogram
TEGDMA
tetraethylene glycol dimethacrylate
TEIB triethyleneiminobenzoquinone
TEL tetraethyl lead
TEM transmission electron microscopy
transverse electromagnetic
triethylenemelamine
TEMED N,N,N,N-tetramethylethylene diamine
temp temperature (also T)
temporal (also t)
temporary
temp dext
the right temple (tempus dextro)
temp sinist
the left temple (tempus sinistro)
TEN total epidermal necrolysis
total excretory nitrogen
toxic epidermal necrolysis
Tenac tenaculum
TENS transcutaneous electrical nerve stimulation
TEP thromboendophlebectomy
TEPA triethylenephosphoramide (also APO)
TEPG triethylphosphine gold
TEPP tetraethylpyrophosphate
TER threefold
transcapillary escape rate
ter rub (tere) (also R)
ter sim
rub together (tere simul)
tert tertiary
TES N-tris(hydroxymethyl) methyl-2-aminoethanesulfonic acid
toxic epidemic syndrome
transcutaneous electrical stimulation
TET tetroxiprim
total exchangeable thyroxine
triethyltryptamine
TETA triethylenetetramine
TETD tetraethylthiuram disulfide
TETRAC
tetraiodothyroacetic acid
TEV tadpole edema virus
TEWL transepidermal water loss
TF tactile fremitus
tetralogy of Fallot (see TOF)
thoroughfare
thymol flocculation
thymus tolerance factor
thymus transfer factor
tissue factor
to follow
total flow
transfer factor
transferrin
transfrontal
tube feeding
tuberculin filtrate
tuning fork
Tf transferrin (also TFN)
TFA total fatty acids
trifluoroacetic acid
TFE tetrafluoroethylene
TFECB Task Force on Emphysema and Chronic Bronchitis
TFH Touch for Health Foundation
TFL tensor fascia lata
TFM testicular feminization mutation
total fluid movement
trifluoromethyl nitrophenol
TFN total fecal nitrogen
totally functional neutrophil
transferrin (also Tf)
TFP treponemal false positive
trifluoperazine (also TFZ)
TFR total fertility rate
total flow resistance
TFS testicular feminization syndrome
TFT thrombus formation time
thyroid function test
transfer factor test
trifluorothymidine
TFZ trifluoperazine (also TFP)

TG testosterone glucoronide
tetraglycine
theophylline-guaifenesin
6-thioguanine (also 6-TG)
thromboglobulin
thyroglobulin
toxic goiter
Toxoplasma gondii
transglutaminase
transmissible gastroenteritis
trigeminal neuralgia
triglyceride (also TGL)
6-TG 6-thioguanine (also TG)
Tg thyroglobulin (also TGB)
type genus
TGA taurocholate-gelatin agar
thyroglobulin antibody (TgAb)
transient global amnesia
transposition of the great arteries
TgAb thyroglobulin antibody (TGA)
TGAR total graft area rejected
TGB thyroid-binding globulin
TGC time-gain compensator (or compensation)
TGD thermal green dye
TGE theoretical growth evaluation
transmissible gastroenteritis of swine
tryptone glucose extract
TGF transforming growth factor
tubuloglomerular feedback
tumor growth factor
TGFA triglyceride fatty acid
TGG turkey gamma globulin
TGL triglyceride (also TG)
triglyceride lipase
TGP tobacco glycoprotein
TGS triglycine sulfate
TGT thromboplastin generation test
thromboplastin generation time
tolbutamide-glucagon test
TGV thoracic gas volume (also VTG)
transposition of the great vessels
TGY tryptone, glucose, yeast
TH Tamm-Horsefall
tetrahydrocortisol (also THF)
theophylline
thyrotropic hormone
topical hypothermia
torcular Herophili
tyrosine hydroxylase
Th T helper
thoracic (also T)
thorium
throat
^{228}Th radioactive isotope of thorium
^{230}Th radioactive isotope of thorium
THA tetrahydroaminoacridine
total hip arthroplasty
total hydroxyapatite
THAM trihydroxymethylaminomethane
tromethamine (also TRIS)
THAN transient hyperammonemia of newborn
THARIES
total hip arthroplasty with internal eccentric shells
THC delta-9-tetrahydrocannabinol
thiocarbanidin
transhepatic cholangiography
THCA trihydroxycoprostanoic acid
THCCRC
tetrahydrocannabinol cross-reacting cannabinoids
THD thioridazine
transverse heart diameter
Thd ribosylthymine (also T)
ribothymidine (also T)
THDOC tetrahydrodeoxycorticosterone
THE tetrahydrocortisone
Ther therapy
THF humoral thymic factor
tetrahydrocortisol (also TH)
tetrahydrofolate
THFA tetrahydrofolic acid
THG 1-N alpha-trinitrophenylhistidine, 12 homoarginine glucagon
THI trihydroxyindole
THIO thioglycolate
THIP 4,5,6,7-tetrahydroisoxazolo-(5,4,-c)-pyridin-3-ol
THM total heme mass
THO tritiated water
THP tetrahydropapaveroline
tissue hydrostatic pressure
total hydroxyproline
THPC tetrabis(hydroxymethyl)phosphonium chloride
THPV transhepatic portal vein
THQ tetroquinone
THR total hip replacement
Thr threonine
THU tetrahydrouridine
THUG thyroid uptake gradiant
THVO terminal hepatic vein obliteration
Thy thymine (also T)
TI temporal integration
therapeutic index
thoracic index
thyroxine iodine
threshold of intelligibility
thymus independent
time information
time interval
tricuspid incompetence
tricuspid insufficiency
trunk index
tumor inducing
Ti titanium
^{44}Ti radioactive isotope of titanium
TIA transient ischemic attack
TIBC total iron-binding capacity
TIC ticarcillin
ticlopidine
trypsin inhibitory capacity
tumor-inducing complex
TICCC time interval between cessation of contraception and conception
TID time interval difference
titrated initial dose
tid three times a day (ter in die) (also td, tdd)
TIDA tuberoinfundibular dopamine
TIE transient ischemic episode
TIF tumor-inducing factor
tumor-inhibiting factor
TIFPB thrombin increasing fibrinopeptide B
TIG tetanus immune globulin
TIH time interval histogram
TIM triose isomerase
tin three times a night (ter in nocte)
tinc tincture (also tr)
TIP translation-inhibiting protein
TIPPS tetraiodophenolphthalein sodium
TIQ tetrahydroisoquinoline
TIR terminal innervation ratio
total immunoreactive

TIS transdermal infusion system
tumor in situ
TISP total immunoreactive serum pepsinogen
TISS Therapeutic Intervention Scoring System
TITh triiodothyronine
TIUV total intrauterine volume
TIVC thoracic inferior vena cava
tiw three times a week
TJ tight junction
triceps jerk
TK thymidine kinase
thymine kinase
tourniquet (also TQ)
transketolase
TKA total knee arthroplasty
transketolase activity
TKD tokodynamometer
TKG tokodynagraph
TKM thymidine kinase, mitochondrial
TKS thymidine kinase, soluble
TL team leader
temporal lobe
terminal limen
theophylline
thermolabile
Thorndike-Lorge
threat to life
thymic lymphocyte
thymus leukemia
time lapse
time limited
tolerance level
total lipids
tubal ligation
tylosin
Tl thallium
^{202}Tl radioactive isotope of thallium
^{204}Tl radioactive isotope of thallium
TLA tissue lactase activity
translaryngeal aspiration
translumbar aortogram
trypsinlike amidase
TLC tender loving care
thin-layer chromatography
total L-chain concentration
total lung capacity
total lung compliance
total lymphocyte count
TLCK tosyl lysine chloromethyl ketone
TLD thermoluminescent dosimetry
thoracic lymph duct
T/LD_{100}
minimum dose causing death or malformation of 100 percent of fetuses
TLE temporal lobe epilepsy
thin-layer electrophoresis
TLI thymidine-labeling index
tonic labyrinthine inverted
total lymphoid irradiation
Totman's Loss Index
trypsinlike immunoactivity
TLQ total living quotient
TLR tonic labyrinthine reflex
TLSO thorocolumbar spinal orthosis
thorocolumbosacral spinal orthosis
TLV threshold limit value
total lung volume
TM tectorial membrane
temporalis muscle
temporomandibular
teres major
term milk
Thayer-Martin
time and modifying
tobramycin
trademark
transcendental meditation
transmediastinal
transmetatarsal
transport maximum
transport mechanism
trimellityl
tubular myelin
tympanic membrane
typanometric
Tm maximum tubular reabsorption capacity
muscle temperature
thulium
tumor-bearing mice
T_m temperature midpoint, Kelvin
t_m temperature midpoint, Celsius
TMA thrombotic microangiopathy
thyroid microsomal autoantibody
trimellitic anhydride
trimethoxyamphetamine
trimethylamine
trimethylxanthine amphetamine
TMAb thyroid microsomal antibody
TMAO trimethylamine oxide
TMAS Taylor Manifest Anxiety Scale
TMB tetramethyl benzidine
tris-maleate buffer
TMBA trimethylbenzanthracene
TMCA trimethylcolchine acid
TMCS trimethylchrolosilane
TME transmissible mink encephalopathy
TmG maximum tubular reabsorption of glucose
TMI transmural myocardial infarction
TMIF tumor migration inhibitory factor
TMJ temporomandibular joint
TMJ-PDS
temporomandibular joint-pain dysfunction syndrome
TML terminal motor latency
tetramethyl lead
TMO trimethadione
TMP ribothymidine 5'-phosphate
thiamine monophosphate
thymidine monophosphate
transmembrane hydrostatic pressure
transmembrane potential
trimethoprim
trimethylpsoralen
TMPAH trimethylphenylammonium hydroxide
TMPD N,N,N'_2N'-tetramethyl-p-phenylene-diammonium
TMP-SMX
trimethoprim-sulfamethoxazole
TMPTA trimethylol propanetriacrylate
TMR tetramethylrhodamine
tissue maximum ratio
topical magnetic resonance
trainable mentally retarded
TMRI tetramethylrhodamine isothiocyanate
TMS tetramethylsilane
thallium-201 myocardial scintigraphy
trimethysilane
TMSI trimethylsilylimidazole
TMSi trimethylsilyl
TMT Trail-making Test
TMTC too many to count
TMTD tetramethylthiuram disulfide
TMU tetramethylurea
TMV tobacco mosaic virus

trachael mucous velocity
TMX trimazosin
TN talo-navicular
tiodazosin
total negatives
trochlear nucleus
true negative
T/N tar and nicotine
T_4N normal serum thyroxine
Tn normal intraocular tension
thoron
TNBP tri-(n-butyl) phosphate
TNBS 2,4,6-trinitrobenzene sulfonic acid
TNCB trinitrochlorobenzene
TNCS Third National Cancer Survey
TND term normal delivery
TNEE titrated norepinephrine excretion
TNF trinitrofluorenone
true negative fraction
tumor necrosis factor
TNG trinitroglycerin
toxic nodular goiter
Tng training
TNH transient neonatal hyperammonemia
TNI total nodal irradiation
TNM primary tumor, regional node, distant metastases
thyroid node metastasis
TNP total net positive
trinitrophenyl
TNR tonic neck reflex
TNS total nuclear score
transcutaneous neural stimulation
tumor necrosis serum
TNT trinitrotoluene
TNTC too numerous to count
TNV tobacco necrosis virus
TO original tuberculin
target organ
telephone order
temperature, oral
Theiler's Original
tincture of opium
total abstruction
triolein
turned on
turnover
TO_2 oxygen transport rate
TOA tuberculin-original-alt
tubo-ovarian abscess
TOB tobramycin
TOCP triorthocresyl phosphate
TOD tracheo-oesophageal dysraphism (also TED)
TOF tetralogy of Fallot
TOL trial of labor
tryptophol
tolb tolbutamide
TONAR the oral to nasal acoustic ratio
TOP temporal, occipital, parietal
termination of pregnancy
tissue oncotic pressure
TOPS Take Off Pounds Sensibly
TOPV trivalent oral poliovirus vaccine
TORCHS
toxoplasmosis, rubella, cytomegalovirus, herpes simplex or syphilis
TORP total ossicular replacement prosthesis
TOS thoracic outlet syndrome
TOTP triorthotolyl phosphate
TOTPAR
total pain relief
Tot prot
total protein
TOV thrombosed oral varix
trial of void
TOVA The Other Victims of Alcoholism
TOWER testing, orientation, work, evaluation, and rehabilitation
Tox toxicity
TP tail pinch
temperature and pressure
temporal peak
testosterone proprionate
tetanus-pertussis
thickly padded
threshold potential
thrombocytopenic purpura
tissue pressure
toilet paper
total population
total positives
total protein
trailing pole
transforming principle
transition point
transpyloric
transverse polarization
transverse process
treatment period
Treponema pallidum
triamphenicol
triazolophthalazine
true positive
tryptophan
tryptophan pyrollase
tube precipitin
tuberculin precipitation
TP5 thymopoietin pentapeptide
Tp tampon
TPA 12-O-tetradecanoylphorbol-13-acetate
tannic acid-phosphomolybdic acid-amido black
tissue polypeptide antigen
total phobic anxiety
Treponema pallidum agglutination
TPAL total pregnancies, premature infants, abortions, living children
TPB tryptone phosphate broth
TPBA prealbumin binding capacity
TPBF total pulmonary blood flow
TPC telopeptide-poor collagen
thromboplastic plasma component
time to pulse height converter
total plasma cholesterol
treatment planning conference
TPCF Treponema pallidum complement fixation
TPCK N-tosyl-L-phenylalanylchloromethyl ketone
TPCP Treponema pallidum cryolysis complement
TPD temporary partial disability
thiamine propyl disulphide (also DTPT)
TPE therapeutic plasma exchange
TPEY telluritepolymixin egg yolk
TPF true postive fraction
TPG therapeutic play group
transplacental gradient
TPH transplacental hemorrhage
tryptophan hydroxylase
TPHA Treponema pallidum hemagglutination
TPHN reduced triphosphopyridine nucleotide
TPI time period integrator
Treponema pallidum immobilization
triose phosphate isomerase

TPIA Treponema pallidum immobilization adherence
TPL triphosphate of lime
TPM total particulate matter
triphenylmethane
TPMT thiopurine methyltransferase
TPN tetrachloroisophthalonitrile
thalamic projection neurons
total parenteral nutrition
triphosphopyridine nucleotide (also NADP)
TPNH triphosphopyridine nucleotide reduced
TPO tryptophan peroxidase
TPP tetraphenylporphyrin
thiamine pyrophosphate
transpulmonary pressure
TPPase
thiamine pyrophosphatase
TPR temperature, pulse, respiration
testosterone production rate
total peripheral resistance
total pulmonary resistance
TPRI total peripheral resistance index
TPS tumor polysaccharide substance
TPT tetraphenyl tetrazolium
time to peak tension
total protein tuberculin
treadmill performance time
typhoid-paratyphoid
TPTX thyroparathyroidectomy
TPTZ triphenyltetrazolium chloride (also RT, TTC)
tripyridyltriazine
TPVR total pulmonary vascular resistance
TQ time questionnaire
tocopherolquinone
tourniquet (also TK)
TR rectal temperature
tetrazolium reduction
therapeutic radiology
time released
total repair
total resistance
total response
trachea
transfusion reaction
tricupsid regurgitation
triradial
tuberculin residuum
tuberculin Ruckland
turbidity reducing
turnover rate
Tr treatment (also TX)
tr tincture (also tinc)
trace
traction
tremor
TRA transaldolase
tumor-resistant antigen
TRAb thyrotrophin receptor antibody
Trach trachea
tracheotomy
TRAJ timed repetitive ankle jerk
TRAM Treatment Rating Assessment Matrix
Treatment Response Assessment Method
TRB terbutaline
TRBF total renal blood flow
TRC tanned red cell
total respiratory conductance
total ridge count
TRCA tanned red cell agglutination
TRCH tanned red cell hemagglutination
TRCHII
tanned red cell hemagglutination inhibition immunoassay
TRCV total red blood cell volume
TRD tongue-retaining device
TREA thoroughness, reliability, efficiency, analytic ability
Trep See T (Treponema)
TRF thyrotropin-releasing factor
TRGI Teacher's Reading Global Improvement
TRH tension-reducing hypothesis
thyrotropin-releasing hormone
TRI Temporary Rules Induction
tetrazolium-reduction inhibition
total response index
TRIAC triiodothyroacetic acid
TRIC trachoma-inclusion conjunctivitis
triCB 2,4',5-trichlorobiphenyl
trid three days (triduum)
Trig triglyderide
TRIS trisamine (also THAM)
tris (hydroxymethyl) nitromethane
trit triturate (triture)
TRITC tetramethylrhodamine
TRK transketolase
TRMC tetramethylrhodamino-isothiocyanate
tRNA transfer ribonucleic acid
TRO tissue reflectance oximeter
TROCA tangible reinforcement operant conditioning audiometry
Troch troche
TRP trichorhinophalangeal
tubular reabsorption of phosphate
Trp tryptophan (also Try)
TrPl treatment plan
TRPT theoretical renal phosphorus threshold
TRS tubuloreticular structure
TrS traumatic surgery
TRT total reading time
TRU turbidity-reducing unit
T_3RU triiodothyronine resin uptake
Try tryptophan (also Trp)
TRZ tartrozine
triazolam (also TZ)
TS Tay-Sachs
temperature-sensitive
terminal sensation
testosterone sulfate
test solution
thermostable
thiosporin
thoracic surgery
tissue space
tocopherol supplemented
total solids
Tourette syndrome
toxic substance
tracheal sound
tracheal spirals
transitional sleep
Transplantation Society
transverse sinus
trichostasis spinulosa
tricuspid stenosis
triple strength
tropical sprue
tubular sound
T/S thyroid to serum ratio
Ts skin temperature
tosylate
T suppressor
TSA technical surgical assistance

Test of Syntactic Ability
Total Severity Assessment
total solute absorption
Tourette Syndrome Association
trypticase soy agar
tumor-specific antigen
tumor-susceptible antigen

T_4SA thyroxine-specific activity
TSAb thyroid-stimulating antibody
TSAG trivalent sodium antimonyl gluconate
Tsaph temperature in the saphenous vein
TSAT tube slide agglutination test
TSB total serum bilirubin
trypticase soy broth
tryptone soy broth
TSBA total serum bile acids
TSBB transtracheal selective bronchial brushing
TSBC Time-Sample Behavioral Checklist
TSC thiosemicarbizide
total static compliance
TSCA Toxic Substances Control Act
TSCS Tennessee Self-Concept Scale
TSD target skin distance
Tay-Sachs disease
theory of signal detection
TSE trisodium edetate
T Sect
transverse cross section
TSEM transmission scanning electron microscopy
TSF tissue coding factor
total systemic flow
triceps skinfold
T suppressor factor
TSH thyroid-stimulating hormone (also TTH)
TSH-RF
thyroid-stimulating hormone-releasing factor
TSI thyroid-stimulating immunoglobulins
triple sugar iron
TSIA total small intestinal allotransplantation
TSL terminal sensory latency
TSP total serum protein
total suspended particulate
tribasic sodium phosphate
tsp teaspoonful
TSPA triethylenethiophosphoramide
TSPP tetrasodium pyrophosphate
TSR theophylline sustained release
thyroid to serum ratio
total systemic resistance
transient situation reaction
TSRBC trypsinized sheep red blood cell
TSS toxic shock syndrome
tropical splenomegaly snydrome
TSSE toxic shock syndrome exotoxin
TSSU theater sterile supply unit
TST total sleep time
transition state theory
treadmill stress test
tumor skin test
TSTA tumor-specific transplantation antigen
TSU triple sugar urea
TSV total stomach volume
TSY trpticase soy yeast
TT tablet triturate
talking task
terminal transferase
tetanus toxoid
tetrathionate
tetrazol
thrombin time
thymol turbidity
tibial tuberosity
tilt table
tine test
token test
tooth treatment
total thyroxine
transferred to
transit time
transthoracic
transtracheal
tuberculin tested
tube thoracostomy
tumor thrombus
turnover time
tyrosine transaminase
TT_4 total thyroxine
TTA tetanus toxoid antibody
timed therapeutic absence
transtracheal aspiration
TTBV total trabecular bone volume
TTC triphenyltetrazolium chloride (also RT, TPTZ)
TTD tetraethylthiuram disulfide
total temporary disability
transient tic disorder
TTF time to failure
TTFD tetrahydrofurfuryl disulfide
TTGA tellurite-taurocholate-gelatin agar
TTH thyrotropic hormone (also TSH)
tritiated thymidine
TTI tension-time index
transtracheal insufflation
TTL total thymic (or T) lymphocyte
TTLC true total lung capacity
TTN transient tachypnea of the newborn
TTNA transthoracic needle aspiration biopsy (also TTNB)
TTNB transthoracic needle aspiration biopsy (also TTNA)
TTP Testicular Tumour Panel (see BTTP)
thrombotic thrombocytopenic purpura
thymidine triphosphate
time to peak
TTPA triethylene thiophosphoramide
TTR transthoracic resistance
type to token ratio
TTS temporary threshold shift
transdermal therapeutic system
TTT thymol turbidity test
tolbutamide tolerance test
total twitch time
TTTT test tube turbidity test
TTV tracheal transport velocity
transfusion transmitted virus
TTVS Transfusion Transmitted Viruses Study
TTX tetrodotoxin
TU testosterone undecanoate
thiouracil
thiourea
thyroidal uptake
Todd unit
toxic unit
transmission unit
transurethral
tuberculin unit
turbidity unit
T_3U triiodothyronine uptake
Tu thulium
^{170}Tu radioactive isotope of thulium

Tuberc tuberculosis (also TB, TBC)
TUDC tauroursodeoxycholate
TUDCA tauroursodeoxycholic acid
TUG total urinary gonadotropin
TUI transurethral incision
TUR transurethral resection
TURB transurethral resection of the bladder
TURBT transurethral resection of bladder tumor
TURP transurethral resection of the prostate
tuss cough (tussis)
TV talipes varus
tetrazolium violet
thoracic vertebrae
tickborne virus
tidal volume
total volume
toxic vertigo
transfer vesicle
transvenous
trial visit
Trichomonas vaginalis
tricuspid valve
trivalent
true vertebra
truncal vagotomy
tuberculin volutin
tubulovesicular
TVA truncal vagotomy plus antrectomy
TVC third ventricle cyst
timed vital capacity
time ventilatory capacity
total volume capacity
transvaginal cone
true vocal cords
TVD transmissable virus dementia
TVG time-varied gain
TVH total vaginal hysterectomy
TVL tenth-value layer
tunica vasculosa lentis
TVP tensor veli palatini
textured vegetable protein
tricuspid valve prolapse
truncal vagotomy plus pyloroplasty
TVR tonic vibration reflex
tricuspid valve replacement
TVT transmissible venereal tumor
TVU total volume urine
TW tap water
terminal web
thymic weight
total water
TWA time-weighted average
Twb wet bulb temperature
TWBC total white blood cells
TWE tepid water enema
TWL transepidermal water loss
TX traction
transplant
treatment (also Tr)
See TC (tuberculin contagious)
TXA_2 thromboxane A_2
TXB_2 thromboxane B_2
Ty type
typhoid
TYR tyramine
tyrode
Tyr tyrosine
TZ terizidone
triazolam (also TRZ)
tuberculin zymoplastiche

U

U kilurane
ulna
uncertain
unerupted
unit
unknown (also UK, UNK)
upper
uracil (also URA)
uranium
Ureaplasma
urecholine
urethra (also UA)
uridine (also Urd)
urinary concentration
urine (also UR)
urology (also urol)
Urtica
uvula
^{232}U radioactive isotope of uranium
^{233}U radioactive isotope of uranium
UI urotensin I
UII uranium-234
urotensin II
UA Ulex agglutinin
ultrasonic arteriogram
umbilical artery
unaggravated
unrelated children raised apart
upper airway
upper arm
urethra (also U)
uric acid
uridylic acid
urine aliquot
uronic acid
uterine aspiration
U/A urinalysis
UAC umbilical artery catheter
UA/EM University Association for Emergency Medicine
UAG uracil-adenine-guanine
UAN uric acid nitrogen
UAO upper airway obstruction
UAP unstable angina pectoris
UAPD Union of American Physicians and Dentists
UAR upper airway resistance
UAS upper abdominal surgery
UASA upper airway sleep apnea
UAU uterine activity unit
UB flumequine
ultimobranchial body
urinary bladder
UBBC unsaturated vitamin B_{12} binding capacity
UBF uterine blood flow
UBI ultraviolet blood irradiation
UC ulcerative colitis
ultracentrifugal
umbilical cholesterol
unchanged
unclassifiable
unfixed cryostat
untreated cell

urea clearance
urethral catheterization
urine culture
uterine contractions
UCB unconjugated bilirubin
UCBC umbilical cord blood culture
UCC United Cancer Council
UCD See UCHD
UCE urea cycle enzymopathy
UCG ultrasonic cardiography
urinary chorionic gonadotropin
UCHD usual childhood diseases
UCL ulna collateral ligament
uncomfortable listening level
upper confidence limit
urea clearance
UCO urethral catheter out
UCP urinary coproporphyrin
urine C peptide
UCPA United Cerebral Palsy Association
UCPP urethral closure pressure profile
UCPREF
United Cerebral Palsy Research and Educational Foundation
UCR unconditioned reflex (also UR)
unconditioned response (also UR)
usual, customary, and reasonable
UCRP Universal Control Reference Plasma
UCS unconditioned stimulus
unconscious
UCT unchanged conventional treatment
UCU urinary care unit
UCV uncontrolled variable
UD underdeveloped
undesirable discharge
urethral discharge
uridine diphosphate
uroporphyrinogen decarboxylase
uterus delivery
ud as directed (ut dictum)
UDC ursodeoxycholate
See UCHD
UDCA ursodeoxycholic acid
UDMH unsym-dimethylhydrazine
UDO undetermined origin
UDP uridine diphosphate
UDPG uridine diphosphoglucose (also UDPGlc)
UDPGA uridine diphosphoglucuronic acid (also UDPGlcUA)
UDPGal
uridine diphosphogalactose
UDPGlc
uridine diphosphoglucose (also UDPG)
UDPGlcUA
uridine diphosphoglucuronic acid (also UDPGA)
UDPGT uridine diphosphoglycyronyl transferase
UDS unscheduled deoxyribonucleic acid synthesis
UDT Underwater Demolition Team
UE uninvolved epidermis
upper extremity
UER unaided equalization reference
UES upper esophageal sphincter
UF ultrafiltration
ultrasonic frequency
unflexed
until finished
urea formaldehyde
UFA unesterified fatty acid
UFC urinary-free cortisol
UFE uniform food encoding
UFR ultrafiltration rate
urine filtration rate
UFV unclassified fecal virus
UG urogenital
uteroglobin
UGD urogenital diaphragm
UGDP University Group Diabetes Program
UGF unidentified growth factor
UGH uveitis, glaucoma, hyphema
UGI upper gastrointestinal
UGIS upper gastrointestinal series
UGIT upper gastrointestinal tract
UGPP uridyl diphosphate glucose pyrophosphorylase
UH unfavorable histology
upper half
UHC ultrahigh carbon
UHF ultrahigh frequency
UHMW ultrahigh molecular weight
UHV ultrahigh vacuum
UI Ulcer Index
uroporphyrin isomerase
UIBC unsaturated iron-binding capacity
UICC International Union Against Cancer (Union Internationale Contre le Cancer) (also IUAC)
UIF undergraded insulin factor
UIP unusual interstitial pneumonitis
usual interstitial pneumonitis
UIQ upper inner quadrant
UK unknown (also U, UNK)
urinary kallikrein
urokinase
UL unauthorized leave
undifferentiated lymphoma
upper limit
upper lobe
utterance length
U&L upper and lower
ULA undedicated logic array
ULL uncomfortable loudness level
ULLL upper lid, left eye
ULN upper limit of normal (also UNL)
ULO chlophedianol hydrochloride
ULPE upper lobe pulmonary edema
ULQ upper left quadrant
ULRE upper lid, right eye
ULT ultrahigh temperature
ult praescript
the last ordered (ultimo praescriptus)
ULV ultralow volume
UM upper motor
UMA urinary muramidase activity
UMANA Ukrainian Medical Association of North America
umb umbilicus
UMN upper motor neuron
UMNL upper motor neuron lesion
UMP uridine monophosphate
UMPK uridine monophosphate kinase
UMS Undersea Medical Society
UN undernourished
urea nitrogen
urinary nitrogen
UNCV ulna nerve conduction velocity
ung ointment (unguentum)
UNICEF
United Nations International Children's Emergency Fund
UNK unknown (also U, UK)
UNL upper normal limit
UNS unsatisfactory

unsymmetrical

UO under observation
undetermined origin

UOA United Ostomy Association

UOQ upper outer quadrant

UOV units of variance

UP ulcerative proctitis
ultrahigh purity
Unna-Pappenheim
upright posture
ureteropelvic
uridine phosphorylase
uroporphyrin (also URO)

U/P urine to plasma ratio

UPC usual provider continuity

UPD urinary production rate

UPET Urokinase-Pulmonary Embolism Trial

UPF United Parkinson Foundation

UPG uroporphyrinogen

UPI uteroplacental insufficiency

UPJ uteropelvic junction

UPN unique patient number

UPOR usual place of residence

UPP urethral pressure profile
urethral pressure profilometry

UPPP uvulopalatopharyngoplasty

UPPRA upright peripheral plasma renin activity

UPS ultraviolet photoelectron spectroscopy
uroporphyrinogen I synthase

UQ upper quadrant

UR unconditioned reflex (also UCR)
unconditioned response (also UCR)
upper respiratory
urine (also U)
utilization review

URA uracil (also U)

URD upper respiratory disease

Urd uridine (U)

URF uterine-relaxing factor

URI upper respiratory infection

URO uroporphyrin (also UP)

UROD uroporphyrinogen decarboxylase

urol urology (also U)

UROS uroporphyrinogen synthetase

URQ upper right quadrant

URSO ursodeoxycholic acid

URTI upper respiratory tract illness
upper respiratory tract infection

US ultrasound
unconditioned stimulus
upper segment

USAID United States Agency for International Development

USAN United States Adopted Names

USCCHO
United States Conference of City Health Officers

USD United States Dispensatory

USDA United States Department of Agriculture

USF United Scleroderma Foundation

USFMS United States foreign medical school student

USG ultrasonography

USMBHA
United States-Mexico Border Health Association

USN ultrasonic nebulizer

USO unilateral salpingo-oophorectomy

USP United States Pharmacopoeia
upper sternal border

USPC United States Pharmacopoeial Convention

USPET Urokinase-Streptokinase Pulmonary Embolism Trial

USPHS United States Public Health Service

USPT United Societies of Physiotherapists

USPTA United States Physical Therapy Association

USR unheated serum reagin

USSG United States Surgeon General

USW ultrashort wave

UT unrelated children raised together
urinary tract
urticaria

UTBG unbound thyroxine-binding globulin

ut dict
as directed (ut dictum)

utend to be used (utendus)

UTI urinary tract infection

UTLD Utah Test of Language Development

UTP unilateral tension pneumothorax
uridine triphosphate

UTS ulnar tunnel syndrome
ultimate tensile strength

ut supr
as above (ut supra)

UU urinary urobilinogen

UUN urine urea nitrogen

UUO unilateral uretal occlusion

UUP urinary uroporphyrin

UV ultraviolet
umbilical vein
urinary volume

UVA ultraviolet A

UVB ultraviolet B

UVC ultraviolet C
Urgent Visit Center

UVJ ureterovesical junction

UVL ultraviolet light

UVR ultraviolet radiation

UWL unstirred water layer

UW unilateral weakness

UWM unwed mother

UX_1 thorium-234

UYP upper yield point

V

V see (vide)
vaccine
valve
vanadium
variable (also Var)
vector
vegetarian
vegetation
Veillonella
vein
velocity
ventilation (also $\dot{V}$, Ve)
ventricle
venule
verbal
vertebral
vertex (also Vtx, Vx)
Vibrio
virulent (also Vi)
virus
vision

voice
volt
volume (also vol)
vomit

$\dot{V}$ gas flow
ventilation (also V, Ve)

^{48}V radioactive isotope of vanadium

^{49}V radioactive isotope of vanadium

v in the evening (vespere)
venous blood

v- vicinal isomer

VA vacuum aspiration
valeric acid
vancomycin
vasodilator agent
ventricular arrhythmia
ventriculoatrial
ventroanterior
vertebral artery
Veterans Administration
viral antigen
visual acuity
visual axis
volcanic ash
volume, alveolar
volume averaging

V_A ventilation, alveolar

va volt-ampere

VABP venoarterial bypass pumping

VAC ventriculoatrial condition
vincristine, actinomycin D, cyclophosphamide
vincristine, doxorubicin (Adriamycin), cyclophosphamide

VACTERL
vertebral, anal, cardiac, tracheal, esophageal, renal, limb

VACURG
Veterans Administrative Cooperative Urological Research Group

VAD virus-adjusting diluent

Vag vagina

VAH vertebral ankylosing hyperostosis

VAHS virus-associated hemophagocytic syndrome

VAIN vaginal intraepithelial neoplasia

Val valine

VALE visual acuity, left eye

VAM ventricular arrhythmia monitor

VAMP vincristine, methotrexate (amethopterine), 6-mercaptopurine, prednisone

VAP variant angina pectoris
vincristine, doxorubicin (Adriamycin), prednisone

VA/Q ventricular to perfusion ratio

VAR visual auditory range

Var variable (also V)
variety

VARE visual acuity, right eye

VAS Venomological Artifact Society
viral analogue scale
visual analogue scale

VASC Verbal Auditory Screening of Children

Vasc vascular

vas vitr
a glass vessel (vas vitreum)

VAT ventricular activation time
Vestibular Accommodation Test
visual action therapy
Vocational Apperception Test

VATD vincristine, cytosine arabinoside, 6-thioguanine, daunorubicin

VATER vertebral, anal, tracheal, esophageal, renal

VATH vinblastine, doxorubicin (Adriamycin), thioTEPA, halotestin

VAV VP-16, doxorubicin (Adriamycin), vincristine

VB vagina bulbi
venous blood
viable birth
vinblastine
vinblastine, bleomycin
voided bladder

VB_1 first voided bladder specimen

VB_2 second midstream bladder specimen

VB_3 third midstream bladder specimen

VBA vincristine, carmustine (BCNU), doxorubicin (Adriamycin)

VBAIN vertebrobasilar artery insufficiency nystagmus

VBAP vincristine, carmustine (BCNU), doxorubicin (Adriamycin), prednisone

VBD vinblastine, bleomycin, cisplatin (DDP) (also VBP)

VBG venous blood gas
veronal-buffered serum with gelatin

VBI vertebrobasilar insufficiency
vertebrobasilar ischemia

VBM vincristine, bleomycin, methotrexate

VBP vinblastine, bleomycin, cisplatin (DDP) (also VBD)

VBR ventricular-brain ratio

VBS veronal-buffered saline

VC color vision
vascular change
vena cava
venous capillary
ventilatory capacity
verbal comprehension
vertebral canal
vincristine (also LCR, VCR)
vinyl chloride
vital capacity
vocal cord
voluntary closing
vomiting center
vowel-consonant

Vc pulmonary capillary blood volume

VCA viral capsid antigen

VCAP vincristine, cyclophosphamide, doxorubicin (Adriamycin), prednisone

VCC vasoconstriction center
ventral cell column

VCDQ Verbal Comprehension Deviation Quotient

VCE vagina ectocervix and endocervix

VCF velocity of circumferential fiber

VCG vectorcardiogram
voiding cystogram

VCIU voluntary control of involuntary utterances

VCM vinyl chloride monomer

VCMP vincristine, cyclophosphamide, melphalan, prednisone

VCN vancomycin, colistin, nystatin
Vibrio cholerae neuraminidase

VCO_2 carbon dioxide production per minute

VCR vasoconstriction rate
vincristine (also LCR, VC)

VCS vasoconstrictor substance
vesicocervical space

VCSF ventricular cerebral spinal fluid

VCT venous clotting time

VCU voiding cystourethrogram (also VCUG)

VCUG voiding cystourethrogram (also VCU)
VCV vowel-consonant-vowel
VD vapor density
venereal disease
volume of distribution
+VD positive vertical divergence
-VD negative vertical divergence
V_D dead space volume
$\dot{V}_D$ dead space ventilation
VDA visual discriminatory acuity
VDAC voltage-dependent anion channel
Vd alv
alveolar dead space
Vd anat
anatomic dead space
VDBR volume of distribution of bilirubin
VDC vasodilation center
VDDR vitamin D dependent rickets
VDEL Venereal Disease Experimental Laboratory
VDG venereal disease, gonorrhea
Vdg voiding
VDH valvular disease of the heart
vascular disease of the heart
VDL visual detection level
VDM vasodepressor material
VDP ventricular premature depolarization
vincristine, daunorubicin, prednisone
Vd p physiologic dead space
VDRL Venereal Disease Research Laboratories
VDRR vitamin D resistant rickets
VDS vasodilator substance
venereal disease, syphilis
Vd shunt
dead space effect of Qs/Qt
VDT visual distortion test
VDU video display unit
Vd/Vt dead space to tidal volume ratio
VE Venezuelan encephalitis
venous extension
ventricular elasticity
ventricular escape
vesicular exanthema
viral encephalitis
visual efficiency
vitamin E
volume ejection
$\dot{V}_E$ ventilation per minute
Ve ventilation (also V, $\dot{V}$)
VEA ventricular ectopic activity
ventricular extopic arrhythmia
VEB ventricular ectopic beat
VECP visual evoked cortical potential
VED ventricular ectopic depolarization
VEE Venezuelan equine encephalomyelitis
V-EEG vigilance-controlled electroencephalogram
vel See V (velocity)
VEM vasoexcitor material
VENP vincristine, cyclophosphamide (Endoxan), Natulan, prednisolone
vent ventral
ventricular
VEP visual evoked potential
VEPA vincristine, cyclophosphamide (Endoxan), prednisolone, doxorubicin (Adriamycin)
VER veratridine
visual evoked response
Ves vesicular
VEWAA Vocational Evaluation and Work Adjustment
VF ventricular fibrillation
ventricular fluid
ventricular fusion
vigil, fatiguing
visual field
vitreus fluorophotometry
vocal fremitus
Vf field of vision
V_f variant frequency
VFA volatile fatty acid
VFC ventricular function curve
VFD visual feedback display
VFP ventricular fluid pressure
VFR voiding flow rate
VFT venous filling time
ventricular fibrillation threshold
VFW velocity wave form
VG Van-Gieson
ventilated group
ventricular gallop
virginiamycin
VH vaginal hysterectomy
venous hematocrit
viral hepatitis
VHD valvular heart disease
viral hematodepressive disease
VHF very high frequency
viral hemorrhagic fever
visual half-field
VI variable interval
vastus intermedius
viscosity index
Visual Imagery
visually impaired
vitality index
volume index
Vi virginium
virulent (also V)
VIA virus-inactivating agent
Vib vibration
VIC vasoinhibitory center
visual communication therapy
voice intensity controller
vic times (vices)
VID visible iris diameter
VIG vaccinia immune globulin
VIH violence-induced handicap
VIN vulvar intraepithelial neoplasm
vin wine (vinum)
VIP vasoactive intestinal peptide
vasoactive intestinal polypeptide
venous impedance plethsmography
voluntary interruption of pregnancy
VIQ verbal intelligence quotient
VIS vaginal irrigation smear
VISC vitreous infusion suction cutter
VISTA Visually Impaired Secretarial Transcribers Association
Vit vitamin
vit ov sol
dissolved in yolk or egg (vitello ovi solutus) (also VOS)
VIVA Visually Impaired Veterans of America
VL vastus lateralis
ventralis lateralis
ventrolateral
visceral leishmoniasis
VLA vanillactic acid
viruslike agent
VLB vinblastine
vinblastine, velban, vincaleukoblastine
VLBW very low birth weight

VLCFA very long chain fatty acid
VLD very low density
VLDL very low density lipoprotein
VLDLC very low density lipoprotein cholesterol
VLDTG very low density triglyceride
VLF very low frequency
VLM visceral larva migrans
VLSI very large scale integration
VM vasomotor
vastus medialis
ventricular mass
ventromedial
viomycin
voltmeter
VMA vanillylmandelic acid
Vmax maximum velocity
VMC vasomotor center
village malaria communicator
vinyl chloride monomer
void metal composite
Von Meyenburg complex
V.M.D.
Doctor of Veterinary Medicine (see D.V.M.)
VMH ventromedial hypothalamus
VMIT Visual-Motor Integration Test
VMN ventromedial nucleus
VMO vastus medialis oblique
VMS visual memory span
VMST Visual-Motor Sequencing Test
VMT vasomotor tone
ventilatory muscle training
VN vesicle neck
vestibular nucleus
virus neutralizing
visceral nucleus
visual naming
VNA Visiting Nurse Association
VNO vomeronasal organ
VNR ventral nerve root
VO verbal order
VO_2 oxygen consumption rate
VOD venocclusive disease
vision, right eye (oculus dexter)
vol volatile
volume (also V)
voluntary (also V)
VOR vestibulo-ocular reflex
VOS vision, left eye (oculus sinister)
vos dissovled in yolk or egg (vitello ovi solutus) (also vit ov sol)
VOT voice onset time
VP vapor pressure
variegate porphyria
vascular permeability
vasopressin
velopharyngeal
venipuncture
venous pressure
venous volume plethysmograph
ventriculoperitoneal
vertex potential
vincristine, prednisone
virus protein
Voges-Proskauer
volume pressure
vulnerable period
V&P vagotomy and pyloroplasty (also P&V)
VPA valproic acid
VPB ventricular premature beat
vinblastine, cisplatin, bleomycin
VPC ventricular premature complex (also PVC)
ventricular premature contraction (also PVC)
volume packed cells
volume per cent
VPCMF vincristine, prednisone, cyclophosphamide, methotrexate, fluorouracil
VPCT ventricular premature contraction threshold
VPF vascular permeability factor
VPG velopharyngeal gap
VPI velopharyngeal insufficiency
ventral posterior inferior
VPL ventralis posteriolateralis
VPM ventilator pressure manometer
ventral posteromedial
vpm vibrations per minute
VPMS Virchow-Pirquet Medical Society
VPO velopharyngeal opening
VPR volume pressure ratio
VPRC volume of packed red cells
VPS visual pleural space
vps vibrations per second
VQ voice quality
V/Q ventilation to perfusion ratio
VR valve replacement
variable ratio
vascular resistance
venous return
ventilation ratio
ventral root
ventricular rate
visual reproduction
vocal resonance
vocational rehabilitation
VRA Visual Reinforcement Audiometry
VRC venous renin concentration
VRD ventricular radial dysplasia
VRE vocational rehabilitation and education
VRI viral respiratory infection
VROM voluntary range of motion
VRP very reliable product
VRS Vocational Rehabilitation Services
VRT variance of residence time
VRV ventricular residual volume
VS vaccination scar
vaccine serotype
vasospasm
venisection
ventral subiculum
ventricular sense
ventricular septum
verbal scale
very sensitive
vesicular sound
vesicular stomatitis
vibration second
vital sign
volumetric solution
Vs voids
vs bleeding (venae sectio)
VSB Volunteer Services for the Blind
vsb bleeding in arms (venaesectio brachii)
VSC voluntary surgical contraception
VSCS ventricular specialized conduction system
VSD ventricular septal defect
VSHD ventricular septal heart defect
VSM vascular smooth muscle
VSP Vision Service Plan
VSR venereal spirochetosis of rabbits

VSS vital signs stable
VSULA vaccination scar, upper left arm
VSV vesicular stomatitis virus
VSW ventricular stroke work
VT tetrazolium violet
tidal volume
total ventilation
vacuum tube
vacuum tuberculin
vasotocin
ventricular tachyarrhythmia
ventricular tachycardia
Vero cytotoxin
V&T volume and tension
VTA ventral tegmental area
VTE ventricular tachycardia event
vicarious trial and error
VTG volume of thoracic gas (also TGV)
VTI volume-thickness index
VTM variegated translocation mosaicism
VTR video tape recorded
VTS vesicular transport system
VTVM vacuum tube voltmeter
Vtx vertex (also V, Vx)
VU volume unit
VUR vesicoureteral reflux
VUV vacuum ultraviolet
VV varicose veins
viper venum
vulva and vagina
vv veins
v/v volume for volume
VVC village voluntary collaborator
VVD vascular volume of distribution
VVI vocal velocity index
VVQ Verbalizer-Visualization Questionnaire
VVS vesicovaginal space
VW vessel wall
v/w volume per weight
VWD Von Willebrand's disease
VWF velocity wave form
vibration white finger
Von Willebrand factor
Vx vertex (also V, Vtx)
VY veal yeast
VZ varicella-zoster
VZIG varicella-zoster immune globulin
VZV varicella zoster virus

W

W tungsten
water
watt
weber (also Wb)
week (also wk)
wehnelt
weight (also wt)
wetting
whole response
widowed
width
wife
Wohlfahrtia
wolfram
Wuchereria
^{181}W radioactive isotope of tungsten
^{185}W radioactive isotope of tungsten
^{187}W radioactive isotope of tungsten
w with (also c)
WA Wellness Associates
when awake
W/A wide awake
WAB Western Aphasia Battery
WAIS Wechsler's Adult Intelligence Scale
WAR Women Against Rape
WARF Wisconsin Alumni Research Foundation
Warf warfarin
WAS weekly activity summary
Wiskott-Aldrich syndrome
Word Atmosphere Scale
WASP World Association of Societies of Pathology
Wass Wassermann
WAT word association test
WB washed bladder
wet bulb
Wb weber (also W)
weight bearing
whole blood
whole body
WBA wax bean agglutinin
whole body activity
WBC white blood cell
white blood corpuscle
white blood count
WBCT whole blood clotting time
WBDS whole body digital scanner
WBE whole body extract
WBF whole blood folate
WBH whole blood hematocrit
WBM whole boiled milk
woman milk bank
WBPTT whole blood partial thromboplastin time
WBR whole body radiation
whole body retention
WBRS Ward Behavior Rating Scale
WBRT whole body recalcification time
WBS Wechsler-Bellevue Scale
wound-breaking strength
WBT wet bulb temperature
WC water closet
wheel chair
white cell
whole complement
whooping cough
work capacity
writer's cramp
WCB Worlmen's Compensation Board
WCC Walker carcinosarcoma cell
white cell count
WCD Weber-Christian disease
WCES Women's Caucus of the Endocrine Society
WCL whole cell lysate
WCOT wall coated open tubular
WCPT World Confederation for Physical Therapy
WCST Wisconsin Card Sorting Test
WD wallerian degeneration
well developed
well differentiated
wet dressing
Wilson's disease
with disease
withdrawal dyskenesia
without dyskenesia
Wolman's disease
wrist disarticulation
Wd word

WDHA watery diarrhea, hypokalemia, fasting achlorhydria
WDI warfarin dose index
WDL well-differentiated lymphocyte
WDLL well-differentiated lymphocytic lymphoma
WDS wet dog shaking
WDWN well developed, well nourished
WE wage earner
wax ester
Western encephalitis
Western encephalomyelitis
whiskey equivalent
WEE Western equine encephalitis
WEG water-ethyleneglycol
WEUP willful exposure to unwanted pregnancy
WF Weil-Felix
Wistar-Furth
Word Fluency
W/F white female
WFA World Federation of Anesthesiologists
WFD World Federation of the Deaf
WFH World Federation of Hemophilia
WFMH World Federation for Mental Health
WFNS World Federation of Neurological Surgeons
World Federation of Neurosurgical Societies
WFOT World Federation of Occupational Therapists
WFP World Food Program
WFPHA World Federation of Public Health Associations
WFR Weil-Felix reaction
WFS Women for Sobriety
WFSS Wolpe Fear Survey Schedule
WG water gauge
Wegener's granulomatosis
WGA wheat germ agglutinin
WH well healed
well hydrated
wound healing
WHA warmed, humidified air
WHAN Wellness and Health Activation Networks
WHF-USA
World Health Foundation, United States of America
WHO World Health Organization
WHOIRP
World Health Organization International Reference Preparation
whp whirlpool (also WP)
whr watt-hour
WHS Werdnig-Hoffman syndrome
WHV woodchuck hepatitis virus
WHVP wedged hepatic venous pressure
WI water ingestion
waviness index
WIA waking imagined analgesia
wounded in action
WIC women, infants, and children
WID widow (widower)
WIQ Waring Intimacy Questionnaire
WIS Ward Initiation Scale
WISC Wechsler's Intelligence Scale for Children
WISC-R
Wechsler's Intelligence Scale for Children-Revised
WIST Whitaker Index of Schizophrenic Thinking
WJ Woodcock-Johnson
wk weak
week (also W)
work
WKD Wilson-Kimmelstiel disease
WKF well-known fact
WKS Wernicke-Korsakoff syndrome
WKY Wistar Kyoto
WL waiting list
wavelength
weight loss
work load
WLE wide local excision
WLF whole lymphocyte fraction
WLI weight-length index
WLM work level month
WLT whole lung tomography
WM warm, moist
whole milk
woman milk
W/M white male
WMA World Medical Association
WMF white middle-aged female
WMM white middle-aged male
WMR work metabolic rate
World Medical Relief
WMS Wechsler Memory Scale
WN well nourished
WNF well-nourished female
WNL within normal limits
WNM well-nourished male
WNV West Nile virus
WO washout
without (also $\bar{s}$)
written order
W/O water in oil
WOAR Women Organized Against Rape
WOB work of breathing
WOHRC Women's Occupational Health Resource Center
WOTB Welfare of the Blind
WOWS Weak Opiate Withdrawal Scale
W/O/W water in oil in water
WP water packed
weakly positive
wet pack
whirlpool (also whp)
white pulp
working point
WPA World Psychiatric Association
WPB whirlpool bath
WPCU weighted patient care unit
WPFM Wright Peak Flow Meter
WPLC Working Party on Leukemia in Childhood
WPN white mucosa with punctation
WPPSI Wechsler Preschool and Primary Scale of Intelligence
WPRS Wittenborn Psychiatric Rating Scale
WPW Wolff-Parkinson-White
WR Wassermann reaction
whole response
work rate
Wr wrist
W/r with respect to
WRAT Wide-Range Achievement Test
WRC washed red cell
water-retention coefficient
WRE whole ragweed extract
WRF World Rehabilitation Fund
WRMT Woodcock Reading Mastery Tests
WRO Welfare Rights Organization
WRST Wilcoxon rank sum test
WRVP wedged renal vein pressure

WS	Waardenburg's syndrome
	water soluble
	water swallow
	wet swallow
	Wilder's silver
	whole response plus white space
ws	watts second
WSA	Western Surgical Association
WSB	wheat soy blend
WSSFN	World Society for Stereotactic and Functional Neurosurgery
WT	wall thickness
	water temperature
	work therapy
wt	weight (also W)
WTD	wet tail disease
WTE	whole time equivalent
W/U	work-up
WV	walking ventilation
	whispered voice
w/v	weight per volume
WW	Weight Watchers
w/w	weight per weight
WWTP	wastewater treatment plant
WX	wound of exit
WY	women years

X

X	cross-section
	decimal scale of potency or dilution
	exophoric, distant viewing
	exposure
	female sex chromosome
	for
	Kienbock's unit (also A)
	magnification
	reactance
	removal of
	sulfadimethoxine
	times
	Xanthomonas
	xanthosine (see Xao)
	xenon (see Xe)
	Xenopsylla
	xerophalmia
$\bar{X}$	mean
X^1	exophoric, near viewing
X^2	chi-square
Xao	xanthosine
XC	excretory cystogram
XDH	xanthine dehydrogenase
XDP	xeroderma pigmentosum (also XP)
Xe	xenon
^{131}**Xe**	radioactive isotope of xenon
^{133}**Xe**	radioactive isotope of xenon
XES	x-ray energy spectroscopy
XF	xerophthtalmic fundus
XH	extra high
XL	excess lactate
XLD	xylose lysine deoxycholate
XLI	X-linked ichthyosis
XLP	X-linked lymphoproliferative
XLR	X-linked recessive
XM	cross matching
XN	night blindness
XO	only one sex chromosome present
XP	xeroderma pigmentosum (also XDP)
XPN	xanthogranulomatous pyelonephritis
XPS	x-ray photoemission spectroscopy
XR	x-ray
XRD	x-ray powder diffraction
XRF	x-ray fluorescence
XRT	x-ray therapy
XS	excess
	corneal scar
	xiphisternum
XSA	cross-sectional area
	xenograph surface area
XSB	Xavier Society for the Blind
XSP	xanthoma striatum palmare
XT	constant exotropia
X(T)	intermittent exotropia
XTE	xeroderma, talipes, enamel defect
XTM	xanthoma tuberosum multiplex
XU	excretory urogram
XX	double strength
Xyl	xylose

Y

Y	male sex chromosome
	ordinate
	year (also yr)
	Yersinia
	young
	yttrium
^{87}**Y**	radioactive isotope of yttrium
^{88}**Y**	radioactive isotope of yttrium
^{90}**Y**	radioactive isotope of yttrium
^{91}**Y**	radioactive isotope of yttrium
YACP	young adult chronic patient
YAG	yttrium-aluminum-garnet
Y/B	yellow/blue
Yb	ytterbium
^{169}**Yb**	radioactive isotope of ytterbium
^{175}**Yb**	radioactive isotope of ytterbium
YBT	Yerkes-Bridges test
YCT	Yvon coefficient test
yd	yard
yd^2	square yard
YE	yeast extract
YEI	Yersinosis enterocolitica infection
YF	yellow fever
YFA	young female arteritis
YHMD	yellow hyaline membrane disease
YHT	Young-Helmholtz theory
YLF	yttrium lithium fluoride
YMA	yeast morphology agar
YNB	yeast nitrogen base
YNS	yellow nail syndrome
YO	year old
YOB	year of birth
YP	yield point
yr	year (also Y)
YRD	Yangtze River disease
YS	yellow spot
	yoke sac
	Yoshida sarcoma
YSIGA	Yellow Springs Instrument glucose analyser
YST	yolk sac tumor
Yt	See Y (yttrium)
YVS	yellow vernix syndrome

Z

Z atomic number (also at no)
benzyloxycarbonyl (also Cbz)
contraction (Zuckung)
impedance
intermediate disk (Zwischenscheibe)
sulfisomazole
Zopfius

Z', Z"...
increasing degrees of contraction

z standard score
zero
zone

ZAP zymosan-activated plasma
ZAPF zinc adequate pair-fed
ZAS zymosan-activated autologous serum
ZAWP zinc adequate weight-paired
ZC zona compacta
ZCP zinc chloride poisoning
ZD zinc deficient
ZEEP zero end-expiratory pressure
ZES Zollinger-Ellison syndrome
ZF zero frequency
ZGM zinc glycinate marker
ZI zona incerta
ZIG zoster immune globulin
ZIM zimelidine
ZIP zoster immune plasma
ZMA zinc meta-arsenite
ZN Ziehl-Neelsen
Zn zinc
^{65}Zn radioactive isotope of zinc
^{69}Zn radioactive isotope of zinc
ZNS Ziehl-Neelsen stain
ZPA zone of polarizing activity
ZPC zero point of charge
ZPG zero population growth
ZPO zinc peroxide
ZPP zinc protoporphyrin
ZR zona reticulata
Zr zirconium
^{95}Zr radioactive isotope of zirconium
^{97}Zr radioactive isotope of zirconium
ZSO zinc suboptimal
ZT Ziehen's test
ZTN zinc tannate of naloxone
ZTS zymosan-treated serum
ZTT zinc turbidity test
Zz ginger (zingiber)